Introduction to
Research in Nursing

Introduction to Research in Nursing

BURTON MEYER, PH.D.

Research Psychologist

AND

LORETTA E. HEIDGERKEN, R.N., ED.D.

Professor of Nursing Education
The Catholic University of America
Washington, D. C.

PHILADELPHIA · MONTREAL
J. B. LIPPINCOTT COMPANY

Second Printing

Distributed in Great Britain by
Pitman Medical Publishing Co., Limited, London

Library of Congress Catalog Card No. 62-11875

Printed in the United States of America

Foreword

Interest in research is high today, and many potential and actual investigators are seeking something more in a research text than the usual methodologies and tools, useful though they may be. Therefore, this work is a valuable contribution to the field.

In the profession of nursing, many leaders, as well as social scientists, are making valiant attempts to formalize a concept of nursing that can be tested scientifically; nurses in clinical practice and in administrative positions are seeking ways and means to improve the nursing care of patients; many projects and studies are being undertaken to find answers to recurrent and current problems; large sums of money are being allocated to the study of the complexities of nursing service and nursing education; nurses themselves are contributing generously to the American Nurses Foundation, the research arm of the American Nurses Association.

To attain any worthwhile professional goal, studies producing insight and answers are required. Research is a strict discipline. Without sound research, new knowledge and improved professional service cannot be advanced in the right direction.

There are few sources available that are of assistance to nurses endeavoring to understand the research process; this text is indeed timely. In it, the experience of the authors is brought to bear on the subject.

The authors emphasize the planning that goes into the production of research design and exemplify the various aspects of a design with illustrations taken from actual studies. They also present a background of progress in research in the field of nursing.

This balanced presentation will have appeal for anyone interested in acquainting students or personnel with fundamental research concepts and with criteria for evaluating research studies.

This text will be a boon for the beginning researcher while, at the same time, it has much to offer to those with some experience in systematic investigations.

Washington, D. C.   Sister Charles Marie, C.C.V.I.

Preface

Research, which smoldered among the embers for years, suddenly has been sparked into activity. It was confined once to the rather exclusive domain of college professors and their students and to isolated recipients of grants. It also was considered to be a secondary pursuit—a pleasurable pastime squeezed into the off-hours and supported by more conventional and profitable sources of livelihood. Now, many people are engaged to practice research on a full-time basis. And the demand for more people, funds and activity has been engendered among governments, industries and universities.

However, in the furor to keep pace with the sudden demand, the meaning has become divorced from the process. The goals seem to be distorted. Often the method is abused. The research worker frequently is cast into an odd assortment of roles from that of a general-problem handyman to that of a highly specialized subject-matter expert. Research has evolved as if it were a panacea for all problems.

This book has been developed in response to the unchanneled enthusiasm. It is an attempt to re-establish meaning in an undertaking that itself must rest on understanding. It is an effort to relocate for the reader the place of research in society.

The book was written in conformity with the belief that research is a unique process with a unique purpose. The format was based essentially on the steps to be followed in research. While recognition was given to other kinds of analysis, such as philosophic inquiry and historical study, research was treated as separate and distinct.

The primary consideration here was "why" rather than "how." Therefore, we sought to elucidate the meaning of each step in the process rather than to compile a source book of the many procedures that already have been implemented to conduct the process. Yet even this limited frame of reference could not narrow the scope of the topic to textbook proportions. In effect, the book touches only the bare elements. The reader is referred to other sources for more extensive details.

A special application of research has been made to nursing. In this regard, we did *not* envision that research would be tailored to the needs of the field. Instead, a general presentation evolved, illustrated by research practices in nursing. In the course of this development, the authors attempted to synthesize some of the problems that are unique to the practice and, accordingly, made recommendations.

The book may be useful to a variety of groups. It was designed especially for graduate students who are beginning to be interested in research. Nevertheless, it may be helpful to some of the more experienced researchers who have started to inquire about their own work habits.

At this point, the authors wish to give special acknowledgment to the numerous researchers in nursing whose studies are used as illustrations. In particular, we wish to thank those whose works were put on display for the sake of the text, although sometimes they have been shown to run counter to the authors' concepts of research in nursing. It would have been desirable to recognize and list all the researchers by name, but there are too many of them. However, the authors can extend their sincere appreciation to the primary printed sources of most of these contributions, the professional nursing journals: *Nursing Research, American Journal of Nursing* and *Nursing Outlook.*

BURTON MEYER
LORETTA E. HEIDGERKEN

Contents

ix

CHAPTER 1

A Point of View

There are many points of view about the nature of research. Each reflects the feelings of the research worker and the manner in which he undertakes an assignment. His point of view even may change as he proceeds from one project to another.

Therefore, research is difficult to define precisely. Several definitions may be equally satisfactory when they are assessed from different points of view. The definition of research that will be employed in the context of this book thus may not be a definition at all, but merely another point of view. (When or whether it is used is a judgment that can be made only by the reader.)

WHAT IS RESEARCH?

It has been said that research "is an intellectual process as ancient as man, changing in purpose and form and currently described as a science."[1] The practice of research is certainly not new and, since the advent of the sputnik, research has multiplied in many directions. People state that they are engaged currently in research, and not entirely for science. Does everyone participate in the same process? Or do some people employ the process in a very special way that is dictated by their own needs?

What is research? Research may be many things. It can be described as a purpose or as an end-result. It can be defined

1

as a method or as a means to an end. Research often is influenced by the character of the person doing it. It is colored by its subject matter or its scope. It is also a reflection of the meaning conveyed to its workers. Research is all these things and many more—and each may be useful when employed as it was meant to be employed.

Research Is Purposeful

According to one point of view, research is purposeful. A research project is not just an aimless endeavor but an activity that is directed steadfastly toward a specific end. We engage in the process for a purpose. Kelley commented, for example, with regard to historical research, "to say that one is engaged in historical research does not define his activity, because the historian always comes to his task, or at least always should come, with a motive."[2]

This point of view characterizes any activity, with the possible exception of the arts or an entertainment, which may be performed for their own sake. To the manufacturer of footwear, the shoe is the primary focus of production. The ultimate aim is not the process but the production of a shoe. The process may be altered when the manufacturer decides to produce something other than shoes.

So it is with research. Each piece of research arises normally from the roots of a particular objective and is maintained within the channels, whether broad or narrow, of that objective. The project may crystallize or dissipate as the purpose is clarified or confused. The primary purpose should direct, and not be directed by, the project. If the purpose is altered, the project also may require modification. On the other hand, if the project is altered without regard to the purpose, the objective also may be modified, but inadvertently.

How has the purpose of research been stated? Many purposes, aims or objectives have been described or can be inferred. Some writers speak in grandiose or profound terms of a general or an underlying purpose. However, the individual research practitioner may not conceive of his assignment in this way. He may have a very specific aim that has little or no bearing upon an ultimate purpose.

To satisfy man's craving for more understanding, to improve his judgment, to add to his power, to reduce the burden of work, to relieve suffering and to increase satisfactions in multitudinous ways— these are large and fundamental goals of research.[3]

This is one of the more general statements that are descriptive of purpose in research. Doubtless there have been very few projects that could not be encompassed by one or more of these aims. But does the individual researcher think along these lines when he initiates his project? These objectives (and there are more than one) are more probably descriptive of the setting into which the general activity is cast. They may serve as the motivating forces by which a society justifies research. In point of time, they extend far beyond the expiration of the initial and single project.

The purpose of research is stated more definitively as "an endeavor to discover, develop and verify knowledge."[4] Research is regarded here as the production of a contribution to knowledge. The statement goes on to imply, however, that not just any piece of knowledge is acceptable—only that which has been verified and has withstood the test of time. The purpose is limited in this sense to what is sought and is not concerned with what can be done or provided for man.

The following phrases have also been employed to depict purpose: "to describe," "to control and predict," "to explain." The purpose, as displayed in this frame of reference, has been refined considerably. These phrases may portray the manner by which this knowledge is sought or the actual form that it may take—a description, a prediction, an explanation. They signify further levels of difference in time and scope. To describe is to observe and record what has happened in the past; to predict is to forecast future occurrences; to explain is to make understandable how an event or a series of events has or could have occurred or could be predicted. It is possible that the purpose of any research project can be stated in one of these three ways.

Lastly, we might examine some individual research reports

and seek to infer the intent or the purpose. Here are the titles
of some masters' theses that were written by nursing students
and abstracted in one of the nursing journals.[5] While the aim
of each of these papers may be characterized by one or more of
the purposes previously listed, they appear also to suggest something more specific.

> Problems referred to head nurses in the seven units of the medical
> and surgical division of a general hospital
> Study of the rate of turn-over among hospital aides
> Diagnosis of a hospital ward situation focused on the human rela-
> tions aspect of nursing service administration
> Some of the teaching needs of normal postpartum patients in a
> specific hospital
> Study of accidents to children occurring in Babies' and Children's
> Hospital, University Hospitals, Cleveland, Ohio, during the years,
> January 1952–June 1954

The researcher, in each case, seems to be probing into an
ongoing or a past operation to determine the areas of difficulty.
She appears to be taking inventory, to be ascertaining a state of
affairs, to be determining the need for action, to be diagnosing.

Deduce and compare the purposes of this group of papers:

> Role of the nurse in the administration of passive exercises
> Guide for teaching administrative concepts and skills in the basic
> nursing curriculum
> Exploratory study to determine a method of improving operating-
> room experience for collegiate students of nursing
> One method of promoting continuity of nursing care to the ma-
> ternity patient
> Proposed program for a clinical experience in nutrition

In these cases, the students apparently intended to propose
and demonstrate a course of action, to provide a solution to a
problem, to treat.

A third group of theses suggests an appraisal of an action
program:

> Appraisal of the program of the Natural Childbirth Associa-
> tion of Milwaukee
> Effects of a listening training program on the listening com-
> prehension of a selected group of nursing students

Study to determine the opinion of nursing students toward the counseling program in a selected school of nursing

Study of the graduates of a selected school of nursing 1949 through 1954

Analysis of competencies derived from affiliations in basic communicable disease and tuberculosis nursing

It is perhaps the purpose of the researcher in these cases to test a proposal, to determine the effects, to evaluate.

Research can be described by a purpose, an aim, a goal or an objective. That is, it can be characterized in terms of the intent of the researcher—what he hopes to derive from his study. Purpose, in turn, may be viewed in a broad or a narrow scope in regard to the product or the contribution to be obtained, or the service provided by the end-result.

RESEARCH IS A METHOD

Research is a method or a means to an end. This point of view is expressed more commonly as part of the definition of research. Most texts tend to be developed in this direction and become, in essence, treatments of research methodology.

Do the authors have any particular method in mind? There is rather common agreement, and research is considered by many as problem-solving.

Research is neither just fact finding nor is it esoteric methods to be used by the genius. . . . Research is outgrowth of the "attempt to solve" . . . problems. When a problem is faced, one procedure after another is tried until a *technique* is found which works.[6]

Research is also defined more descriptively in terms of the problem-solving process itself, as "purpose, theory, verification of hypothesis by observation and/or experiment."[7]

However, there are some differences in regard to the specific application of the problem-solving method to research. One school of thought, for example, which considers the end-result or the purpose as the verification of knowledge, follows a more idealistic approach. It would stress the rigorous manner and the care with which research studies are to be undertaken.

The progress of man in solving problems suggested in terms of the unknown has been concomitant with the discovery and development of methodological procedures making the research process itself more rigorous, more discriminatory and more dependable. This program has been further enhanced by an attitude of dedication to research as the best way to study problems as well as to improve decisions and actions in respect to them.[8]

The statement that follows is a rather concise, though detailed, summary of this point of view:

When man faces problems he sooner or later seeks a solution. Solutions to some problems are psychological and take the form of adjustments within the individual—a change of purpose, a new understanding, a different kind of reaction. Other solutions take the form of a change in the external environment so that a different situation obtains. In any case, rationally derived solutions give man dependable power over relationships, call for an understanding of the nature of the situation and the factors governing it.

If, in seeking this understanding, man is content to devise and accept intriguing stories based on the ideology of the common lore, he may find explanations that satisfy his surface curiosity, but which are not likely to afford efficient control. . . . If he questions his explanations, the stage is set for research. If he goes further and challenges the methods by which he arrives at his conclusions; if he critically and systematically repeats his observations; if he tests the reliability and validity of these tools and evaluates his data in other ways; if he scrutinizes the thought processes by which he passes from one step of his logic to another; if he gradually refines his concept of what he is trying to explain and considers anew the necessary and sufficient conditions for proof; if at every step he proceeds with the utmost caution, realizing that his purpose is not to arrive at an answer which is personally pleasing, but rather one which will stand up under the critical attacks of those who doubt his answer—if he can meet these criteria and steadfastly hold to his purpose, then he is doing research.[9]

There has arisen more recently a school of research realism that suggests that the process should be considered in terms of the actual operation itself. Its adherents do not subscribe to the rigorous, systematic, logical picture that often is given of the research process. Instead, they feel that this approach is more characteristic of the final product than of the operation.

They recommend that the researcher look more realistically at the actual day-by-day task of getting the job done.

Actually, the process of doing research . . . is a rather informal, often illogical and sometimes messy-looking affair. It includes a great deal of floundering around in the empirical world, sometimes dignified by names like "pilot studies" and "exploratory research." Somewhere and somehow in the process of floundering, the research worker will get an idea. In fact, he will get many ideas. On largely intuitive grounds he will reject most of his ideas and will accept others as the basis for his extended work. To make the picture even less amenable to rational understanding, the ideas he accepts and cherishes and in which he invests his time and resources will sometimes even fly in the face of "known facts."[10]

This school of thought is concerned primarily with the task of educating the research worker. The emphasis, therefore, is upon the person as a research worker rather than upon the product of the work—the experience rather than the rules.

The importance of methodology of research and logic in training teachers to consume and produce research shouldn't be underestimated. However, the equation of research with logic is an erroneous and misleading assumption. It is true that logic plays an important role in research, but not the only important role. The research experience is as much a process of *feelings and personal behavior* as it is a process of logic.[11]

Research, then, can be explained as a method. However, as in the case of purpose, there are different schools of thought. The ideal, the manner by which research should be done, is one expression of methodology. The practical, the realistic concept of getting the job done, is another.

RESEARCH IS A PERSON

Can one identify a single approach or process that is applicable to all research activities? Perhaps there is one, but it may not be possible to learn it from an examination of the researcher at work. How successful people go about doing research has been considered by an inquiry board of psychologists.[12] They concluded that there seems to be little uniformity and great diversity in the way individuals engage in research—especially the more creative aspects.

Research, therefore, often is equated with the particular person who engages in this activity. Each project is considered as a special problem requiring a solution that is determined in some manner or form by the individual worker. There are no stock answers that can be drawn upon on the proper occasions. Instead, the research worker often must create a solution and the means by which it can be tested.

Research may be described as a person. The approach toward learning research is to study the person. Thus, the numerous biographic sources of great research personages can be more illustrative of the research process than their actual studies. The doctoral student learns as an apprentice—observing, following, working with his master.

What are the characteristics of this person? Is he different from the other breeds of professionals? There are strong reasons to believe that he is. The research assignment is such that some of the more common attributes of man may not suffice to carry it through. Furthermore, occasions may arise in which some forms of deviant behavior are necessitated. The researcher becomes, in some measure, a special kind of person.

The researcher is highly intelligent. This does not necessarily imply that he is a genius, because the field then would be the exclusive property of a very limited few in each generation. Unfortunately, biographic studies single out and concentrate upon the geniuses, the Einsteins, the Freuds, the Darwins, the Newtons. While these men have produced some of the greatest ideas of the ages, the bulk of research is carried on by more ordinary folks. On the other hand, a minimum level of high intelligence has been suggested. It also has been pointed out that high intelligence alone does not suffice to produce a good research person.[12] As a matter of fact, it does little to differentiate the research worker from other workers in the field.[12]

The researcher is highly creative. This is a special attribute of intelligence that grants the researcher wide latitude in devising new solutions or technics for testing solutions. Guilford considers it to be a "divergent thinking" kind of ability in which a variety of responses is produced.[13] Winston Churchill is reported to have a high degree of this quality. He always seems to have about ten ideas for any problem that confronts him.

Research is an activity that demands this kind of productive thinking. Variability is a basic feature. One may be required to devise different technics with each new research experience.

Every aspect of research requires some degree of creativeness—the conception of the idea, the formulation of the hypothesis, the development of the procedures for testing, the interpretation of the results, and the writing-up. Stein assumed that some men may be creative in a single aspect of research and others in all phases.[14] It can be inferred from Kelley's study of eminent men of science that creativity in many phases is more characteristic: He concluded that, without exception, each one possessed creative ability in most aspects of research. They were "apt at drawing inferences," "ingenious in making hypotheses," "inventive in the matter of techniques," and "rich in (the) variety and number of hypotheses."[15]

The researcher is also, as Kelley concluded, "persistent on the trail of a discovery."[16] He not only creates the idea, but sees it through to completion. He nourishes the thought, establishes and tests the hypothesis, and, in the face of failure, will begin anew with another idea. The history of research is replete with classic examples of persistence in the pursuance of an idea. Paul Ehrlich developed a compound for the treatment of syphilis that he named 606—to signify 605 failures. It was related that Newton withheld announcement of one of his laws for 20 years because he was not completely satisfied with his experimental verification. Persistence denotes the ability to surmount repeated frustration or failure and, in addition, the ability to avoid premature closure.

Other equally important traits, such as "the ability to think in a logical and consistent manner," "independence of thought," and "the willingness to take a chance," have been listed.[15] Each signifies the character of the research assignment, on the one hand, and the kind of person needed to fulfill the obligation, on the other hand. We deal in research with abstract matter, unobservable relationships; the researcher must be of reasonably high intelligence to comprehend this material. We deal in research with the novel, the unknown, the to-be-discovered; the researcher must be ready to use materials of which he is not yet aware and to invent technics for uncovering them. We recognize in research that events unfold in a logical and consistent manner; the researcher must be able to think and reason accordingly, to derive and specify the nature of these relationships. We accept from research only that which has been verified by reason and empiric testing; the researcher does not necessarily accept previous offerings despite their referral authenticity—he questions the authority, he scrutinizes his own work carefully. We seek new areas of investigation, and the contradictory in research; the researcher has confidence in his ideas and is willing to take a chance. We are subjected by research to continuous frustration, to a sequence of study that may span more than one lifetime; the researcher has a high frustration tolerance level, he is willing to persist at his activity until he is satisfied that the specified criteria have been met—he may even persist beyond that point.

The ledger is replete with descriptions of this kind. Whether the nature of the work or of the person was entered first is difficult to determine. It appears that one side must be balanced by the other. The type of research often is determined by the type of person who engages in it.

Research Is Subject Matter

The subject or the scope of an investigation is presented sometimes as an example of research. In this regard, research has been categorized and labeled as "basic, fundamental or pure" as opposed to "practical or applied." The classification system is by no means definitive, since the line of progression between the two categories may be interpreted in various ways.

The initiating events, the points toward which the process is focused, the kinds of knowledge to be produced, may describe, at times, the nature of the research. Good made the following comparison:

In pure research the investigator may attack any problem that appeals to his fancy. After he has selected his problem he need only apply scholarly methods to its solutions and publish the results, with no concern about any practical social use of his findings. In practical research the problem is localized within practice, and the results are to be applied to the improvement of practice.[17]

The National Science Foundation has distinguished further between basic and applied research. They observed that, in applied research, effort is concentrated upon the unexpected problem.[18] This problem is considered as a negative factor, causing delay and presenting obstacles to be overcome as quickly as possible. "Knowledge is needed," as one engineer observed, "not too much knowledge, just sufficient to solve the problem." The practical goal and the time element are always factors to be considered in applied research.[18] The basic researcher, on the other hand, does not deal directly with the practical problem, nor is time an important commodity to him. His aim is to provide solutions for problems to come, to have available an accumulation of knowledge that can be applied ultimately to the appropriate problem situation as it arises. The problem is important primarily as a vehicle through which he can derive and test the knowledge to be acquired. In applied research, the subject matter becomes the knowledge that is immediately available to satisfy the requirements of the problem at hand. In basic research, the subject matter is knowledge that may have applicability for problems yet to come.

We may follow this same train of thought and focus upon another aspect of subject matter, the problem itself. It may be conceived that the knowledge is to be derived with reference to three kinds of problems: a specific, a common, and an underlying problem. The specific problem is unique in the sense that it occurs in a single situation to a single person—the nursing student has the problem of talking to a patient; the teacher has the problem of motivating her students. The common problem occurs more repetitively and spans a number of specific situations—many nursing students may have difficulty in conversing with patients; teachers, in general, must stimulate their students. The underlying problem transcends the specific and the common problem situations. The general problem of dealing with stress reactions, for example, may be the concern of nursing students with their patients, parents with their children, counselors with their clients, trainers with their animals. The general problem of motivation in learning also will occur universally.

The basic researcher is concerned primarily with the acquisition of knowledge derived from underlying problems. His quest for knowledge may begin with any type of problem but is directed ultimately toward the underlying problem. However, this type of problem is really an abstraction of any number of specific problems. The basic researcher, therefore, must utilize the specific and concrete problem situation as the testing ground for the knowledge resulting from his study.

The applied researcher also may consider each of the three types of problems as his subject matter. However, he will employ them in different ways. His activities will be initiated by and culminate in knowledge applicable to specific or common problems. Nevertheless, he may turn to knowledge that has been derived from some underlying problem and apply it to his own specific situation. It is possible also that knowledge derived from applied research could culminate in more basic research.

There has arisen in recent years a branch of applied research that concentrates upon the specific problem. It is known commonly as "action research"—perhaps because the results are applied immediately. Corey, one of the leaders of this group, has defined and contrasted "action" with "basic" research.

Action research is conducted to improve practices while fundamental research is usually conducted to establish broad generalizations. Fundamental research is done by outside specialists while action research is done by people who want to evaluate their own work situation.[19]

Thus, it is conceived as an endeavor performed by practitioners (not necessarily research people), who apply research technics to aid them in the solution of their own specific problems. Their activities begin and end with a specific problem.

The subject matter of the different schools of research also may focus upon the depth to which the researcher intends to probe. The teacher, for example, may be satisfied to learn simply that tests can serve to motivate her students. She may not be concerned about the fact that tests have both a favorable and an unfavorable effect upon students and may motivate some to advance and cause others to regress. The question is: At what point in the inquiry does the investigator become satisfied with the knowledge that he has accumulated?

Research may be looked upon as the unfolding of cause-and-effect relationships. The nature of cause and effect may be regarded as a series of successive steps wherein an effect becomes an antecedent condition or cause and produces another consequent event or effect. Thus, one event may have stemmed from a long series of successive causes. Several events may have stemmed from the same underlying causal condition or series of conditions. In the process of establishing cause-and-effect relationships, therefore, it would seem that the more stable or fundamental conditions are those that occur earlier in the sequence or train of events. The subject matter for the basic researcher is the discovery of these fundamental conditions. The applied researcher, by contrast, may be satisfied to probe only to the point at which his findings solve his immediate problems.

The lines of progression between the subject matter of the two types of research workers sometimes become thin and merge. Even the basic researcher must begin at the point at which he is able to discover a relationship. Furthermore, despite his immediate concerns, the interests of the applied researcher do not have to be divorced from the discovery of more basic truths. Shumsky, for example, states that "action research is not solely action technique at solving a practical problem, but is rather an attempt to help the teacher arrive at generalizations by investigation of his own field problems."[20]

Research Is Meaningful

If we scrutinize the foregoing points of view carefully, it can be observed that they really do not conflict. As in the case of the blind men of Indostan,* they merely represent the observation of different parts of the elephant at the same time. However, each proposal must be regarded from the vantage point of its proponent, if it is to be at all meaningful to another observer.

Any definition of research, its purpose or its method of procedure should be meaningful if it is to be useful, and each of the definitions can be useful at one time or another. They will not, however, all be satisfactory all the time. Since the problem-solving situations may vary considerably, there is no general panacea to be offered. We cannot issue a single set of rules that will be applicable in all cases or in the same way. As a matter of fact, the research worker may find it necessary at times to invent some rules of his own. In any case, these rules should be meaningful to the person who uses them. They should not be used blindly without regard to the kinds of situations for which they were prepared. Each research project is a meaningful whole. The rules should be integrated accordingly and woven interrelatedly one into the other.

RESEARCH AS PROBLEM-SOLVING—
A POINT OF VIEW

The point of view to be emphasized in the context of this book is that research is problem-solving. Therefore, a general method of problem-solving will be developed and considered as a process for research. It will not be the intent, however, to judge all problem-solving as research. The specific application of problem-solving to those problems that satisfy the over-all purpose of research will be regarded as being within the province exemplified by this point of view.

What Is Problem-Solving?

According to Black, a problem-solving situation is one "in

* See page 338.

which an answer is required to a question, in the absence of reliable information concerning the appropriate procedures to be adopted."[21] Problem-solving is the process or the steps taken to provide a satisfactory solution to the question at hand. Each question may require the development of a special and, perhaps, unique set of procedures designed to bring forth the best possible answer. The general steps to be followed in deriving the answer, however, are not unique and can be described.

Let us begin by examining a problem-solving situation. Here is the report of a nursing supervisor regarding a problem and its solution:

Floor X contains the busy surgical service of a 200-bed general hospital. It consists of three 2-bed and six 4-bed rooms. A variety of surgical cases, ranging from the simple to the complex, is cared for normally. The unit is staffed during the day by a head nurse, three professional and two practical nurses, and two auxiliary nurses.

On this particular day, two of the professional nurses were ill and failed to report for duty. As the patient load throughout the hospital was quite high, replacements could not be obtained from other units in the hospital. To complicate matters further, three of the patients, who were in two of the rooms, had had extensive surgery the previous day and were still critically ill. A fourth patient was expected back from the surgical suite momentarily, after having undergone extensive surgery.

How could the head nurse assign her limited staff? The four critically ill patients required constant observation. Should each of the practical nurses have two of these patients assigned to her? Professional nurses would have to supervise them from time to time, while attempting, with the aid of the two auxiliaries, to provide routine care for twenty other patients.

Suddenly an idea occurred to the head nurse. Why not group the critically ill patients in a single room with a professional nurse? The two practical nurses could be released then to provide the kind of care they were well suited to perform for the other patients. The head nurse remembered having read that other hospitals had found this kind of arrangement to be quite satisfactory.

The situation is initiated by the existence of a problem. What is a problem? Dewey described it as "a felt difficulty."[22] This feeling arises when an obstacle is thrust in the pathway to a goal. The goal is an objective—the fulfillment of an assignment (as in the example just given); the satisfaction of some need; the attainment of an end. The obstacle is a block to the goal fulfillment that may be real or unreal, physical or nonphysical. The problem is how to circumvent or overcome the obstacle and attain the goal, and it becomes apparent as soon as the individual perceives or feels its presence.

The first step in problem-solving is to locate and define the problem. A "felt difficulty" had arisen. What was the cause of this feeling? In these cases, Dewey states, "there are necessary observations deliberately calculated to bring to light just what is the trouble, or to make clear the specific character of the problem."[23] The head nurse was disturbed, as she must have been on many other occasions. However, in order to ease the disturbance, she had to determine specifically just what it was that disturbed her. She was required to identify and define her problem.

To define a problem, according to Black, is to be aware of and understand "the kind of answer that is needed."[24] The head nurse's goal was not only to staff her unit adequately but to do so on that particular day. The problem was: How was she going to do it? Her critically ill patients could not wait until the absent nurses returned to duty, and there were no other nurses to serve as replacements. Therefore, in redefining her problem the head nurse had to consider a solution that would enable her to make use of the nurses who were available on that particular day.

Once a problem has been established clearly, the actual process of finding a solution may emerge. The next step involves the derivation of possible answers. Dewey calls them suggestions, but they also may be described as suppositions, guesses, conjectures or tentative hypotheses. This phase of problem-solving essentially comprises the thinking process.

It involves going from what is present to something absent. . . . Its control is indirect, on the one hand, involving the formation of habits of mind which are at once enterprising and cautious; and on the other hand, involving the selection and arrangement of the particular facts upon perception of which suggestion issues.[25]

We must think of the answers. In this regard, it is considered profitable to spread before ourselves all possible solutions or tentative hypotheses, many of which subsequently will be eliminated.

The head nurse first considered the proposition of securing replacements from other hospital units. This was rejected when she learned that replacements could not be obtained. She then proposed that practical nurses be employed for the care of the critically ill patients. This idea soon was rejected on the ground that the assignment was more properly the concern of the one professional nurse who was available. Then she thought of regrouping her critically ill patients in a single room under the care of the professional nurse. This seemed to be the most promising solution to the problem.

It should be observed in the example just given that each solution or proposition is tested and is, as a consequence, rejected or maintained. The process of corroborating the answers is 2-fold. First, as displayed in the example, each solution is sifted through the reasoning process and a more creditable hypothesis is established. Second, each hypothesis is confirmed in the actual situation.

The reasoning process is a most important step in problem-solving. It not only enables us to narrow down the number of tentative solutions, but also assists in establishing the remaining hypotheses in more suitable and testable form.

> Even when reasoning out the bearings of a supposition does not lead to rejection, it develops the idea in a form in which it is more apposite to the problem.[26]

It is possible that all solutions can be rejected at this point. The process of reasoning then may suggest or aid in establishing other, more tenable hypotheses.

Black considered several adjuncts to the reasoning process. The use of previous knowledge can be applied to both the formulation and the testing of tentative hypotheses.[27] We seldom undertake a problem whose solution has not been attempted by others in some way or form. We can and should draw upon the other experiences in this regard. "The part played by deduction" in the elimination of suitable hypotheses is illustrated in the example. "The recognition of relevance" also is regarded as an important factor and was exemplified when the head nurse considered the relationship of the role of the professional nurse to the care of the critically ill patient and of the practical nurse to more routine nursing care. Finally, Black mentioned the use of subsidiary assumptions, of which he stated:

> It is impossible to explore every possibility which might be relevant to the solution of a problem. The only feasible procedure is to take the truth of a number of assumptions for granted, and to concentrate attention upon the testing of the *main* hypotheses.[28]

The final step in problem-solving is to confirm or verify the remaining hypothesis by further observation. The head nurse actually would have to move her critically ill patients into a single room, assign her nurses accordingly, and let things happen. If it worked—assignments completed and patients satisfied—she probably would feel pretty good about the solution and perhaps try it again some other time. If it did not work, she would either have to find out why and make adjustments or consider other hypotheses.

The various steps of problem-solving may be summarized briefly:

1. The appearance of a problem—"a felt difficulty"
2. The location and definition of the problem
3. The determination of solutions
4. The testing and the elimination of solutions by reasoning
5. The testing of the remaining solution in actual practice.

Is All Problem-Solving Research?

If it is proposed that all research is problem-solving, is all problem-solving research? The point of view to be adopted here is negative in this regard. It will be contended that the solution of problems is not the primary purpose of research but is merely a vehicle or a means by which some other purpose is satisfied. Therefore, research does not attempt to solve just any problems, but selects only those that further this other purpose.

If it were possible to trace the origin of research, we probably should learn that it began with man's crude attempts to solve highly specific problems. In the course of these endeavors, no doubt, man found that he could apply some of the solutions derived in the past to his current problem-solving activities. This was a time-saving device; he did not have to engage in a number of fruitless trial-and-error procedures. He may have learned further that, by pooling past solutions, he would have a valuable reservoir from which to draw solutions for many future problems. Could we consider that man might apply himself deliberately to the creation and the development of such a resource?

When it was stated previously that the purpose of research was to make a contribution to knowledge, perhaps this point of view was implied. That is, if we conceive that knowledge consists of a pool or a resource of solutions to past problems that can be applied to future problems, could we not state that it is the purpose of research to develop such a resource? Our attention is turned then not upon the problem but upon the solution, not upon the past but upon the future. Furthermore, our sights are set not upon specific problems but upon common or underlying problems, because the solutions of these have wider application. Problem-solving becomes the method by which solutions are derived. The specific problem becomes the vehicle through which the solution is tested. Research becomes problem-solving with a purpose: to contribute to the pool of knowledge.

The development of a pool of knowledge is, furthermore, a gradual process in which the results of one research project are added to those of others to yield additional knowledge. It is rare that a single effort will make more than a minor dent in the over-all number of contributions. To be of maximum effectiveness, the researcher might well consider the total needs of the area to which research is to be directed. A framework could then be developed, specifying the required research and the relationship of projects to each other and to the total framework. Thus, while the effects of the single study may be hardly perceptible, the results of the concentration of the studies within the framework are apt to be significant. The purpose of any research study may be justified readily when it is cast in such a framework.

If we continue this trend of thought, the research problem becomes special in another sense. Once the nonresearch problem is solved, the instigator is satisfied and may or may not continue to pursue the problem or any aspect of it. The research problem, on the other hand, when cast into a specific framework often will open the gates to further avenues of study. The development of a field of knowledge is a never-ending process and the research worker should be aware of the implications of his study to future inroads in his field. Frequently one study leads to other studies. Thus Kelley suggested the following addendum to the general problem-solving steps formulated by Dewey:

> After the solution has been found to work there is a mental looking forward, the general purpose of which is to appraise this new solution in the light of possible future needs.[29]

The point of view is expressed, therefore, that *not all problem-solving is research*. While this text will be developed in accordance with the point of view that research is problem-solving, it will be modified to satisfy the requirements of the second proposition. The problem-solving process, as set forth previously, is amended to include the following:

1. A statement of the purpose and its justification
2. The derivation and the statement of the problem
3. The derivation of hypotheses
4. The confirmation of the hypotheses
5. The consideration of future avenues of study.

The context of this book will be cast accordingly.

RESEARCH IN NURSING—A FELT DIFFICULTY

The phenomenal growth in the scope and the specialization of research has become apparent in nursing. The tremendous interest of nurses in research is evidenced both nationally and internationally by the continually increasing number of research reports in the nursing literature and the large attendance of nurses at the meetings devoted to research. The research conferences have been sponsored by nursing organizations at the local, the state, the national and the international levels. Nursing is beginning to "come of age" in this regard. When a profession undertakes research, it takes a step toward maturity and the assumption of its social responsibilities.

Despite the interest and the rapid progress in recent years, many problems still are coming to the fore. Research in nursing is suffering growing pains. Numerous obstacles have strewn the pathway and can be regarded as "felt difficulties." There is a high degree of consensus among the members of the nursing profession regarding the values of research. There is also a lack of clarity as to what would be the most fruitful or significant line of development to pursue.

Considerable time and financial and personnel resources are being poured into research. In the rush to push forward, however, nursing needs to pause to ask some pertinent questions:

1. Is nursing really doing research? What is its point of view? Has nursing research been fact-finding? Problem-solving? Basic? Applied? Action?

2. What is the purpose of research in nursing? Has a purpose been stated? Are there many purposes?

3. What is the subject matter of research in nursing? The nurse? The patient? The profession? Technic? Tools? The sciences?

4. What is the method of the nurse researcher? The case study? The survey? Is there overemphasis upon method?

5. Who are doing the research? Are they adequately prepared?

6. Is research in nursing meaningful? To the nurse practitioner? To the leaders? To the nurse researcher? To the consumer of nursing services?

A basis for answering these questions will be sought by examining the history of nursing research to date in the light of the points of view expressed in the previous section.

A Short, Short History of Research in Modern American Nursing

The development of research in nursing parallels the growth and the development of nursing practice itself. The emergence of the profession reflects directly upon the character and the course of the project undertaken. A brief review of research cast in the perspective of nursing history may uncover the problems that underlie the current stage of development.

No doubt the history of research in nursing started long before the years of modern practice. It covers the evolution of the scientific principles that are applied continuously in nursing today but may have been discovered as much as a thousand years ago. It should include also the many informal but unrecorded research activities that began when the nurse and her colleagues encountered their first problem. Most histories (including this one) of necessity must utilize as their primary source of data the events of the past that have been observed and preserved, recorded and reported. This short, short history of nursing research will review only the formalized activities during the reign of modern nursing practice.

Research in modern nursing may be divided into three periods. Each period may be described by different purposes, subject matter, research personages and methodology. The periods range as follows:

1. From 1860 to the First World War
2. From the First World War to the Second World War
3. From the Second World War to the present.

From 1860 to the First World War

This period, which spans approximately 60 years, marks the beginning of modern professional nursing. It was a period of emergence, signifying the onset of nursing as a profession. It was also a movement founded upon the works of a small number of great personages. The history of research during these years parallels the emergence of the profession and is intertwined with the contributions of the nursing leaders.

The emergence of nursing as a profession resulted from two coexisting developments. A formal program of nursing education was initiated and fostered throughout this span of years. There was effected, in addition, a wide and diversified body of procedures that could be integrated into the order known as nursing practice.

Until the middle of the nineteenth century, nursing was performed by women who were not specifically trained as nurses. The first formal school of nursing was established in 1860 at St. Thomas's Hospital in London. The aims of the school were to train hospital nurses, to train nurses to train others, and to train nurses for the sick poor.[30] In 1873, the first three schools of this order were established in the United States.[31] The schools multiplied rapidly thereafter, increasing from 35 to 432 during the single decade 1890 to 1900. In 1910, Sutton's Hospital and Institutional Directory recorded 1,630 training schools for nurses.[32]

The work of both the physician and the nurse changed considerably during this era. The health field and the practices of medicine and nursing were altered by numerous discoveries and technical developments. The gradual control of the great pestilential diseases, the discovery of anesthesia, and the development of antiseptic and aseptic practices added to the duties and the responsibilities of both the physician and the nurse.[33, 34] The doctors began to delegate more and more of the technical responsibilities to the nurse. The advent of new diagnostic and treatment procedures required the nurse's assistance in the hospital wards, the operating rooms, the doctors' offices and the x-ray and pathologic laboratories.[35] As developments in preventive medicine progressed, the nurse was required to assume new and important responsibilities in the field of public health practice.[36] In 1900, there were 200 nurses engaged in what is now called public health nursing. By 1912, 3,000 nurses were so engaged.[37]

The two movements of nursing education and nursing practice reached a milestone in the development of the nursing profession with the formation of the professional societies. The directors of the American training schools for nurses organized in 1893 into a group known first as the American Society of Superintendents of Training Schools for Nurses and later as the National League of Nursing Education. The graduates of these programs established in 1897 a society called initially the Nurses Associated Alumnae, which was renamed the American Nurses Association in 1911. The International Council of Nurses, organized in 1900, provided an affiliation of nursing organizations throughout the world. In 1912, the National Organization for Public Health Nursing came into being, differing from the other organizations in that its membership was open to lay people interested in public health nursing. This organization combined with the National League of Nursing Education in 1952 to form the National League for Nursing.

Each of the societies issued annual reports of articles published in periodicals, giving a fairly comprehensive account of the technical and the educational developments in nursing. Beginning in 1900, the *American Journal of Nursing,* issued monthly to a wide body of nurses, has provided a record of the movements in nursing and nursing education.

Spearheading the movements was a small group of nurses who initiated the programs, stimulated activities in other groups, and prepared extensive reports depicting the nature of the activities and the ensuing problems. Florence Nightingale was perhaps the most influential in this regard. She was active in every sphere of nursing. It was Miss Nightingale who founded the first school of modern nursing at St. Thomas's Hospital. She also prepared papers on nursing resources for the British Army, and on nursing practice.[38] Three American nurses and one social worker of the period were outstanding: Isabel A. Hampton, Mary Adelaide Nutting, Lavinia L. Dock and Abby Howland Woolsey. Miss Hampton was one of the first nurse educators to recognize the problems inherent in a system that was expanding so rapidly.[39] Miss Dock and Miss Nutting wrote numerous articles and pamphlets, and two volumes on the history of nursing.[40] Miss Dock expanded the record of the history of nursing by writing Volumes III and IV several years later.[41] Abby Woolsey prepared a report on a survey of nursing that she made in Europe and in the United States entitled *A Century of Nursing.*[42] The publications recorded the story of the nurse's struggle for self-government and educational opportunities.

These few personages contributed much of what might be classified as the research studies of that period. The papers that evolved related to the major problems of nursing education and practice and professional growth. They considered the difficulties of rapid and diversified growth. They pinpointed the need to define and qualify the nature of what was going on.

Nursing Education. Nursing education had progressed with such rapidity that many poor practices were instituted in the schools. Miss Hampton raised the issue at a meeting of the training school superintendents in 1893: "A trained nurse 'may' mean then anything, everything, or next to nothing . . . and public criticism is frequently justly severe on our shortcomings."[43] The subject of "training versus education" occupied much of the early literature. Adelaide Nutting summarized the feelings of the time as part of the first comprehensive survey of the situation in American nursing, entitled *The Educational Status of Nursing,* which was published in 1912 by the U. S. Bureau of Education:

. . . it seems tolerably clear that the principle of dependence upon the student body for all of the actual nursing work, and for a very considerable amount of other work, some purely domestic in nature, some supervisory and executive, is so universally accepted and so deeply rooted as to render hospitals unwilling to tolerate any conditions which affect this principle and which require a modification or frank abandonment of the plan and system upon which it is based.[44]

While hospital and training school are fundamentally interdependent, there is no more reason why the hospital should own and control the training school than the medical school. The basis of relationship should be one of close and efficient cooperation.[45]

Nursing Practice. Emanating from the wide range of poor practices in the nursing care of people in the hospital or in their homes was the need to define and describe nursing. Florence Nightingale contributed a definitive report on the subject in 1859: *Notes on Nursing: What It Is and What It Is Not.*[46] She later made a functional analysis of qualifications and duties for nurses, which was used to develop the training program for nurses at St. Thomas's Hospital. This list, with some modifications, was employed frequently by the American schools founded on the Nightingale system.[47] In 1893, another report on nursing practice, prepared by Miss Nightingale, was read by Isabel Hampton at the International Congress of Charities, Correction, and Philanthropy in Chicago.[48]

Five systems of nursing prevailing in different countries are described by Abby Woolsey in *A Century of Progress*. She observed that progress in hospital reform was accompanied by efforts to recruit and retain in the nursing service women of good character who are fitted for their work. She stated:

> Nursing is a serious business; it signifies the proper use of fresh air, light, warmth, cleanliness, quiet, the proper selection and administration of food, close observation, and report of symptoms and the most scrupulous fulfillment of medical orders, and all with the greatest economy of the patient's strength.[49]

Two other sources contained much of the literature giving detailed descriptions of nursing in America. They can be grouped in two categories: (1) articles on nursing as reported in the periodicals and convention summaries and (2) textbooks on nursing. Most of these source materials are rather sketchy and pertain to the training of nurses. Nevertheless, they give the best available descriptions of American nursing practices of the time.

Articles on the care of typhoid fever, pneumonia, tuberculosis, mental illness and infant feeding appeared in the journals. One of these has been described by the editors of the *American Journal of Nursing* as one of the finest articles ever to appear on nursing.[50] This article revealed how, in 1901, 396 of 500 pneumonia patients were successfully cared for in their homes by visiting nurses. It was a story of achievement based on a study of records at a time when records were not stressed.

Descriptions of nursing practices also can be found in the early textbooks written by nurses. During the first 12 years of nursing education, fifteen such texts were identified.[51] Clara Weeks wrote the pioneer book on nursing in 1885.[52] Like Osler's book in medicine, it served as an institution for 25 years. She was "the first nurse to dare make the distinction between true nursing care and execution of . . . doctors' orders."[53] Isabel Hampton wrote another text in 1893 that influenced the development of nursing for many years.[54] Lastly, the rapid expansion of public health nursing necessitated the development of guides for action. In response, Mary Gardner developed a text in 1916 (revised in 1924 and in 1942) that has continued to serve as a guide to public health nurses.[55]

Nursing Profession. It is rather difficult to separate the growth of nursing education and practice from the development of the profession. Thus, each of the early reports contributed materials about the slowly evolving profession of nursing. The Woolsey study urged that nursing be rescued from the hands of the ignorant, from unfaithful drudges, and made into an educated and honorable profession. The Nutting report discussed some of the present-day issues of professionalism. The author spoke of the movement toward education for the profession, citing the establishment of a Department of Nursing at Teachers College, Columbia University, at which graduate nurses could prepare for teaching, administration and public health nursing. She considered the relationship between hospitals and training schools, observing that nursing in hospitals was performed by students. She noted also that graduate nurses were employed by the hospitals in administrative posts or as private duty nurses, but rarely as staff nurses.

Many of the early articles reflect the concern of the nursing leaders for sound professional growth. One can recognize the character of these reports by their titles: "Is the Profession Overcrowded?"[56]; "Is Nursing Really a Profession?"[57]; "How To Lift Your Business Into a Profession"[58]; "The Limitations of the Nursing Profession."[59]

The literature records the major struggles in the attainment of self-direction and independence. The movement was opposed particularly by hospital and medical men. Thompson compiled a brief report on 22 new schools of nurses at the end of the 1st decade, commenting that:

> The old nurses were good enough . . . the new nurses would be overtaught . . . they would soon think they knew as much as or more than the doctors . . . the educated nurse would lose interest and consequently efficiency in performing monotonous and menial duties. . . .[60]

The famous Shattuck report of 1850, on the other hand, offers the reflections of a few men who could visualize the potential of nursing. The report suggested that nursing often may do more to cure disease than the physician himself and, in regard to the prevention of disease and the promotion of health, it is of equal or even greater importance.[61]

A small body of materials that might be called research in nursing resulted from this period. They dealt with the major problems of the age and were compiled by the nursing leaders who conducted the research.

Could these reports really be classified as research? If so, what point of view do they represent? Let us regard a sample of the reports from each of the points of view that were presented previously. The reports that will be analyzed briefly include:

Florence Nightingale: *Notes on Nursing: What It Is and What It Is Not,* 1893.[62]

Abby H. Woolsey: *A Century of Nursing,* 1893.[63]

Adelaide M. Nutting and Lavinia L. Dock: *A History of Nursing, Vols. I & II,* 1907.[64]

Adelaide M. Nutting: *Educational Status of Nursing,* 1912.[65]

What Was the Purpose of the Research? Three types of purposes characterized these works:

1. To describe a state of affairs
2. To isolate problem areas
3. To determine solutions for problems.

Three of the studies were essentially descriptive. Woolsey described and compared the contemporary systems of nursing in Europe and America. Dock and Nutting traced the evolution and the development of nursing systems from the earliest times to the foundation of the first English and American training schools for nurses. Nutting surveyed the status and the progress made in nursing education.

Why did they describe? Nutting employed her information to identify and isolate problem areas. The persistence of low standards of admission and "unrestricted development of training schools as a part of their (hospitals and sanitaria) working organization (which) has led to a very large demand for students essentially for utilitarian purposes" were two of the major problem areas that she identified.[66] The reconstruction of nursing education was imperative for, according to Nutting, "it is out of right relationship with the thought and methods of education to-day."[66]

Nutting also used her materials to indicate the changes needed in the nursing education system and to suggest the direction of the changes. She suggested that the control of the school be moved from the hospital to educational institutions or that the education be on an independent basis in a hospital. In the latter case, the school would have freedom to plan and administer a program whose objectives were truly educational. The descriptive materials collected by Miss Woolsey were utilized ultimately to lay the groundwork for future planning. She identified hospital reforms and the principles guiding the reforms. She evolved a plan for the establishment of a training school for nurses.

The Nightingale report was primarily an embodiment of principles or generalized solutions for problems of nursing. Miss Nightingale provided information on and principles for health and sanitation that were applicable to the care of the ill. She gave many illustrations of poor observations by nurses and suggestions for training nurses in better observation skills. For example, she observed that the question "How is your appetite?" frequently really meant "How is your digestion?"

Though interrelated, the two questions have different meanings. She noted that there are four different causes of "poor appetite," any one of which will produce the same result: poor cooking, the choice of diet, the time of the meal, and the actual lack of appetite. "Yet, all of these are generally comprehended in the one sweeping assertion that the patient has 'no appetite.' "[67] Florence Nightingale suggested that a much closer distinction in observation was required; the remedies appeared to be as diverse as the causes.

Miss Nightingale made a distinction between simple observation and observation distorted by imagination. Both observers may fully intend to speak the truth. The information of the first is defective simply in that the answers are imperfect—he has never really observed. The second has observed just as little but describes the whole thing merely from imagination, being perfectly convinced all the while that he has seen or heard it. It was inferred that the observers were unaware of what was seen or not seen, remembered or forgotten.

She gave numerous suggestions for the improvement of the skill of observation:

If you find it helps you to note down such things on a bit of paper in pencil, by all means do so . . . if you cannot get the habit of observation one way or other, you had better give up the being a nurse, for it is not your calling, however kind and anxious you may be.[68]

I think that few things press so heavily on one suffering from long and incurable illness, as the necessity of recording in words, from time to time, for the information of the nurse, who will not otherwise see, that he cannot do this or that, which he could do a month or a year ago. What is the nurse there for if she cannot observe these things for herself?[69]

What Was the Method of the Research? The methodology employed by the writers of the reports listed consisted of the age-old technics of recording, reporting and armchair thinking. It was definitely not a period of experiment and testing.

The library review was used extensively throughout each of the papers. Materials from Europe and America were collected over a period of 15 years and compiled into the two volumes of the history of nursing. The reports by Woolsey and Nutting were also replete with literature of this kind. Several technics actually contributed to their reports. Woolsey secured her data by visiting hospitals and training schools in France, Germany, Russia, Switzerland, Italy, England and the United States. Although her report does not specify the procedures she followed, it indicates that she interviewed nurses, doctors and others interested in nursing. She supplemented her report with facts obtained from other reports, such as the Nightingale one. Nutting collected facts about nursing practice and education. These included facts on hospitals—type, size, finances, types and census of patients; on schools—number of schools and students, types, administration and control, curricula, facilities, faculty, and the like; and status and standards for state registration. Many of these facts had been collected previously by the U. S. Bureau of Education but were employed by Nutting, with additional information.

The treatise on nursing by Florence Nightingale was compiled through the process of logical thinking. Starting with the general principle that "all disease, at some period or other of its course, is more or less a reparative process, not necessarily accompanied with suffering,"[70] Florence Nightingale logically developed the contribution that nursing can make to this reparative process. She states:

. . . the symptoms or the sufferings generally considered to be inevitable and incident to the disease are very often not symptoms of the disease at all, but of something quite different—of the want of fresh air, or of light, or of warmth, or of quiet, or of cleanliness, or of punctuality and care in the administration of diet, of each or of all of these.[70]

From this statement, Florence Nightingale proceeds to show how nursing can contribute to each of these factors and what the want of attention to each will cause. She observes:

The very elements of what constitutes good nursing are as little understood for the well as for the sick. The same laws of health or of nursing, for they are in reality the same, obtain among the well as among the sick.[71]

In her conclusion, she states that sanitary nursing is prevention through the accurate observation of and attention to fresh air, ventilation, light, warmth, cleanliness, quietness and nutrition, and that the care of the patient is the responsibility of all nursing regardless of whether the patient is surgical or medical, child or adult, male or female.

What Was the Subject Matter of the Research? Some common problems of nursing practice and education, and indirectly of the nursing profession, were considered in the Nutting and the Woolsey reports. Woolsey attempted to describe the systems of nursing in other countries as well as in the United States. Nutting confined her attention to the system of nursing education in the United States. Both were concerned with the problem of control of the education of nurses. The existing system of hospital control resulted in extremely wide variations in admission standards to the schools, and the dependence upon students for the staffing of the hospitals for nursing care. Some of the other problems analyzed by Nutting included:

1. Multiplication of hospitals and sanitoria with the unrestricted development of the training of nurses as part of the nursing staff of the institutions

2. Persistence of low standards for admission

3. Paucity of clinical resources for an adequate training program for nurses. (Very small hospitals, including such specialized ones as psychiatric and pediatric hospitals, were operating schools.)

4. The lack of a qualified faculty

5. The lack of adequate facilities.

Woolsey, on the other hand, was concerned primarily with the steps and the procedures for initiating reform in the current nursing service in hospitals and in devising new programs for the training of nurses. Since much of her report dealt with nursing in Europe, where most of the nursing was done either by or under the auspices of religious orders, she considered the relationship between and the control of government agencies and religious groups as a problem area.

The subject matter in Nightingale's report concerned the problem of simple health knowledge ("sanitary nursing," as she termed it), which every woman must have at some time or other, either in the care of her own family or of other people. Thus she was solving a problem that was common to all those who are interested in healthful living. It was a common problem in nursing, for nursing was concerned basically with restoring an individual to health, maintaining a certain state of health, and preventing a state of absence of health.

Nightingale delineated a series of problems inherent in this broad common problem:

1. Fresh air and ventilation, particularly in the sick room
2. Nutrition and appetite
3. Environmental sanitation—cleanliness, water, drainage, sewerage
4. Management problems regarding personnel (servants in homes, nurses in hospitals) in providing healthful environment, prevention of accidents, lessening noise, and the like.

In addition to the problems relating to health, she also analyzed problems that were more specific to the nursing care of patients. The "influence of mind over body," as she termed it (the psychosomatic principle of today), and what the nurse could do to help to provide pleasant surroundings, diversion and recreation, were discussed in detail.

Who Did the Research? The research of the day was performed by the leaders of the period. They were few in number, although versatile in the pursuit of their activities. We may question the character of the research reports they developed, measured by current standards. We also may conclude, upon a cursory examination of their traits, that they would have emerged as the research personages of today.

Florence Nightingale (1820-1910) was born to relatively wealthy English parents, while they were traveling in Florence, Italy,[72-74] and died in London at 90 years of age. Well educated for a woman of her day, she spent much of her early life in travel and social affairs. At 31 years of age, she managed to fulfill a persistent ambition by entering and completing a short-term nurse-training program. A series of careers followed that shaped her into the figure with which we are so familiar.

At 34 years of age, Florence Nightingale was called to the Crimean War by Sir Sidney Herbert, the British Secretary of War. She began her campaign for improvement in the hospital upon her arrival in Scutari. Within 8 months the death rate had been reduced to 2 per cent, and the earlier opposition to a woman in medical affairs had been overcome. She also initiated action that was to result in the complete reform of the Army medical system.

Upon her return from the Crimea, she began a career as a sanitarian. Inspection tours of military hospitals were initiated, and the future sanitary standards of the Army were shaped. Her work in this area culminated with a comprehensive report on the sanitary conditions of the Indian Army.

The movement to establish a training school for nurses began while Florence Nightingale was still in the Crimea. A fund was raised in appreciation of her services. Although a semi-invalid upon returning from the Crimea, she led the movement that founded the modern art and practice of nursing.

Florence Nightingale was *highly persistent.* She tried at 25 to become a nurse but met with stern opposition from her parents, who took her on an extensive foreign tour, so that she would forget nursing. She persisted in her determination, overcame the resistance, and some 6 years later visited Kaiserswerth, where she studied nursing and the life of the deaconess nurses.

She had *considerable foresight.* She was dissatisfied with the nursing of her day. She recognized the need for a national foundation and for a sound educational system. Above all, she was able to translate her thoughts into action.

She was a *systematic thinker.* Florence Nightingale was the first nurse to prepare a report on what might be called research. This report on the health and the efficiency of the hospital administration of the British Army during the Crimean War was well documented from her experiences and replete with statistics.

Mary Adelaide Nutting (1859-1948) was born in a small town in the Province of Quebec, Canada. Although socially prominent and gifted with talent in painting and music, she resisted the lure of conventional life and, at 30 years of age, entered into nursing as a way of life.[75, 76]

Many "firsts" mark the life of Miss Nutting. She was graduated in the first class in nursing at Johns Hopkins Hospital. She was selected by the first university (Teachers College, Columbia University) ever to offer special work for graduate nurses. She was the first nurse to be appointed to a professorship on any college or university faculty.

In recognition of her work in nursing education, Yale University bestowed upon her an honorary Master of Arts degree in 1921. She was characterized at the time as "one of the most useful women in the world."[77]

Miss Nutting was *highly persistent*. Although reared in an isolated pioneer village, she trudged through the storms of many severe Canadian winters to the academy where she got her first schooling. There she found the intellectual stimulation that patterned her life to be.

She was *highly creative*. She was at home in painting, music, literature, history, philosophy and politics, as well as in nursing and education.

She had *considerable foresight*. Between the years of her graduation from Johns Hopkins in 1891 and her retirement as Director of Nursing Education at Teachers College in 1925, Miss Nutting systematically shaped a new concept of preparation for nursing. She was able to characterize the entire system before it actually existed. Some 50 years ago she depicted in her writings the problems that are faced by nursing students today.[78, 79]

Lavinia L. Dock (1886-1956) was born in Harrisburg, Pennsylvania, into a family that included six other children. She was well educated and quite mature when she entered Bellevue Hospital to study nursing.[80, 81]

Upon graduation, she moved into a variety of positions.

After becoming the first nurse to be employed for home nursing by the United Workers, a pioneer social organization of Norwich, Connecticut, she became assistant principal at Johns Hopkins Hospital. She pursued her career in nursing education as principal of the Illinois Training School for Nurses, and then returned to home nursing with Lillian Wald at the Henry Street Settlement House.

Her career ultimately took her into national and international affairs and into the field of writing. Miss Dock was one of the organizers and the first secretary of the Society of Superintendents. She served the I.C.N. in the same capacities.

She wrote profusely. Her publications included a textbook on nursing and a history of nursing in four volumes.

Miss Dock was *highly creative.* She was an accomplished musician. She also was skilled in painting and was a student of languages, including German, French and Italian. Her first publication, *Materia Medica for Nurses,* was employed as a textbook for 50 years. Her histories, it was stated, were "a revelation of American research in nursing, and the work has no rival in any language."[82]

Miss Dock had *considerable foresight.* She recognized at an early date the significance of the oncoming world health movement that would emphasize prevention and the need for nurses to have preparation in public health nursing. She foresaw the importance of developing nursing through organizations on the national and the international levels. Through her work at the Henry Street Settlement House, she demonstrated the relationship between poor social conditions and health problems. She also published a small book on hygiene and morality many years before venereal disease could be mentioned in public.

From the First World War to the Second World War (1918-1945)

The second period of this brief history lies between two great wars. It was a period during which the public had become aware of the value of nursing care and had created a demand for service. A marked growth in the number of nurses, hospitals and schools of nursing resulted. The leadership was transferred from the person to the organization, which became the directing agent for an outflow of studies. It was during this period that governmental agencies became participants in nursing activities.

The continued growth in the numbers of nurses, hospitals and schools is reflected in the table that follows. The different rates of growth that can be observed for each group indicate that the factors present in the period affected the nurse, the hospital and the school of nursing in different ways.

An increased demand for nursing services can be observed during the 1st decade following World War I. This may have resulted in part from the organization of the American Red Cross and the Public Health Nursing agencies and the need to provide care for World War I veterans. Growth continued

TABLE 1. GROWTH IN THE NUMBERS OF PROFESSIONAL NURSES, HOSPITALS AND SCHOOLS OF NURSING DURING THE PERIOD BETWEEN WORLD WAR I AND WORLD WAR II*

YEAR	NUMBER	
	NURSES AND STUDENTS	RATIO
1920	149,128	1 per 708 people
1930	294,189	1 per 416 people
1940	371,066	1 per 357 people
	HOSPITALS	BEDS
1918	5,323	612,251
1928	6,852	892,934
1938	6,166	1,161,380
1945	6,511	1,738,944
	SCHOOLS OF NURSING†	ENROLLMENT
1920†	1,775	55,000
1930†	1,900	83,000
1940	1,311	85,156
1945	1,295	126,576

* Facts About Nursing, American Nurses' Assn., New York, 1935, 1945 and 1947 editions.

† Estimates are given: the records were not accurate, as the schools did not always report the enrollment figures.

during the next decade, but at a slower rate. These were the depression years when many graduate nurses, as well as other people, were unemployed. World War II, which followed, brought a considerable change. The demand for nurses to meet military and civilian needs far exceeded the number of nurses available. As a result, other workers, such as practical nurses, nurse's aides and voluntary workers, were brought into the hospitals and other health agencies to assist and, in some cases, to replace the graduate nurses.

The number of hospital beds increased gradually during the 1st two decades of this period, and then rose substantially at the conclusion of World War II. There was a rather sharp increase in the number of hospitals, on the other hand, during the decade following World War I. Apparently a number of these hospitals closed during the depression years and reopened after the war. The disparity between the two sets of figures— hospitals and hospital beds—suggests a reversal of the trend from the smaller, perhaps proprietary type of institution, to larger hospitals. The effect of this event upon nursing practice today may be pictured.

If the growth of nursing education is measured by the increase in the number of schools, an erratic course may be plotted. The expansive forces created during the latter part of the previous century continued to operate. A peak was reached in 1926, when there were 2,155 schools of nursing registered.[83] Then the forces were reversed. Over 850 schools were eliminated during the next two decades. In 1945, 1,295 schools of nursing were listed.[84]

The student enrollment is perhaps a more accurate index of growth. In this regard, the growth curve paralleled the changes taking place in the numbers of nurses and hospital beds. In other words, the schools, like the hospitals, were getting larger.

The three national nursing organizations—the American Nurses Association, the National League for Nursing Education, and the National Organization for Public Health Nursing —acquired full status in 1921, when they established a national headquarters in New York City.[85] They took a strong leadership role in bringing about a more detailed appraisal of the schools and the establishment of standards for practice.

Each of the organizations undertook special functions. In 1932, the National League for Nursing Education established a Department of Studies to provide factual materials for developing standards and guides.[86] The American Nurses Association organized the National Information Bureau, which published the first issue of *Facts About Nursing* in 1935.[87] The Joint Orthopedic Nursing Advisory Service was organized in 1942 under the sponsorship of the National Organization for Public Health Nursing and the National League for Nursing Education.[88] This was one of the first programs to concentrate upon the patient rather than upon the nurse and her activities.

Many of the studies reported during the period were initiated, sponsored and conducted by the national nursing organizations. An extensive system of national committees was employed for this purpose. The committees often were assisted by representatives from state agencies. Individuals directed the studies and collected and analyzed the data; the committees usually made the recommendations.

The work of the committees was essentially fact-finding, the development of guides for study and the establishment of standards. The movement toward the accreditation of schools was an outgrowth of these studies. The first effort in this direction by a professional nursing organization initiated a program for approving university programs in public health nursing.[89] By this time, state accreditation had been accepted in all the states. In 1937, the National League for Nursing Education began its study and development of a co-operative plan for accreditation with schools of nursing.[90] The first list of schools accredited by the National League for Nursing Education appeared in 1941. Seventy schools were included on the list.

The need for education on the college level for positions in public health nursing and nursing education was emphasized by the studies of the previous era. The first collegiate program in basic nursing leading to a baccalaureate degree was started in 1916. Growth was rapid. By 1929, 105 schools of nursing reported some affiliation with colleges.[91] However, only 32 of these schools offered programs leading to a degree. Many of the others did not offer any collegiate courses in nursing. The Association of Collegiate Schools for Nursing was organized in 1932 to develop standards and criteria to stem the growth of the poorly developed, so-called collegiate programs.[92]

In response to the growing demand for nursing services, the federal government made its first real contribution to the advancement of nursing during this period. Limiting itself at first to the field of public health nursing, in 1936 the U. S. Public Health Service undertook the task of maintaining a census of public health nurses.[93] In 1940, this agency undertook a national inventory of all registered nurses in co-operation with the state nursing associations.[94] A National Nursing Council was organized in 1940 to consider the role of the nurse and of nursing in the program of national defense and to unify all nursing activities directly or indirectly related to it.[95] It was reorganized in 1942 and in 1945, at which time it broadened its function to establish long-range plans for nursing.[96]

The most direct contribution by the federal government was the Bolton Bill of 1943.[97] This piece of legislation established the U. S. Cadet Nursing Corps to augment the number of students in the schools of nursing. It provided students with books, uniforms, tuition and other fees, and monthly stipends. By this bill, the federal government offered financial support for basic nursing education for the first time. At the same time, the Bolton Bill also provided aid for the short-term training of teachers.

The 2nd period of this historical treatise was thus an era of growth, evaluation and stabilization. Fact-finding studies in the area of nursing practice predominated and suggested the requisites for training in nursing education. Curriculum guides were developed accordingly.

Nursing Education. Public health nursing was the first nursing group to become aware of the need for better preparation of nurses. A conference was called by the Rockefeller Foundation in 1918 to consider the problem. The conference members soon realized that the entire problem of nursing education required study. The committee therefore was broadened to include representatives from nursing, medicine, public health and the public. A comprehensive study, directed by Josephine Goldmark, was undertaken and financed by the foundation. The final report, entitled *Nursing and Nursing Education in the United States,* was published in 1923.[98]

This survey, which resulted in the reiteration of many of the recommendations of earlier leaders of nursing, gave impetus to a 5-year series of studies designed to bring about the needed reforms in nursing education. The studies culminated in another report, *Nursing Schools Today and Tomorrow,* in which the results of the overproduction and the undereducation of nurses pointed to the need for a radical change in the system of nursing education.[99] The studies did effect some change, as, following them, a number of poor schools were eliminated.

Several other fact-finding studies were undertaken to obtain data for the development of standards and guides for collegiate education for nursing. Two of the studies of major interest for public health nursing include *Survey of Public Health Nursing Administration and Practice* by Tucker and Hilbert,[100] and *An Analysis of First Level Public Health Nursing in 10 Selected Organizations,* by McIver.[101] Petry directed her attention to the basic professional curricula in nursing, leading to a baccalaureate degree.[102] Oates contributed a study of the advanced curricula.[103]

The fact-finding studies led to the development of standards and guides for action. The most extensive and far-reaching of the guides published during the period were the Curriculum Guides of the National League for Nursing Education. The first guide, published in 1917, was entitled *A Standard Curriculum for Schools of Nursing.*[104] The 1923 survey of nursing provided data that were employed for the revision of this guide in 1927.[105] The guide was revised again in 1937, the revision being based upon information received from the Grading Committee reports and other studies.[106] This edition was presented as a suggested guide rather than as a standard curriculum pattern.

The Grading Committee also provided information concerned with the costs of nursing education, *Nurses, Patients and Pocketbooks*.[107] The first systematic study in this regard, however, was not performed until 1940, when Pfefferkorn and Rovetta devised a system for cost analysis that could be used by schools of nursing and hospitals in assessing the costs of nursing service and education.[108]

Nursing Practice. The fact-finding studies, such as those performed in public health nursing by Tucker and Hilbert, and McIver, while they were directed toward education, actually explored nursing practice. Among other studies of this type were the Commonwealth Fund Child Health demonstration in 1927.[109] These studies were conducted for the purpose of measuring the nurse power of the public health nurse and attempted to determine how the public health nurse's time was distributed among her required activities.

The first systematic effort to study the practice of hospital nursing was performed by Pfefferkorn and Rottman at Bellevue Hospital.[110] They sought to provide a quantitative index, a nurse-patient ratio, of nursing care. Several years later, Johns and Pfefferkorn attempted to describe what "good nursing care" is. They categorized the patient-condition requisites of nursing care in hospital and public health nursing, and classified nursing activities accordingly.[111]

The increased employment of the graduate staff nurse in giving care to patients in hospitals was the cause of a major study by three of the national agencies.[112] To facilitate this movement and encourage the effective use of the staff nurse, the American Nurses Association and the National League for Nursing Education, in co-operation with the American Hospital Association, undertook a study of general staff nursing. This study consisted of two parts. The first dealt with the salaries of general staff nurses. The second investigated personnel policies concerning housing, hours of work, physical examinations, illnesses, vacations and opportunities for professional development. It was a factual report and did not make any recommendations.

Nursing Profession. The major efforts of the profession as a whole were directed toward the need to maintain an adequate number and an efficient body of nursing resources. Various surveys were conducted during this period to determine the movement of people in and out of the profession.

The National Organization for Public Health Nursing completed its first census of public health nursing services in 1922.[113] This survey was repeated in 1930. The U. S. Public Health Service began its census of public health nurses in 1936, and conducted these surveys biennially thereafter.[114]

A report on an appraisal of all nursing resources was published in 1940 under the title of "A National Inventory of Nurses."[115] The ensuing role of the U. S. Public Health Service and the National Nursing Council, discussed previously, in combating the impending shortage of nurses, resulted in the publication of "A Comprehensive Program for Nationwide Action."[116] This blueprint for the future of nursing marked the culmination of several years of study. Nursing was credited by the Surgeon General of the U. S. Public Health Service as the first profession to undertake a critical analysis of its problems and to formulate a constructive program for action.[117]

Some attention also was directed by the profession toward the determination and the description of the qualifications of nurses engaged in nursing practice. The National Organization for Public Health Nursing began this trend in 1925 by describing the minimum qualifications for public health nursing.[118] The National League for Nursing Education, recognizing the need to attract and select adequate candidates for the schools of nursing, described in 1932 "The Characteristics of a Nurse Able To Adjust Well to Nursing Situations."[119]

The nursing leaders also recognized the place of research in nursing. Isabel Stewart considered the need for a research approach to problems of nursing and concluded:

We nurses pride ourselves on being practical people, keeping our feet on the ground, getting things done and not bothering our heads very much with speculations and theories. But there are times when serious, concentrated thinking about aims and meanings and relative values in life is a much more profitable exercise than bustling about and getting ahead with the work.[120]

One of the first references regarding research as an activity for nurses was published by Marvin in 1927.[121] She pointed out that the research activity would enable nurses to find new facts and principles and to apply known facts and principles to the problems of nursing. Other articles of this type followed within the next few years.[122-124] The writers discussed research as it related to nursing practice. They stressed the need of nurses to find safer and sounder nursing procedures based upon experimentation. The ultimate place of research in nursing was summarized in 1943 by Sister Mary Therese.[125] Citing the views of the National Nursing Council, she stressed that the full stature of nursing as a profession is contingent on a broad educational base—nurses will be educated who can contribute to the expansion and the refinement of the body of knowledge upon which the practice of nursing is based.

An increasing body of factual material that might be called research in nursing resulted during this period. The material reflects the efforts made by nurses to specify and define the problems further, to gather data for the setting of standards, and to develop guides that would help in improving nursing practice and nursing education. They were conducted under the sponsorship of the nursing organizations.

Could these reports be classified as research? If so, what point of view do they represent? Let us regard a sample of the reports from each point of view that was presented previously. The reports, which will be analyzed briefly, include:

Josephine Goldmark: *Nursing and Nursing Education in the United States,* 1923.[126]

Ethel Johns and Blanche Pfefferkorn: *An Activity Analysis of Nursing,* 1934. [127]

Kathryn Tucker and Hortense Hilbert: *Survey of Public Health Nursing Administration and Practice,* 1934.[128]

A Curriculum Guide for Schools of Nursing, Committee on Curriculum, National League of Nursing Education, Isabel Stewart, Chairman, 1937.[129]

What Was the Purpose of the Research? Four types of purposes characterized these works.

1. To describe a state of affairs
2. To isolate problem areas
3. To determine solutions for problems
4. To analyze standards and guides for action.

Three of the studies were essentially descriptive. The Goldmark report described in detail the status of the entire field of nursing occupied by the nurse and other workers of a related type. Tucker and Hilbert described the status of public health nursing. Johns and Pfefferkorn analyzed and described nursing activities.

Why did they describe? The Goldmark report sought to determine the ingredients essential for the establishment of sound and minimal educational standards for each type of nursing service. In essence, it was a search for criteria, performed in a reasonably objective fashion. It attempted to describe the nursing service of the day in order to develop concepts of the tasks to be performed and the qualifications necessary for their execution.

The ultimate goal of the Tucker and Hilbert survey also was the establishment of criteria. The researchers sought to determine the extent to which the generally recognized standards enumerated by the National Organization for Public Health Nursing were adequate and accepted in practice. They desired to provide a basis for the revision of the current standards and the addition of new criteria. They uncovered problem areas. They sought to determine solutions for problems.

An analytic study of nursing activities to provide information that could be used in the development of curricula was the purpose of the Johns and Pfefferkorn study, which attempted to answer the questions: What is good nursing care? What do nurses do? How can they be taught to carry out these activities? How can the activities be classified so that they can be employed by a faculty in the development of courses and the selection of clinical learning experiences?

The immediate purpose of the curriculum project was to prepare a guide that could be used by the faculties in basic schools of nursing to study their own educational problems and to revise or develop curricula for their own schools. It also had the indirect effect of stimulating, clarifying and crystallizing group thinking regarding educational aims and standards for schools of nursing.

What Was the Method of the Research? The methodology employed by the writers of these reports consisted of the commonly used technic of recording, analyzing and reporting. The studies did not attempt to test or experiment. They were concerned primarily with observing and describing.

The Goldmark project and the public health survey engaged in extensive field studies. In the former situation, a pair of investigators (a nurse and a general educator) visited schools, hospitals and public health agencies. They followed students in the classrooms, on the floors and in their living areas. Similar procedures were followed in the public health survey. Public health nurses were interviewed and observed in clinics, homes, schools, agencies and industry. Questionnaires and observation check lists also were used.

Johns and Pfefferkorn relied heavily on data from other studies. These were analyzed and compiled into lists of nursing activities and disease conditions that could be used as a source for curriculum development.

The participants in the curriculum project gathered, evaluated and presented ideas and practices on curriculum development in basic nursing. The materials employed had been used successfully in the past or were judged by committee members to be suitable and practical for use. Data from previous studies such as those of the Grading Committee were utilized throughout. Surveys and job analyses were performed to supplement these courses.

What Was the Subject Matter of the Research? Problems common to the broad fields or areas of nursing were the concern of each of the studies. They considered the problem of what constitutes the best nursing practice wherever it is needed—in the home, the hospital, the clinic. They dealt with the question of the kind of education that can best prepare the nurse practitioner.

What is required of the nurse practitioner at each level of practice, and the educational progress necessary to develop these people, were the major problems considered by the Goldmark report.[126] These evolved into a series of specific questions:

1. Can individuals with training in hygiene and health education meet the increasing educational needs related to public health programs, or does this require individuals prepared as nurses, with some additional preparation in public health nursing?

2. To meet the shortage of nurses, should admission standards be lowered so that more individuals will enter nursing, or is there a minimum line of safety regarding the educational preparation that should be required of all graduate registered nurses?

3. What nursing and related activities can be safely assigned to subsidiary personnel, and how can this assignment be regulated? How can personnel best be trained to perform these activities safely?

4. What is the result if an agency (hospital), whose aim must be the best type of patient care at a minimal cost, operates a school of nursing whose educational program is largely of an apprenticeship nature?

5. How can nursing education programs at all levels be financed?

6. Do administrative and nursing personnel need educational preparation beyond the basic nursing course?

Tucker and Hilbert were concerned with the problem of assessing public health nursing practice, personnel and education. The public health movement had progressed beyond its earlier objectives of community sanitation and control of the contact-borne diseases by isolation and vaccination. It had advanced to objectives that included active public participation in health matters. Thus, the function of the public health nurse changed in emphasis to include patient, family, and community education. Were the public health nurses actually performing the practice suggested by this function? How could they learn to do so adequately? The writers inquired what the public health nurse actually was doing. How was she prepared?

The Johns and Pfefferkorn study and the curriculum project had similar objectives: to provide materials or a guide for curriculum development. However, they proceeded differently. The approach of Johns and Pfefferkorn was to ask what the nurse actually was doing. As a result, they developed lists of nursing activities pertaining to specific nursing functions and lists of common disease conditions. The latter group was concerned with the problem of what constituted good nursing practice, and they evaluated nursing activities accordingly. They extended their results into guides that suggested curriculum patterns, content, and learning experiences.

Who Did the Research? Most of the research projects described during this period were carried out under the auspices of a committee, which typically consisted of from 9 to 15 members. The members usually represented the various fields in nursing: education, service, public health. General education and medicine, as well as private and governmental agencies, were also represented on the committee. Often a lay member was included to speak for the consumer of nursing services.

The following might describe a nurse member of this committee:

She was a middle-aged woman who had been in the field of nursing for about 20 years. After graduating from a diploma school of nursing, she had progressed from a series of staff-level positions to instructional and supervisory positions. At the time of her appointment, she occupied the joint position of director of nursing service and education of a large midwestern hospital.

Although she had not actually given nursing service for at least 10 years, she was well acquainted with the problems of nursing and was relatively dissatisfied. In an effort to improve her own standards, she had managed to accumulate, over a number of years, sufficient credits for a baccalaureate degree. In an effort to improve the job situation, she had participated first in the activities of her local nursing group and later in those of state and national agencies. She had participated previously in committee projects.

This person brought to the committee an intense desire to improve the standards of nursing education and/or practice. She had a few ideas about what could be done; most of these, however, were centered about her own job situation. She would have liked to engage in the research project itself, but, frankly, did not have the time, the preparation or the ability to do so adequately.

The committees did not conduct the investigations but served primarily in an advisory capacity as subject-matter experts. A research investigator conducted the studies.

Another nurse may have been a typical investigator. She, too, graduated from a diploma school of nursing but persisted long enough to obtain baccalaureate and master's degrees in fields other than nursing. Although she was interested in nursing, she engaged in nursing practice only during her days as a nursing student. She was never employed in a staff-level position.

She went to work for a national agency soon after obtaining a baccalaureate degree. She progressed gradually from a series of small fact-finding studies to the rather grandiose project in which she was presently engaged.

Since persons like herself were relatively scarce, she had relatively little formal preparation as a research worker. She learned, in essence, by the "brute force" method. Being highly creative, persistent, and a good organizer, she was able to obtain considerable proficiency in her work. She had to—there wasn't any one to whom she could turn. Since her background as a staff nurse was nil, on-the-job problems did not stand in her way. She was able to conceive of problems in their broader scope, of the interrelationship of nursing and other fields, of the future of nursing.

Most of the studies conducted during the period were surveys. A statistician usually was employed to assist in the collection and the tabulation of data. Simple data collection and analytic procedures were used. The statistician was therefore not highly trained but usually had a working knowledge of nursing problems.

From the Second World War to the Present

It might be considered that the momentum generated shortly before the turn of the century and progressing slowly during the years between the two world wars suddenly burst into full force during the current period of observation. The enormous social upheavals and technologic developments had their effect upon nursing—practice, education and professional growth. And as a concomitant effect, research in nursing assumed a recognized position.

Dr. Wearn, in a report on medical education, considered the many factors influencing the medical profession as an outgrowth of World War I.[130] He listed among the strains and stresses laid upon medicine: the demands of the civilian population; the development of medical research, particularly in surgery; the demands upon physicians to meet the new medical and psychological problems in the war theater; and the economic and social changes within society itself. Nursing was subjected to the same pressures. It was required to develop or invent new practices to compensate for the inadequacies of previous practices and the demands imposed by new developments. It was required to prepare more personnel at each level of practice. It was required, in view of the impending growth, to re-examine its professional structure and institute appropriate modification.

The term "nursing practice" has grown to mean things other than "ministering to the needs of patients under the direction of a physician." Within its boundaries have been included "planning and organizing," "administering a department," "supervising other nurses," "consulting," "teaching nurses," "teaching patients and their families," and even "engaging in research." When and how these practices were assumed it is difficult to state. Nevertheless, they have suggested such questions to the various professional groups as: What is the nurse doing? and What should the nurse be doing? They have instigated studies of the nurse and her co-workers. They have provoked investigations of the surroundings into which the nurse is cast—the general and the psychiatric hospitals, the public health nursing agencies, and the home. Above all, they have initiated studies of the consumer of nursing care, the patient.

The continued expansion and extension of nursing services has caused the demand for the "registered nurse" to far exceed the supply. Changes in traditional educational patterns have been coupled with pressure from administrative personnel for nurses to assume administrative and advisory roles, for which the majority are not prepared. At the same time, they have received pressure from physicians to assume traditional patient care roles, which the work situations themselves often make impossible. All of this has led to confusion and the cry of "shortage of nurses." Whether this extension of nursing service away from the bedside resulted from a shortage of nurses or in a shortage of nurses is an academic issue. There has existed to date a very definite shortage, having impact in many directions.

In order to compensate for the lack of the necessary "hands and feet," many other people have been brought into the nursing care situation. The term "nurse" is applied currently to the nurse-aide trained on the job, the practical nurse, the hospital-school-trained nurse and the collegiate-trained nurse. A hierarchy of functions has developed from the physician to the professional nurse, to the practical nurse and, ultimately, to the nurse aide. As the nurse assumed higher-level functions, she relinquished her lesser functions to her subordinates. A hierarchy of personnel also has been established, which necessitated an administrative and a teaching order and their related practices. Subsequent shortages have resulted in various other categories of this person called "nurse."

In order to alleviate the nursing shortage, efforts have been directed toward the development of programs at each level of practice. The growth of practical nurse education has been very rapid. Federal and state support has increased the number of vocational schools offering practical nurse programs. The National Association for Practical Nurse Education has been actively supporting and promoting licensure. The National League for Nursing has established a consultation service for practical nurse schools. Each movement has been directed toward better acceptance and greater utilization of the practical nurse.

Several types of programs have been instituted at the professional level. The junior college movement to develop the so-called "bedside nurse" in an educational setting has provoked much interest and concern. At the other extreme has been the development of graduate education for nurses. Master's-degree and, in a limited number of cases, doctoral programs in nursing have been inaugurated to alleviate one of the most critical shortage areas in nursing—the need for leadership personnel.

The accreditation activities established during the previous period have kept pace with the growth of professional nursing education. A joint committee was appointed in 1946 to plan for a single professional body for accrediting.[131] The committee engaged Dr. George Works, an accreditation expert in general education, to bring together patterns of organization that would centralize common policies and procedures. Under the direction of this committee, a tentative statement of policies and standards was drawn up and submitted to nursing representatives throughout the country. There emerged, in 1948, a National Nursing Accrediting Service whose principal function was to provide a means for accrediting all categories of nursing education—basic and advanced professional and practical nursing programs.[132] The purpose of the service was to assist nursing educational institutions to improve their own programs and services.

In 1941, the National League for Nursing Education's committee on measurement and guidance developed a testing program as an additional service to the schools. The program began with a part-time secretary, much volunteer service, and some borrowed funds. By 1946, the service had grown to such an extent that a permanently staffed Department of Measurement and Guidance was established.[133] The growth and the development of this department in the number and the kinds of services rendered to schools, individuals and state board examiners have been outstanding. Some of the projects included the Pre-Nursing and Guidance Test Service, Achievement Tests, State Board Test Pool Licensure Examinations for

Professional and Practical Nurses, and the Graduate Nurse Qualifying Examinations.

As the practice of nursing service and education multiplied and became more diversified, the demands upon the guiding forces—the national organizations—also increased manyfold. As a consequence of the past train of events and in anticipation of future activities, research gained in strength and became more active.

An effort to co-ordinate nursing organizations in the United States began in 1939. During the next 10 years several committees from the six major national nursing organizations met, a study ensued, and there ultimately evolved a satisfactory plan for the emergence of just two organizations, the American Nurses Association and the National League for Nursing. This plan was adopted by the nursing profession in 1952.[134]

Research simply erupted during this period. It grew from the part-time activity of a few interested persons to an integral segment of the movement toward professionalism. Many different kinds of personages engaged in this research. Studies flourished in almost every component of the nursing activity.

The national organizations did much to foster the development of research. They conducted studies with their own staffs and provided or procured funds for studies by others. They developed media for reporting research. They encouraged the establishment of programs to educate nurses for research activities.

The publication of *Nursing Research* in June of 1952 marked a milestone in nursing history. It was a dream come true, for several nursing leaders had long recognized the need for such a periodical. This journal provided a medium for the publication of completed research and kept nurses informed of research in progress.

The growth of other professions, particularly in the social sciences, has influenced the growth of research in nursing. Researchers from the field of social science have invaded the health field, and a discipline of medical social science has developed.

This period of our short history finds the first real attempt to develop a theory of nursing. A few nurses were beginning to ask: Is there a body of substantive knowledge that can be called a science of nursing? Johnson, in tentatively developing some concepts regarding the nature of a science of nursing, stated: "Certainly no profession can long exist without making explicit its theoretical bases for practice so that this knowledge can be communicated, tested and expanded."[135]

Governmental agencies also have taken some leadership in initiating and stimulating research in nursing. The Division of Nursing Resources of the U. S. Public Health Service has conducted its own research and has provided grants-in-aid for research projects to individuals and institutions. The grants-in-aid have made possible studies that otherwise would not have been undertaken.

The interrelationship between the ongoing events in nursing practice and education and the research activities can be examined as research in nursing education, in nursing practice and in the nursing profession is reviewed.

Nursing Education. The coexisting needs to provide trained nurses at each level of practice and, at the same time, to improve the quality of their education stimulated studies in this area. These studies were performed for each of the programs, ranging from the training of practical nurses to graduate education for professional nurses.

The rapid rise of practical nurse programs provided much cause for concern. Schmitt studied the effectiveness of practical nurse education in Michigan after 5 years of operation.[136] She noted considerable confusion and unrealistic objectives; there was little relationship between the objectives and the learning experiences. McGlothlin and Souza made a 5-state study of 5 years of practical nurse education. They identified some of the qualifications and the characteristics of successful practical nursing.[137] They also reported that the practical nurse was not fully accepted, nor utilized to full capacity.

The Institute of Research and Service in Nursing Education

of Teachers College undertook a co-operative research project in 1952 to develop and test the junior college program in professional nursing. The project extended over 5 years and involved the co-operation of seven junior and community colleges and one hospital school in different sections of the United States. The final report describes the process and the progress of junior college education for nurses and the effectiveness of the graduates on the job.[138]

In an effort to speed the improvement of nursing education for beginning positions in professional nursing, the National Committee for the Improvement of Nursing Services undertook a study of schools that were classified by levels of quality.[139] The classification was based upon organization, enrollment, student health, curriculum, clinical resources, instruction, state board test results and costs. This report paints an interesting picture of nursing education at the mid-century.

Criteria were required to implement the programs of the National Accrediting Service for Nursing. A document, *The Manual of Accrediting Programs in Nursing,* was prepared, which contained conflicting and outdated material, much of which was not based on systematic study.[140] In recognition of the need for establishing more suitable criteria, a series of curriculum conferences was instituted. The first was held in 1950 to review, co-ordinate and organize the various activities relating to curriculum development in the different national nursing organizations.[141]

A few curriculum studies appeared in the literature during this period. The University of Washington undertook a project to answer two fundamental questions: (1) How can the time required to prepare a competent professional nurse be reduced? and (2) How can the instructional program in basic nursing be improved?[142] This was an action research project involving the entire faculty. Another project, commonly referred to as "the abilities study," was carried out under the aegis of the National League for Nursing.[143] The purpose of this study was to discover to what extent nurses, especially nurse educators, give verbal acceptance to the idea of attempting to develop certain qualities and skills in the basic professional program.

The importance of nursing education at the collegiate level was reiterated at this time. Studies emphasizing the urgency of this need include *Nursing for the Future*,[144] a report of the American Medical Association on nursing problems,[145] and a report of the Committee on the Function of Nursing that is commonly referred to as "the Ginsberg report."[146]

Margaret Bridgman, the dean of Skidmore College, was invited first by the Russell Sage Foundation and later by the National League for Nursing to serve as a counselor for collegiate programs of nursing education. Based on visits to 80 colleges in all parts of the United States, she prepared a report considering the supply of nurses for different kinds of assignments and the standards for the organization of hospital and collegiate programs.[147] She outlined principles that can be employed by colleges interested in developing nursing programs.

Graduate education became the subject of considerable attention in 1952. A conference, called by the National League for Nursing to consider criteria for graduate nurse programs, resulted in the *Report of Work Conference on Graduate Education*.[148] This report discussed trends in graduate nurse education and the problems and the issues relating to both baccalaureate and master's-degree programs. The conference agreed that the baccalaureate programs should prepare the student for general professional nursing, the master's-degree programs for specialization.

The first national conference devoted entirely to graduate education was held in 1954.[149] This conference attempted to formulate some tentative guiding principles as criteria for the development and the improvement of graduate programs. Other activities that followed over the years culminated finally in two documents that present a series of statements of principles, policies and practices characteristic of sound education at each level of preparation.[150, 151]

There has been an increasing interest evidenced by nurses in education at the doctoral level, particularly for the faculties in university programs and for research. The question has been discussed frequently as to whether this kind of preparation should be offered by one of the related disciplines having well-established research doctoral programs, or by doctoral programs in nursing. Two research projects on this matter are currently in progress. They concern the development of experimental programs.[152, 153]

Nursing Practice. The field of nursing service also has been surveyed extensively. Studies of the nurse, the patient, nursing care and nursing practices at various levels in varying situations comprise the range of exploration.

The nurse, rather than the patient, recently has been studied extensively. Henderson, a member of a research team, after locating, classifying and evaluating research completed in nursing during the past decade, asked, "Research in Nursing Practice—When?"[154] In a brief report of the research studies up to 1956, she stated that studies of the nurse outnumbered investigations on the practice of nursing by more than ten to one.[155]

Studies of nurses included an analysis of their social origin, mobility, geographic location, family background, education, personal characteristics and leisure time activities. Findings regarding these factors are reported by Hughes *et al.* in *Twenty Thousand Nurses Tell Their Story.*[156] The critical shortage of nurses prompted researchers to seek the factors relating to job satisfaction. Bullock was one of the first investigators to attempt to answer this question.[157] He uncovered many problem areas, particularly in intergroup relationships. Other researchers have sought information that might be helpful in the recruitment of students in the field of nursing.[158]

Efforts to ascertain the "status" of the nurse in the opinion of the doctor, the patient and the public were made first in 1945.[159] A series of additional studies on this matter was published in 1955.[160]

Psychiatric nursing has contributed much to the limited studies of the patient. Ward behavior of the mental patient,[161] perception by the patient of the interactive process,[162] and the identification and the application of psychotherapeutic principles to psychiatric nursing[163] are some of the topics investigated. Nurse researchers have studied the nurse-patient interaction in detail to demonstrate the therapeutic value of the nurse in the care of the psychiatric patient.[164-166]

Fifteen studies sponsored by the American Nurse Association attempted to determine the functions of the nurse.[167] They sought information on how nurses spend their time and what activities are performed by the different levels of nursing personnel. One of the more consistent findings reported was the great variation in practice. In addition, they learned that, while the registered nurse was spending more time away from the bedside, the practical nurse was providing more direct patient care.[168]

In view of the nursing shortage, the problem of staffing has been a topic of considerable interest. One of the first experimental studies in this regard was conducted by Bredenberg in 1949.[169] She established a design, in which the proportion of professional to nonprofessional members of the nursing team varied. George and Kuehn investigated various staffing patterns in order to provide service at a minimal cost for a nonsegregated medical and surgical ward of a 335-bed general hospital.[170]

Recent studies have attempted to obtain more adequate criteria for evaluating the different nurse staffing patterns. Abdellah and Levine related the hours of nursing care available per patient per day to the expressed feeling of patients regarding the adequacy of nursing service.[171] The investigators of another study sought to answer the question, "Is there an optimum number of nursing hours of care?"[172] Two factors were considered in answering the question: the shifting ratio of the nursing hours of care available to the patients, and the shifting ratio of graduate nurses to the total nursing personnel on the units.[172]

A small series of independent studies has been evolving to synthesize gradually the vast array of projects listed previously. While the latter have dealt with descriptions of what nursing is doing, the former sought to establish a basis or a rationale for understanding. They considered the process rather than the action.

Kreuter asked the question, "What is good nursing care?"[173] She then developed a classification system of functions, which was based upon what the patient required rather than upon what the nurse was doing. Three types of nursing care were defined—elementary, technical and professional. They were requisites for moving the patient from a state of complete dependency upon the nurse to self-reliance.

Johnson defined nursing as a professional discipline that gives social service.[174] It was said to provide a direct service to individuals, offering comfort, gratifications and assistance at times when they are under stress. The function of the nurse was conceived in this frame of reference as the assessment of the situation and the implementation of a course of action designed to resolve nursing problems.

Peplau, seeking an understanding of psychiatric nursing, concentrated upon the study of interpersonal relations in nursing.[175] She identified some concepts and principles that underlie interpersonal relationships and the transformation of nursing situations into learning experiences. Four phases of the nurse-patient relationship were hypothesized: orientation to the problem; identification with the nurse as a helping person; exploitation of the situation, leading to improvement in interpersonal relations; and resolution, or independence from identification with helping persons.

In recognition of the changing character of the position of the nurse, research also was directed to the other-than-care functions of the nurse. Particular emphasis was given to the problems of nursing service administration. A seminar, supported by the W. K. Kellogg Foundation, was held in 1951 to define nursing service administration and to suggest content materials for educational programs. Finer, the seminar director and advisor on administration, prepared a written analysis of nursing services based upon the discussions of the seminar.[176] A final survey, detailing the programs developed by the faculties of 14 participating universities, was presented by Mullane.[177]

Four of the universities conducted projects designed to consider various aspects of nursing service administration. They directed their efforts to studies of teaching by the case method[178]; engineering technics and industrial management applied to nursing service[179, 180]; and human relations in nursing service administration and in-service education for the development of team-nursing assignments.[181]

Lastly, studies were performed to consider the environment or the setting in which the nurse must work. The status, the roles and the relationships of various hospital personnel became the subjects of inquiries. Studies such as *Change and Dilemma in the Nursing Profession,*[182] *The Give and Take in Hospitals,*[183] and *Human Problems of a State Mental Hospital*[184] provide information on the problems faced by nursing in the complex and changing character of the modern hospital.

Nursing Profession. The period following World War II was a time for self-evaluation. The nursing profession studied its organizations and asked: Is this the kind of structure we want? They also examined their total educational system and asked: Is it doing an adequate job?

Raymond Rich Associates, a private research organization, was employed to study the structure of the nursing organizations.[185] The over-all purpose of this study was to discover what revisions were required to enable the nursing organizations to best serve the rapidly expanding needs of nurses and of the nation. The needs considered were: (1) to develop and enforce optimum standards in recruitment, preparation and practice of the profession, its specialties and auxiliaries; (2) to promote and protect the social and economic welfare of qualified nursing practitioners; and (3) to make adequate qualified nursing service readily and economically available to care for all the individual and general health needs of the American people. The merger of the various nursing organizations occurred in 1952 as a result of this study.[186]

World War II and its tremendous strain upon nursing once again focused attention upon the existing system of nursing education. This system was unable then to provide the amount of qualified general nursing care that was required by the expanding health services, much less the nurses with specialized preparation who were needed for public health nursing, supervision, administration, teaching and research. The nursing profession again concluded that there was something drastically wrong with a system of education that could not meet the demands of society for qualified nursing personnel in adequate numbers. Once more it decided to study the situation. Lucile Esther Brown, a social scientist, was engaged to find answers to the questions of who should organize, administer and finance professional nursing schools.[187] In order to be able to answer these questions, however, she required information regarding the future health needs of the nation, the resultant demands upon the nursing profession, and the kinds of educational programs needed to prepare nurses for the essential services.

The mandate given to Brown was to focus on the community at large, its health and nursing needs. In contrast with the study on structure, it did not consider the needs of nurses, but instead what was needed for nurses to serve the public. The report, *Nursing for the Future,* published in 1948, was direct and frank.[188] Brown projected a system of education that was divorced from the agency giving the service. Her recommendations were not new, but they did serve to stimulate new activity, such as national accreditation.

The professional organizations continued to collect facts to be used for various purposes: research, programs, estimations of needs, etc. In 1948, the National Security Resources Board asked the American Nurses Association to initiate and conduct a count and a classification of professional registered nurses. The results were published in 1949 and again in 1951.[189] The National League for Nursing collects and publishes facts on schools, students, teachers, curricula and other matters pertaining to schools and nursing service agencies. In 1957, in an attempt to estimate educational requirements 5, 10 and 15 years hence, the National League for Nursing's Committee on the Future issued a report forecasting professional nursing needs up to 1970.[190]

In this brief account of the continued development of nursing since World War II, a rather substantial increase in the activities relating to research can be observed. It can be noted that much of the research has been conducted by individuals. In addition, the studies have been designed to do somewhat more than describe. Some testing and experimentation have been carried out. There has been a moderate shift in emphasis from the complete concentration on the nurse to the determination of the patients' requirements for nursing care.

What points of view do these studies represent? Let us examine a sample of the reports from each point of view that was previously presented. The reports, which will be analyzed briefly, include:

Lucile Esther Brown: *Nursing for the Future.*[191]

Robert P. Bullock: *What Do Nurses Think of Their Profession?*[192]

Ole Sand: *Curriculum Study on Basic Nursing Education.*[193]

Marion S. Lesser and Vera R. Keane: *Nurse-Patient Relationships in a Hospital Nursing Service.*[194]

What Was the Purpose of the Research? Five types of purpose characterized these studies:

1. To describe a state of affairs
2. To isolate problem areas
3. To determine solutions for problems
4. To determine cause-and-effect relationships
5. To predict.

The Brown report represented another of the monumental studies in nursing that seem to arise in each generation, e.g., the Nutting report and the Goldmark study. The purpose was to provide source material to accelerate the changes and the reforms needed in the nursing educational system. Specifically, it sought, first, to predict the probable nature of the health services and the concomitant nursing services that would be required in the 2nd half of the twentieth century. The requisite programs of education needed to prepare nurses to render the various kinds of nursing services could then be derived.

Bullock was interested in determining the relationships between job satisfaction and attrition in the field of nursing. It was his purpose to describe the social and the occupational roles of the nurse and to determine the correlates of low morale, irritations, frustrations and inefficiency with departure from the profession.

Sand defined the purpose of the curriculum project at the University of Washington School of Nursing as being 2-fold:

1. To determine the most effective program of basic nursing education consistent with essential professional competency and patient safety to prepare students for bedside nursing in the shortest possible time

2. To describe the tasks upon which the faculty was engaged and the manner in which they worked together.

The project was made up of a series of small interrelated studies that were designed to develop and test creative learning experiences in the clinical situation and to increase the faculty's understanding of evaluation and research.

Lesser and Keane pinpointed their activities on the needs of the maternity patient. It was their purpose to describe dissatisfactions in the care of these patients and to determine the sources. What did patients expect? Did they receive the kind of nursing care they expected? Did the nurses feel that they were administering the kind of care expected by patients?

What Was the Method of the Research? Approximately two thousand people took part in the Brown study, although Brown herself was entirely responsible for the analysis, the conclusions and the recommendations of the report. Three advisory committees—a professional nursing committee, a lay advisory committee (composed of representatives of the public interests) and a committee of allied professionals (hospital administrators, doctors, social workers)—served in a consultant capacity to Brown.

Brown made an extended field trip over the United States to interview professional and lay people and to visit schools, hospitals and public health agencies. A workshop was held early in the study to consider the probable nature of the nursing services that would be needed in the future. Three regional conferences were conducted also to consider nursing problems and education. Each of the sources contributed to the final report.

Bullock engaged in an observation-interview program as an exploratory step to clarify potential areas for study and to formulate hypotheses to be tested. This consisted in three types of activities: (1) informal observations of nursing activities in a hospital; (2) systematic interviews with 115 nurses; and (3) the collection of standardized descriptions of nurse stereotypes and of characteristics of the nursing profession. As a result of these activities, eight hypotheses were formulated.

Scales to measure factors influencing job satisfactions were constructed and pretested. The scales and schedules were given to a representative sample of registered nurses and nursing students. Statistical analyses were performed and conclusions were drawn.

The University of Washington curriculum study was conducted under the direction of Sand as an action research project of the faculty. Observations, individual and group interviews, questionnaires and library reviews were used in the planning and the development stages. A number of small studies related to the over-all project were carried on concomitantly by individual investigators. Frequent group conferences and faculty workshops were employed to help the faculty to participate more effectively.

Ten major hypotheses were evolved from the faculty deliberations. They were tested in the actual situation. A variety of evaluation procedures was planned to assess the curriculum. Follow-up evaluations of graduates also were performed.

Lesser and Keane employed the intensive interview technic

to obtain data from nurses and patients. They ascertained the nurses' and the patients' perceptions of the nursing care received, and determined whether the two groups were in agreement or in conflict.

What Was the Subject Matter of the Research? While the broad common problems so characteristic of research during the earlier periods are represented here, there has been a marked tendency to consider problems that are narrower in scope but broader in application. It will have been observed that, in the preceding discussion, consideration was given to problem areas that also are characteristic of and applicable to fields of endeavor other than nursing.

The primary problem that Brown was commissioned to study was: Who should finance, organize and administer professional schools of nursing? This problem, of course, was common in professional nursing education in the United States. The answers to this question were drawn from information supplied in answer to other common problems. They referred to the problems of determining society's needs for nursing and to its present resources of nurses and educational facilities for nurses. Brown examined society's present and probable needs, assessed the status of practice and education, and recommended the kinds of preparation required to meet these needs.

The common problem of morale as a determinant of effective performance in staff nursing in the hospital was the subject matter of Bullock's study. This situation can be construed as a problem common to many other fields of human endeavor; it is not peculiar to nursing. He isolated a series of factors that were descriptive of job satisfaction or morale and influenced the attitudes of nurses toward nursing and the nursing profession. The knowledge gained regarding these factors might have application also to fields other than nursing.

Although the forces initiating the curriculum project and the study of maternity patients were generated largely by nursing problems, they dealt in part with some of the underlying problems of man. The Sand study considered the nature of learning. It asked specifically how nursing students learn, but the question could have been directed to any student anywhere. There evolved ultimately a curriculum applicable to the area of basic nursing education.

Lesser and Keane were concerned with the problem of perception and its influence upon interpersonal relationships. They studied the problems of nurse-patient relationships as perceived by maternity nurses and patients in a hospital maternity service. It was common to maternity nursing, but might have application to other areas of nursing and, possibly, to areas outside nursing. The influence upon interpersonal relationships of such factors as the perception each person has of himself, what he believes others think of him, what his role is, and whether or not he is fulfilling his role made up the subject matter of this study.

Who Did the Research? In this period of our brief history, an increasingly larger number of persons have been engaged in the practice of research. These people come from a variety of settings and disciplines. Among the group, the following individuals were found: a social scientist, a statistician, a nurse leader, a nurse researcher, a nurse practitioner, and a nurse student. Each of these will be classified hypothetically.

Social Scientist
By comparison, the social science member on the nursing research team was perhaps its youngest member. He was certainly the best educated—prepared at the doctoral level with a major in psychology, sociology or anthropology. He was also the least experienced member of the team. He may never have been in a hospital before he became involved in nursing research.

This researcher had only a secondary interest in nursing. He was interested primarily in making a contribution to the knowledge and the technics of the social sciences. He looked not at the patient, but at the behavior of the person in a state of stress; not at the nurse, but at a therapist teacher; not at the hospital, but at a complex organization of substructures, of horizontal and vertical lines of communication; not at nursing, but at a diverse occupational group in a state of transition.

The social scientist was perhaps the team member most knowledgeable in the methods and the technics of research. Therefore, he was employed more frequently as the chief investigator. Because of his diverse interests, he was often in conflict with other members of the team. Because of his secondary interest in nursing, he was more objective, more far-sighted. Because of his primary interest in social science, he could have done his work in a field other than nursing. He popped in and out of the nursing scene from time to time.

Statistician

By comparison with the social scientist, this person may have been an older, more acceptable member of the nursing research team. He was, in part, a holdover from the previous generation when fact-gathering studies on nursing resources were particularly in vogue. Nurses developed a working relationship with this kind of individual. He knew nursing; fact-gathering in nursing was of particular interest to him.

This person also could have been a social scientist, a psychologist, an economist or one trained in public health methods. In this regard, he belonged to a newer generation. He was more highly trained than the old-line statistician, more diversified in his pursuits, and he held a peer rather than a subordinate relationship to his nursing component. Unlike the nonstatistician social scientist, he generally was more specialized in the nursing or, at least, in the health fields. He probably remained with nursing for a longer period of time.

Nurse Leader

From the time nursing first engaged in formal research practice, a nurse leader has been assigned a role. At first she was the total research person: the idea man, the data collector, the writer. She later assumed a seat on a committee, initiating studies, offering consultation, implementing results. As the body of research people grew about her, she stepped more quietly into the background, offering support when needed, keeping peace among the conflicting disciplines. More than anyone else, she recognized the limitations of current practice, the needs of the nursing future. Her voice was heard above the crowd when the wheels of progress came to a halt.

In part, she was a prototype of the Florence Nightingales, the Mary Adelaide Nuttings, the Lavinia Docks. She was well educated and experienced in each aspect of nursing. She was equally at home in nursing practice and in nursing education. Unlike many of her lesser compatriots, she conversed well with members of other disciplines; she felt at home in their company; she invited their participation.

Nurse Researcher

This was a new breed of person—created to fill a void between the nurse practitioner and the professional researcher. The need for this kind of person readily became apparent during the period following World War II. She was the younger person. Educated in professional nursing, she pursued her studies beyond the minimal requirements. She obtained a master's and, perhaps, a doctor's degree. Her studies may have taken her into fields other than nursing, particularly the social sciences.

She was a restless individual, aggressive and independent. She moved quickly from nursing practice, to teaching, to further study and research. Ultimately she found a place in an organization whose principal occupation was nursing research—governmental, nonprofit, private or university. She engaged in a variety of studies at first, but often moved steadily toward areas of particular interest: nurse-patient relationships, patient teaching, the nursing team concept.

In many respects the professional nurse researcher was a master of nursing practice but a neophyte in research methodology. She knew the technical language of nursing; she was aware of its current problems; she was knowledgeable in related practices. At the same time, she lacked many of the technical skills required of the competent research person—a knowledge of statistics, experimental design, theory building, data-gathering technics. If she was headstrong and did not take the time to learn, she employed the older available technics and relied heavily upon the statistician. In this regard, she was not fully aware of the implications of her study. If, on the other hand, she took the time to learn, she was able to work in a more complementary fashion with other members of the research team. She became the more complete researcher.

Nurse Practitioner

Since many of the studies were performed in the field—the home, the hospital, the clinic—the nurse practitioner often became a necessary participant in research studies. This was the staff nurse, the head nurse in the general hospital, the psychiatric hospital, the public health service agency. She did not have any formal training in research but learned in accordance with the requirements of the particular study. Usually she was quite co-operative; however, there were times when she was an unwilling participant.

This person contributed to the research project in many ways. She may have been the observer or the observed. She was asked to perform old practices and invited to learn or to develop the untried new practices. She was asked to interview and to be interviewed. She was asked to work alone and with others. She served as a control and as a guinea pig.

Nurse Student

With the increased emphasis upon graduate education in nursing, many nurses, willingly or otherwise, became nurse researchers. A research project, the master's thesis, frequently was offered in partial fulfillment of the requirements for graduation. The nurse student researcher, therefore, came from many avenues of nursing. She was quite young or relatively old; she was inexperienced or highly experienced. She was a public health nurse, a nursing administrator, a supervisor, a clinical instructor, a head nurse, a staff nurse, a nurse researcher, a psychiatric nurse.

The nurse student generally was unsophisticated in the matter of research. She had to learn from the beginning in a relatively short period of time. If she was a willing learner and had the necessary potential, she may have developed a significant contribution to the research literature. If she was not sufficiently capable or motivated, she merely went through the exercise and made a contribution to a long list of repetitive studies.

THE QUESTIONS

This overview, brief as it is, will permit us to re-examine the questions that were posed initially. The writers will not answer the questions. Instead, they will pose other questions. There are no clear-cut answers to these questions. The reader himself must decide ultimately upon the most appropriate answers.

1. **Is Nursing Really Doing Research?** A variety of projects have been observed in the course of this review. They began with general questions covering broad areas in nursing: What is nursing practice? How should nurses be trained? What are nurses doing? The reports that evolved were based essentially upon experience, although they were developed in a systematic fashion. Could these projects be classified as research?

There developed a series of fact-finding studies: What are nurses doing? Where are they being educated? How are they being educated? How many nurses are there? These were statements of what is and of what happened in the past. Were these research projects?

Suddenly there was a barrage of studies—the same broad, general statements, the same fact-finding studies. In addition, there evolved many problem-solving and descriptive studies— the highly specific and the more generalized. There also appeared a few attempts to characterize nursing in terms of the components of more basic knowledge. Which of these studies constituted research? What is your point of view?

2. **What Is the Purpose of Research in Nursing?** Practically all the early studies and most of the later studies can be classified as descriptive analyses. There have evolved in addition the so-called action-research studies, the development and the testing of principles, the search for understanding. Can one state that the major purpose of research in nursing is to describe; that nursing also is striving by action research to solve problems, and by principle development to predict and to understand? What should be the purpose of research in nursing?

3. **What Is the Subject Matter of Research in Nursing?** The early studies attempted to describe the nurse, what she was doing and how she should be trained. The rather broad problems common to nursing were, therefore, the principal subject matter of research during this period. The second period concentrated upon fact-finding studies of nursing resources and curriculum development. The subject matter, though somewhat different in content, also consisted of common problems. Common-problem analysis persisted into the final period and, in addition, concerned itself with the problems of the nurse as a person, the patient, the nurse-patient relationship, methods of collecting data, job satisfaction and a variety of other topics. These problems bridged nursing as well as allied areas. Very specific and broad underlying problems also became the subject matter for study. There was an attempt to include the problems underlying the social sciences. That is, nursing problems were considered as problems universal to man. Are these the proper subject matter of research in nursing?

4. **What Is the Method of the Nurse Researcher?** Initially, the nurse leader researchers utilized their experiences, surveyed various situations and existing literature and pieced together in a logical fashion their broad descriptive statements. The later researchers became more sophisticated in fact-finding technics, employing some of the better-developed data-collection technics and methods of analysis. The more recent studies have employed a greater variety of the survey-research and observational technics. They have utilized the data-processing technics of other disciplines. The beginning of experimentation has appeared. Much of the work, in fact, has been concentrated upon the development of appropriate methodology and technics. Has there been an overemphasis upon method? What should be the method of research in nursing?

5. **Who Is Doing the Research?** The research assignment has passed from the nurse leader to the committee, to the nursing research team. The last-named has included the social scientist, the statistician, the professional nurse researcher, the nurse leader and the nurse practitioner. These people vary in proficiency, in research and in knowledge of the subject matter. Should the social scientist who has a fringe knowledge of nursing engage in nursing research? Should the nurse researcher who lacks sophistication in research methodology engage in nursing research?

6. **Is Research in Nursing Meaningful?** There has been a tremendous response to research in nursing. The expenditure of time, money and personnel is large. It has threatened to become larger. What is the ultimate meaning? Why does the nurse engage in research? What is she trying to do? Is research in nursing meaningful to you?

REFERENCES

1. McLure, W. P.: Educational research: a new view, Phi Delta Kappan 35:3, 1953.
2. Kelley, T. L.: A Scientific Method: Its Functions in Research and Education, p. 14, Columbus, Ohio State Univ. Press, 1929.

3. Good, C. V., and Scates, D. E.: Methods of Research, p. 15, New York, Appleton-Century-Crofts, 1954.
4. Rummel, J. F.: An Introduction to Research Procedures in Education, p. 2, New York, Harper, 1958.
5. Studies in nursing, Nurs. Res. 5:40-43, 1956.
6. Smith, H. L., and Smith, J. R.: An Introduction to Research in Education, pp. 2-3, Bloomington, Ind., Education Publications, 1954.
7. Cornell, F. G.: Research and Science in Education, Report of the First International Conference on Education Research, Educational Studies and Documents, No. 20, Paris, UNESCO, 1956.
8. Rummel, J. F.: *Op. cit.* (see Ref. 4), p. 2.
9. Good, C. V., and Scates, D. E.: *Op. cit.* (see Ref. 3), p. 11.
10. Education for research in psychology, Amer. Psychologist *14*: 169, 1959.
11. Shumsky, Abraham: The Action Research Way of Learning, p. 1, New York, Bureau of Publications, Teachers College, Columbia Univ., 1958.
12. Education for research in psychology: *Op. cit.* (see Ref. 10), pp. 169-179.
13. Guilford, J. P.: The relation of intellectual factors to creative thinking in science *in* Research Conference on the Identification of Creative Talent, Salt Lake City, Univ. Utah Press, 1956.
14. Stein, M. I.: A transactional approach to creativity *in* Research Conference on the Identification of Creative Scientific Talent, Salt Lake City, Univ. Utah Press, 1956.
15. Kelley, T. L.: *Op. cit.* (see Ref. 2), p. 182.
16. *Ibid.*
17. Good, C. V.: Introduction to Educational Research, pp. 7-8, New York, Appleton-Century-Crofts, 1959.
18. National Science Foundation: Basic Research, pp. 1-10, Washington, D. C., U. S. Govt. Printing Office, 1957.
19. Corey, S. M.: Curriculum development through action research, Education Leadership 7:147-153, 1949.
20. Shumsky, Abraham: *Op. cit.* (see Ref. 11), p. 100.
21. Black, Max: Critical Thinking, An Introduction to Logic and Scientific Method, pp. 247-248, New York, Prentice-Hall, Inc., 1946.
22. Dewey, John: How We Think, p. 72, New York, Heath, 1910.
23. *Ibid.*, p. 74.
24. Black, Max: *Op. cit.* (see Ref. 21), p. 249.
25. Dewey, John: *Op. cit.* (see Ref. 22), p. 75.
26. *Ibid.*, p. 76.

27. Black, Max: *Op. cit.* (see Ref. 21), pp. 248-249.
28. *Ibid.,* p. 251.
29. Kelley, T. L.: *Op. cit.* (see Ref. 2), p. 24.
30. Nutting, M. A., and Dock, L. L.: History of Nursing, vol. II, New York, Putnam, 1907.
31. Woolsey, A. H.: A Century of Nursing: Report to the Standing Committee on Hospitals of the State Charities Aid Association, New York, 1876, New York, Putnam, 1950.
32. Nutting, M. A.: Educational Status of Nursing, Bulletin No. 7, No. 475, p. 23, U. S. Bureau of Education, Washington, D. C., U. S. Govt. Printing Office, 1912.
33. Medicine in the Changing Order: Report of the New York Academy of Medicine Committee on Medicine and the Changing Order, New York, Commonwealth Fund, 1947.
34. Sullivan, Mark: The Turn of the Century, vol. 1 (1900-1904) *in* the series Our Times—The United States, 1900-1925, New York, Scribner, 1926.
35. Bayne-Jones, Stanhope: The role of the nurse in medical progress, Amer. J. Nurs. *50*:601-604, 1950.
36. Ravenal, Mazyck (ed.): A Half-Century of Public Health; Jubilee Historical Volume, Am. Public Health Assn., New York, 1921.
37. Roberts, M. M.: American Nursing, History and Interpretation, p. 83, New York, Macmillan, 1954.
38. Nightingale, Florence: Notes on Matters Affecting the Health, Efficiency and Hospital Administration of the British Army: A Report Published at the Request of the Secretary of State for War, London. Published in 1858.
39. Hampton, I. A., *et al.*: Nursing of the Sick—1893. Paper and Discussions from the International Congress of Charities, Correction and Philanthropy, Chicago, 1893, published under the sponsorship of the National League of Nursing Education, New York, McGraw-Hill, 1949.
40. Nutting, M. A., and Dock, L. L.: *Op. cit.* (see Ref. 30).
41. Dock, L. L.: History of Nursing, vols. III and IV, New York, Putnam, 1912.
42. Woolsey, A. H.: *Op. cit.* (see Ref. 31).
43. Hampton, I. A., *et al.*: Op. cit. (see Ref. 39), p. 5.
44. Nutting, M. A.: *Op. cit.* (see Ref. 32), p. 24.
45. *Ibid.,* p. 51.
46. Nightingale, Florence: Notes on Nursing: What It Is and What It Is Not, London, Harrison, 1859; Philadelphia, Lippincott, 1946.
47. Hampton, I. A., *et al.*: *Op. cit.* (see Ref. 39), pp. 24-43.

48. *Ibid.*
49. Woolsey, A. H.: *Op. cit.* (see Ref. 31), p. 112.
50. Hitchcock, J. E.: Five hundred cases of pneumonia, Amer. J. Nurs. *3*:169, 1903.
51. Chayer, M. E.: The trail of the nursing textbook, Amer. J. Nurs. *50*:606-607, 1950.
52. Weeks, C. S.: A Textbook of Nursing for the Use of Training Schools, Families, and Private Students, published in 1885; latest revision, New York, Appleton-Century-Crofts, 1916.
53. Chayer, M. E.: *Op. cit.* (see Ref. 51), p. 606.
54. Hampton, I. A.: Nursing, Its Principles and Practices for Hospital and Private Use, New York, Saunders, 1892.
55. Gardner, M. S.: Public Health Nursing, New York, Macmillan, 1916 (revised 1924 and 1942).
56. Editorial: Is the profession overcrowded? Amer. J. Nurs. *2*:976, 1902.
57. Worcester, A.: Is nursing really a profession? Amer. J. Nurs. *2*:908, 1902.
58. Sewall, M. W.: How to lift your business into a profession (editorial), Amer. J. Nurs. *6*:81, 1906.
59. Lockwood, E. B.: The limitations of the nursing profession (editorial), Amer. J. Nurs. *9*:939, 1909.
60. Thompson, G.: Training Schools for Nurses (Summary of the Work of 22 Schools), New York, Putnam, 1883. *Quoted in* Stewart, I.: Education of Nurses, p. 94, New York, Macmillan, 1943.
61. Shattuck, L., *et al.*: Report of the Sanitary Commission of 1850 (reprint), p. 224, Cambridge, Harvard, 1948.
62. Nightingale, Florence: *Op. cit.* (see Ref. 46).
63. Woolsey, A. H.: *Op. cit.* (see Ref. 31).
64. Nutting, M. A., and Dock, L. L.: *Op. cit.* (see Ref. 30).
65. Nutting, M. A.: *Op. cit.* (see Ref. 32).
66. *Ibid.*, p. 13.
67. Nightingale, Florence: *Op. cit.* (see Ref. 46), p. 62.
68. *Ibid.*, p. 63.
69. *Ibid.*, p. 66.
70. *Ibid.*, p. 5.
71. *Ibid.*, p. 6.
72. Cook, Sir Edward T.: The Life of Florence Nightingale, London, Macmillan, 1942.
73. Nightingale, Florence: *Op. cit.* (see Ref. 38).
74. ———: Evidence on the Evidence Contained in the Stational Reports Submitted to the Royal Commission on the Sanitary

State of the Army in India, Reprinted From the Report of the Royal Commission Appointed to Enquire into the Regulations Affecting the Sanitary State of the Army, London, Harrison, 1858.

75. Yost, E.: M. Adelaide Nutting, *in* American Women of Nursing, pp. 3-21, Philadelphia, Lippincott, 1947.

76. Nutting, M. A.: As known by friends, students and co-workers, Amer. J. Nurs. *25*:445-454, 1925.

77. Editorial: Amer. J. Nurs. *25*:207, 1925.

78. Nutting, M. A.: A Sound Economic Basis for Schools of Nursing, New York, Putnam, 1926.

79. ———: *Op. cit.* (see Ref. 32).

80. Pennock, M. R.: Makers of Nursing History, New York, Lakeside Pub. Co., 1940.

81. Roberts, M. M.: Lavinia Lloyd Dock—nurse, feminist, internationalist, Amer. J. Nurs. *56*:176-179, 1956.

82. Robinson, Victor: White Caps—The Story of Nursing, Philadelphia, Lippincott, 1946.

83. Burgess, M. A.: Nurses, Patients and Pocketbooks, New York, National League of Nursing Education, 1928.

84. Facts About Nursing, 1945, New York, Nursing Information Bureau, American Nurses Assn., 1945.

85. Roberts, M. M.: The national nursing organizations establish headquarters *in* American Nursing History and Interpretation, pp. 201-211, New York, Macmillan, 1954.

86. Report of the Committee on Studies: Proceedings of the Thirty-eighth Annual Convention of the National League of Nursing Education, San Antonio, Texas, 1952.

87. Facts About Nursing, 1935, New York, American Nurses Assn., 1935.

88. Joint Orthopedic Nursing Advisory Service, Amer. J. Nurs. *42*:313-314, 1942.

89. Leone, L. P.: The national nursing accrediting service, Amer. J. Nurs. *49*:362-363, 1949.

90. Report of the Committee on Accrediting: Annual Report and Proceedings of the 43rd Convention of the National League of Nursing Education, 1937.

91. Leone, L. P.: Basic professional curricula leading to degrees, Amer. J. Nurs. *37*:287-297, 1937.

92. Goodrich, A. W.: Association of Collegiate Schools for Nursing, Amer. J. Nurs. *33*:239, 1933.

93. Census of public health nurses, 1937, Public Health Nurse *29*:648-652, 1937.

94. A national inventory of nurses, Amer. J. Nurs. *40*:1246, 1940.

95. Nursing Council on National Defense, Amer. J. Nurs. *40*:1013, 1940.
96. Nursing councils for war service, Amer. J. Nurs. *42*:1413, 1942.
97. Public Law No. 74, 78th Congress (June, 1943).
98. Goldmark, Josephine: Nursing and Nursing Education in the United States: Report of the Committee for Study of Nursing Education, New York, Macmillan, 1923.
99. Nursing Schools Today and Tomorrow: Report of the Committee on the Grading of Nursing Schools, New York, National League of Nursing Education, 1934.
100. Tucker, K., and Hilbert, H.: Survey of Public Health Nursing Administration and Practice, New York, Commonwealth Fund, National Organization for Public Health Nursing, 1934.
101. McIver, Pearl: An Analysis of First Level Public Health Nursing in Ten Selected Organizations, New York, National Organization for Public Health Nursing, 1935.
102. Leone, L. P.: *Op. cit.* (see Ref. 91).
103. Oates, Louise: Advanced professional curricula, Amer. J. Nurs. *38*:287-297, 1938.
104. A Standard Curriculum for Schools of Nursing, New York, National League of Nursing Education, 1917.
105. The Curriculum for Schools of Nursing, Committee on Nursing Education, New York, National League of Nursing Education, 1927.
106. A Curriculum Guide for Schools of Nursing, Committee on Curriculum, New York, National League of Nursing Education, 1937.
107. Burgess, M. A.: *Op. cit.* (see Ref. 83).
108. Pfefferkorn, B., and Rovetta, C. A.: Administrative Cost Analysis for Nursing Service and Nursing Education, Chicago, American Hospital Assn. and the National League of Nursing Education, 1940.
109. Winslow, E. A.: The measurement of nurse-power, Public Health Nurse *19*:492-498, 1927.
110. Pfefferkorn, B., and Rottman, M.: Clinical Education in Nursing, New York, Macmillan, 1932.
111. Johns, E., and Pfefferkorn, B.: An Activity Analysis of Nursing, New York, National League of Nursing Education, 1934.
112. Personnel Practices for General Staff Nurses, Sponsored by American Hospital Assn., National League of Nursing Education, American Nurses' Assn., 1944.
113. Activities of the Organization for Public Health Nursing, Public Health Nurse *15*:146-148, 1923.
114. Census of public health nurses, 1937, *Op. cit.* (see Ref. 93).

115. A national inventory of nurses, *Op. cit.* (see Ref. 94).
116. A comprehensive program for nationwide action, Amer. J. Nurs. *45*:707, 1945.
117. Roberts, M. M.: American Nursing, History and Interpretation, p. 468, New York, Macmillan, 1954.
118. Tucker, K., and Hilbert, H.: *Op. cit.* (see Ref. 100), pp. 230-237.
119. Eads, L. K.: The characteristics of a nurse able to adjust well to nursing situations, Amer. J. Nurs. *36*:705, 1936.
120. Stewart, I. M.: The philosophy of the collegiate school of nursing, Amer. J. Nurs. *40*:1033-1034, 1940.
121. Marvin, M. M.: Research in nursing, Amer. J. Nurs. *27*:331-332, 1927.
122. Goodell, Frances: Research of, by and for the nurse, Amer. J. Nurs. *32*:1019, 1932.
123. Beck, Sister Bernice: Underlying Scientific Principles in Nursing Practice, p. 118, Proceedings of the 40th Annual Convention, National League of Nursing Education, 1934.
124. Beckwith, T. D.: The University, p. 125, Annual Report and Proceedings of the 42nd Annual Convention, National League of Nursing Education, 1936.
125. Sister Mary Therese: Why College Education? p. 203, Annual Report of the Proceedings of the 49th Annual Convention, National League of Nursing Education, 1943.
126. Goldmark, Josephine: *Op. cit.* (see Ref. 98).
127. Johns, E., and Pfefferkorn, B.: *Op. cit.* (see Ref. 111).
128. Tucker, K., and Hilbert, H.: *Op. cit.* (see Ref. 100).
129. *Op. cit.* (see Ref. 106).
130. Wearn, J. T.: Background and philosophy of experiment, J. Med. Educ. *31*:515, 1956.
131. Petry, Lucile: The national accrediting service, Amer. J. Nurs. *49*:362-363, 1949.
132. *Ibid.*
133. National licensing examinations, Amer. J. Nurs. *45*:1035, 1945.
134. McIver, Pearl: Nursing moves forward, Nurs. Outlook *52*:821-823, 1952.
135. Johnson, Dorothy: The nature of a science of nursing, Nurs. Outlook 7:291, 1959.
136. Schmitt, Mary: Facts About Practical Nurse Education in Michigan, Lansing, Mich., Department of Public Instruction, 1957.
137. McGlothlin, W. J., and Souza, M.: Five States Study: Five Years of Practical Nurse Education, Battle Creek, W. K. Kellogg Foundation, 1956.
138. Montag, Mildred: Community College Education for Nursing, New York, McGraw-Hill, 1959.

139. Nursing Schools at the Mid-Century, New York, National Committee for the Improvement of Nursing Services, 1950.
140. The Manual of Accrediting Programs in Nursing, New York, National Accrediting Service, 1949.
141. Nursing Organization Curriculum Conference, Curriculum Bulletin No. 1, New York, National League for Nursing, 1950.
142. Sand, Ole: Curriculum Study on Basic Nursing Education, New York, Putnam, 1955.
143. Shields, M. R.: A project for curriculum improvement, Nurs. Res. *1*:4-31, 1952.
144. Brown, L. E.: Nursing for the Future, New York, Russell Sage Foundation, 1948.
145. Report of the Committee on Nursing Problems, J. A. M. A. *137*:878-879, 1948.
146. Ginsberg, Eli, *et al.*: A Program for the Nursing Profession, New York, Macmillan, 1948.
147. Bridgman, Margaret: Collegiate Education for Nursing, New York, Russell Sage Foundation, 1953.
148. Report of Work Conference on Graduate Education, New York, National League for Nursing, 1952.
149. Report of the Meeting of Administrators of Graduate Programs in Nursing, New York, National League for Nursing, 1954.
150. Criteria for the Evaluation of Educational Programs in Nursing Leading to a Diploma, New York, National League for Nursing, 1958.
151. Criteria for the Evaluation of Educational Programs That Lead to Baccalaureate or Masters' Degrees, New York, National League for Nursing, 1960.
152. Henle, Robert (S. J.), and Kohler, Carol: A Doctoral Program in Health Organization Research, St. Louis Univ., 1958.
153. Development of a Doctoral Program, Mimeographed Report, School of Nursing, Univ. California, 1959.
154. Henderson, Virginia: Research in nursing practice—when? Nurs. Res. *4*:99, 1956.
155. ———: An overview of nursing research, Nurs. Res. *6*:61-71, 1957.
156. Hughes, Everett, *et al.*: Twenty Thousand Nurses Tell Their Story, Philadelphia, Lippincott, 1958.
157. Bullock, R. P.: What Do Nurses Think of Their Profession? Columbus, Ohio, State Univ., Research Foundation, 1954.
158. Bressler, M., and Jephart, W.: Career Dynamics: A Survey of Selected Aspects of the Nursing Profession, Harrisburg, Pennsylvania State Nurses Assn., 1957.

159. The nurses' contribution to American victory, Amer. J. Nurs. *45*:683-686, 1945.

160. A Study of the Registered Nurse in a Metropolitan Community (in 6 parts), Part I. The Evaluation of Nurses by Male Physicians, Part II. Public Images of the Nurse, Kansas City, Community Studies, Inc., 1955.

161. Boyd, R., Baker, T., and Greenblatt, M.: Ward social behavior: an analysis of patient interaction at highest and lowest extremes, Nurs. Res. *3*:77-79, 1954.

162. Carter, F. M.: The critical incident technique in identification of the patient's perception of therapeutic patient-patient interaction on a psychiatric ward, Nurs. Res. *8*:207-211, 1959.

163. Hayes, Sister Immaculata: Some selected psycho-therapeutic principles applied to psychiatric nursing care, Nurs. Res. *53*: 27-35, 1953.

164. Stevens, F. B., and Halpert, P. W.: The nurse's Thursday in a psychiatric ward, Nurs. Res. *6*:29-34, 1957.

165. Tudor, G. W.: A socio-psychiatric nursing approach to interaction in a problem of mutual withdrawal on a mental hospital ward, Psychiatry *15*:193, 1952.

166. Mellow, June: An Action Study of Ways of Improving Nursing Service Through Intensive Supervised Clinical Experiences With Psychotic Patients. Unpublished Study, Mimeographed, Boston, Massachusetts Mental Health Center, 1959.

167. Hughes, E., et al.: Op. cit. (see Ref. 156).

168. Ibid., p. 135.

169. Bredenberg, Viola: Nursing Service Research, Philadelphia, Lippincott, 1949.

170. George, F., and Kuehn, R. P.: Patterns of Patient Care, New York, Macmillan, 1955.

171. Abdellah, F. G., and Levine, E.: Effect of Nurse Staffing on Satisfaction With Nursing Care, Chicago, American Hospital Assn., 1958.

172. New, P. K., et al.: Nursing Service and Patient Care: A Staffing Experiment, Kansas City, Community Studies, Inc., 1959.

173. Kreuter, Frances: What Is Good Nursing Care? Viewpoints on Curriculum Development, pp. 40-45, New York, National League for Nursing, 1957.

174. Johnson, Dorothy: A philosophy of nursing, Nurs. Outlook *7*: 198, 1959.

175. Peplau, H. E.: Interpersonal Relations in Nursing, New York, Putnam, 1952.

176. Finer, Herman: Administration and the Nursing Service, New York, Macmillan, 1952.

177. Mullane, M. K.: Education for Nursing Service Administration, Battle Creek, W. K. Kellogg Foundation, 1959.
178. Faculty and Graduate Students: Case Studies in Nursing Service Administration, Boston, Boston Univ. Press, vol. I, 1954, vol. II, 1956.
179. George, F., and Kuehn, R. P.: *Op. cit.* (see Ref. 170).
180. Anderson, H. E., and Owens, B. W.: Report of the Research Study in Methods Analysis Application in the Hospital, Seattle, Univ. Washington, 1955.
181. Barnowe, T. J.: Human relations involved in administering nursing service in a large modern hospital, Nurs. Res. *6*:72-74, 1957.
182. Reisman, L., and Rohrer, J. H.: Change and Dilemma in the Nursing Profession, New York, Putnam, 1957.
183. Burling, Temple, *et al.*: The Give and Take in Hospitals, New York, Putnam, 1956.
184. Belknap, Ivan: Human Problems of a State Mental Hospital, New York, McGraw-Hill, 1956.
185. Raymond Rich Associates: Report on the structure of organized nursing, Amer. J. Nurs. *46*:648-661, 1946.
186. McIver, Pearl: Nursing moves forward, Nurs. Outlook *52*:821-823, 1952.
187. Brown, L. E.: *Op. cit.* (see Ref. 144).
188. *Ibid.*
189. Inventory of Professional Nurses, New York, American Nurses Assn., 1949; 1951.
190. Nurses for a Growing Nation, New York, National League for Nursing, 1957.
191. Brown, L. E.: *Op. cit.* (see Ref. 144).
192. Bullock, R. P.: *Op. cit.* (see Ref. 157).
193. Sand, Ole: *Op. cit.* (see Ref. 142).
194. Lesser, M. S., and Keane, V. R.: Nurse-Patient Relationships in a Hospital Nursing Service, St. Louis, Mosby, 1956.

CHAPTER 2

The General Purpose of Research

Research has been defined in this book as an order of problem-solving directed by a special purpose. What is purpose? What is the purpose of research? Are there many purposes of research? Or can a single purpose be isolated that characterizes all research?

A purpose is an aim or an objective. It is a goal or a thing desired. Describing a purpose is like taking a trip. A project of any kind is analogous to a journey. There are reasons for going, a point of departure, a means of conveyance, a route to be followed, interim stops along the way, and a final destination. The ultimate purpose or objective of this journey is the final destination. It is not the reason for going, for that is the initiating cause. It is not the means of conveyance or the routes to be followed, for the destination may be attained through other means or routes. It is not any one of the interim stops, although the traveler may confine himself for a time to one of these more immediate goals. The purpose is really the end-result, which varies from something almost immediate to something quite remote in time.

The purpose of research is the end-result of the single study or the series of studies. It is not the problem, for that is often the point of departure; nor is it the method, for that is the means of conveyance. The purpose of the researcher is his objective or goal. It may be his final destination, but probably will involve a series of interim stops.

The purpose of research may seem to be many-sided. That is because we sometimes view research as a point of departure or a means to an end. If we confine our observations to the interim stops along the way, there would appear to be more than one specific purpose of research. If we extend our point of view to the final destination, an ultimate purpose may come into focus.

This chapter will seek to develop the point of view that there is a general or ultimate purpose of research. It will be conceived as an underlying current that generates the power of the research project—any research project—before its birth, throughout its life, and thereafter. It is impersonal and will extend from research worker to research worker, research project to research project. This chapter will not offer detailed guidelines for the specific project. It is very unlikely that the specific project will designate the underlying purpose. Instead, the chapter has been conceived to provide a philosophic basis for research—a reason for engaging in research—and, perhaps, should comprise the unstated purpose of any project.

WHAT IS THE GENERAL PURPOSE OF RESEARCH?

What does a person try to do when he engages in research? Why go through all the difficulties that usually confront the researcher and always face the possibility that the end-result might be negative? Why stress exactitude? Why should anyone have to justify his studies? Why the care, the refinement, the numerous tests? These are some of the many questions confronting the research worker each time that he engages in a study. They may be summarized in the question: Why do research?

Let us reappraise the very specific situation presented in Chapter 1 of the head nurse and her problem of making assignments (see p. 15). This situation was conceived and offered as an example of problem-solving. It was suggested further that it was not research because it lacked a purpose. Could it have been conceived also as a project for research? If so, what would be the purpose of undertaking such a project?

To Satisfy Curiosity

A researcher may have been tempted out of sheer curiosity to learn the best possible combination of nursing personnel for this assignment. The situation could have intrigued him. He could have asked himself: "What are all the possible combinations? What would be the effect of each upon the patients in the area? What basis do I have for deriving and selecting each of the combinations beforehand? Is there some scheme or gimmick that would specify in advance the best possible combination?"

It might be conceived that there resides in some men an almost insatiable drive to learn the nature of the world about them, the old and the new. They are not satisfied with the *status quo,* with what they are told, with what they can see. They wish to look beyond, to discover how or why things happen, to probe for better solutions. They seek to learn for the sake of learning—to acquire knowledge as its own reward. Could we state that these men engage in research because they are curious?

This proposition implies that there lie before us myriad phenomena signifying the solutions to the problems of mankind. Some are natural—they are the end-products of nature's problem-solving attempts. We observe that plants and animals exist harmoniously. The plant utilizes the carbon dioxide emitted by animals; the animals utilize the oxygen given off by plant life. We perceive how the birds and the animals will gather, protect and nourish their young until they can help themselves. We observe the child growing, the learning process, the healing process. Is this the way that nature has provided for man?

Other solutions may be man-made, perhaps contrived from nature but suggestive of something utilitarian. Man has studied the power-producing qualities of the organism to construct engines that are infinitely more powerful. Man has discovered the healing potentials of certain bacteria and molds, broken them down into their components and reproduced them in larger quantities. And man's curiosity forces him to inquire how we can live longer; how we can fly faster; how we can harness the atom; what lies on the moon, on Venus, on Mars; what lies beyond the sun; what the secret of life itself is.

Every age is represented by a small group of men who are driven to seek out these solutions. They yearn to discover and describe phenomena. Some of the more inquisitive even may desire to understand the processes employed by nature or man in attacking their problems. They ask: Why these solutions and not others?

But how does the drive to learn, the yearning to satisfy curiosity, help the head nurse and her patients? Must she wait until some bright young researcher is attracted by curiosity to her kind of problem? This forces research into the realm of chance: by chance someone will happen along whose curiosity is drawn to this area. And chance itself implies a lack of purpose. This approach to research makes the undertaking a personal affair and confines the activity to those who are both interested and capable. The quality of curiosity may be one of the characteristics that distinguishes the research person from other kinds of people. It may motivate him to seek out research work. It may be a reason for undertaking his journey. But can we justify doing research on this basis alone? Is it the ultimate purpose of research to satisfy man's craving to learn? While curiosity arouses the spirit of man and stimulates research activity, is it also the principal objective of the activity itself?

To Solve Problems

It is more than likely that the head nurse will not wait for her researcher. As was indicated, she will move ahead and solve the problem herself. Her patients and her nurses cannot wait for a more definitive and perhaps better solution. They require a solution within minutes. Is it the purpose of research to assist the head nurse or others like her to solve their own problem?

The point of view was adopted in Chapter 1 that research

is a special order of problem-solving. Also, the subject matter was described in terms of the kinds of problems considered by the different levels of research. We will learn further that research often is generated by the problems of government, business, industry, education and daily living. Can it be stated that the *general* purpose of research is to solve problems?

Action research apparently is directed toward this end. It has been described simply as "research . . . based on concrete problems in actual situations."[1] This mode of practice originated in the school situation to enable the teacher to become more adept and less dependent upon others in problem-solving. Since the practitioner (the school teacher) is confronted daily with many problems, her position would be enhanced if she applied a more precise approach to her problem-solving activities. It was suggested in these cases that the practitioner should become a researcher also.

The head nurse may not be very different from the teacher in this regard. Could she not learn the more precise technics that the researcher applies to his problem-solving activities? Would these technics have enabled her to arrive at a better solution? If problem-solving is the purpose of research, it would appear that the main difference between the non-research-trained nurse, the research-trained nurse, and the expert nurse researcher is one of degree. Furfey, for example, felt that the same mental abilities and processes that are employed in the more systematic research projects also are used in everyday or common-sense problem-solving.[2] The difference is one of degree. Both nurse and researcher solve problems. Then does everyone who engages in problem-solving conduct some degree of research? If not, at what point along this continuum does problem-solving become research?

The question also is asked: What happens as a result of research aimed strictly at solving problems?

First of all, when action research has been completed, its results are quickly utilized by the teacher and put into practice. The teachers then either find some other area for research, or go back to teaching school. The important follow-up questions, such as what happens to a teacher *after* action research results have been put into practice, are seldom asked.[3]

The head nurse solves her problem and may feel satisfied with the solution. The nursing personnel have managed to complete their assignments and the patients are content. It is unlikely, unless she was curious, that the head nurse would pursue her problem further.

Is problem-solving a sufficient purpose? If this is the case, the general purpose again becomes confining. Each project will begin and end with the problem. The major difference between research and general problem-solving activities becomes essentially one of technics and abilities. To the non-research person, this will be a practical endeavor, because it applies the best possible technics to problems as they arise. Research will become extensive and diversified among the many different problems occurring in the field of practice. It will become a job specification of the practitioner to engage in research. But the research will be limited in application to the problem that is posed. It may benefit solely the individual or the small group of individuals immediately involved—the head nurse, her co-workers and the patients—and the situation at hand. But what about society at large, other nurses, other patients? The research will be limited in point of time to the immediate period. But what about the problems to come?

The questions are actually questions of expediency. Is it expedient to expend the practitioner's time and efforts to develop and test exact solutions to each problem as it occurs? Could she possibly engage in this pursuit? Does she actually have the time and the resources? Is it expedient to pursue such arduous activities that are beneficial to so few? In the meantime, societies at large—for example, the general population of nurses—share many grave problems and yearn for common answers. Is it expedient to demand solutions for problems that are past and will never recur in exactly the same way? We can be certain that the future will be laden with recurrent unsolved problems.

On the other hand, the feeling has been voiced that research does not necessarily begin with the problem nor end with its specific solution. Instead, like the problem-solving process, the problem itself may be merely a vehicle to obtain some other end, some other final destination. The situation of assigning nurses will lend itself to the derivation of something else.

This feeling also has been extended to action research, and it has been stated that:

Action research is not solely an action technique aimed at solving a practical problem, but is rather an attempt to help the teacher arrive at generalizations by investigating his own field problems. The purpose of these generalizations is to guide and enrich the teacher's educational work.[4]

Perhaps the nurse, too, can look beyond the specific situation.

To Collect Facts

"Let's get the facts!" the cry goes out. "Provide us with sufficient evidence! What is the truth?" A major source of research activity is fact-finding, the collection of data. Is it the general purpose of research to collect facts?

A large expenditure of governmental, industrial and private agency funds and personnel is made to collect facts. This activity is performed hourly, daily, weekly, monthly, annually, biennially, every 5 or 10 years, etc. People, animals, insects, opinions, diseases, accidents, events, stocks, bonds, elements, household items, buildings, money, and numerous other items are counted periodically by large teams of highly trained experts, by semiskilled and relatively unskilled personnel, by individuals and by small agencies. Facts are collected in bulk with regard to a small number of specific items, or there may be a highly detailed report containing many items.

Every 10 years the Census Bureau of the United States collects, summarizes and reports facts about the population of this country.[5] This agency also periodically collects more detailed accounts of specific areas.[6] Other governmental agencies collect numerous facts. The Public Health Service gathers information on the number of health personnel and the incidence of disease.[7] The Office of Education makes a biennial count of students and teachers of all grade levels and lists the educational programs that are in use.[8] The Labor Department maintains a record of employment figures and prices.[9] The Weather Bureau notes and records the daily changes in temperature throughout the nation.[10] The Atomic Energy Commission measures the amount of Strontium 90 in the atmosphere.[11]

These governmental activities are supplemented by the projects of the private agencies. Many professional societies maintain records of their membership, practitioners and/or clientele.[12, 13] Other nonprofit organizational groups annually collect large quantities of statistics. The American Hospital Association gathers and reports information periodically on the number and the types of hospitals, beds, personnel, facilities, expenditures, etc.[14] The National League for Nursing accumulates annual figures on the number of schools of nursing and students admitted and graduated.[15] The National Education Association prepares estimates of the number of teachers needed and the number of teachers available, at all educational levels.[16]

Industrial groups employ scores of research personnel whose primary activity is to keep track of marketing conditions. They maintain records on the sales of products and the buying habits of consumers. Newspapers survey and report daily changes in the prices of stocks and bonds. Specific research groups keep track of the television programs that people listen to, the automobiles that they own, the people for whom they vote, the sizes of their families, their education, the jobs that they hold.

Private individuals also collect facts. The physician may keep a detailed record of his patient's progress on a day-by-day basis. Many of these case studies are reported in the medical literature. The patient may maintain his own records, as Clifford Beers did in *The Mind That Found Itself*.[17]

Is it the purpose of research to collect facts? If so, of what use are the facts that have been collected? That is, what can be done with the facts once they are collected?

Facts can be utilized to isolate areas of difficulty, to diagnose a problem. The doctor employs his facts—the patient's signs and symptoms—to assist in the diagnosis of what is wrong with the patient. Population statistics may pinpoint areas of expanded or depressed growth, either of which may suggest problems.

Organized facts are employed also to make predictions. The Weather Bureau forecasts future climatic conditions on the basis of the facts accumulated. Market analysts survey product sales to determine future consumer buying habits. The physician makes a prognosis on the basis of his diagnosis and suggests treatment accordingly.

Finally, facts are employed to evaluate a course of action. The head nurse, for example, may wish to assess her solution by collecting facts pertaining to the reactions of patients and personnel. The physician will continue to observe signs and symptoms to note the effects of treatment. The sponsor will determine how many people actually listen to the television program he subsidizes.

It would appear that we collect facts for some other end: to diagnose a problem, to prescribe a course of treatment, to evaluate. The ultimate objective or purpose is not the collection of facts. Fact-gathering itself may be described more appropriately as a means to an end—a method to establish a problem or to verify that a particular course of treatment is trustworthy. It may be regarded as a means of denoting the true state of affairs.

To Contribute to Knowledge

Three points of view have been explored in the attempt to establish an underlying purpose for research. It was suggested that we engage in research because we are curious; to satisfy a curiosity drive, however, was regarded as a personal experience, a motivating force, a means of getting started and not as the ultimate goal. To solve problems was then considered as the possible objective of research, of any research project; but problem-solving seemed to be more characteristic of a means to an end, a mode of conveyance, a vehicle to reach some further goal. To collect facts was offered as a third alternative. This, too, was considered to be a means to an end, a method to establish some element of truth, but not the end itself. Then what is the end, the underlying purpose, of research?

Consider again the head nurse and her problem. What would be the most valued contribution that research or any other undertaking could make to this person? A technic to be employed in solving problems? This would be valuable in the sense that she would be free of the bonds of dependency. She would be more flexible and need not rely upon other people to solve her problems. But problem-solving is time-consuming and uncertain—the investigator is not always sure that he will arrive at the correct or the most appropriate solution. A more desirable contribution, perhaps, is not the process, but the end-result—the solution itself. If a pool of predetermined solutions, tested and true, were available to the head nurse, she could scrutinize this resource and select from it the most applicable solution. Her problem would be solved and she could return to other activities. If we were to re-examine the case (see p. 15), we would learn that this is exactly what the head nurse did. It was stated:

Why not group the critically ill patients in a single room with a professional nurse? The two practical nurses could be released then to provide the kind of care they were well suited to perform for the other patients. The head nurse remembered having read that other hospitals had found this kind of arrangement to be quite satisfactory.

Is it general practice to borrow solutions in the process of solving problems? If so, where do these solutions come from in the first place?

Let us concede that it is the purpose of research to isolate, determine or provide solutions of this kind and contribute them to a pool or resource where they can be held in readiness for the appropriate problem. Let us define this pool or resource as a body of knowledge and seek to demonstrate that it is the underlying purpose of research to contribute to knowledge.

The authors recognize that there are other more profound definitions of knowledge. The reader should not reject these in favor of the one that is offered in this text. Instead, he should regard this definition as a working definition—one that may be useful to us in deriving the purpose of research.

Three questions will be posed in the process of demonstrating that a contribution to knowledge should constitute the underlying purpose of research: Why accumulate knowledge? What are the attributes of knowledge? What is the role of research in the accumulation of knowledge?

Why Accumulate Knowledge?

A number of very practical illustrations of the employment of knowledge occur daily in the lives of most people. For instance, recently one of the authors had occasion to purchase a pair of shoes for his 1½-year-old son. He watched the shoe salesman fitting the youngster. The man measured the boy's right foot first with a standard foot-size indicator. Why the right foot? Because it is common knowledge in the shoe business that the right foot generally is larger than the left. The salesman then slipped a shoe on this foot and depressed the toe with his thumb. "We generally allow a thumbnail's length for growth," he said.

Here was an example of knowledge employed independently of any problem. The shoe salesman, indeed, had anticipated problems that might occur. Knowledge exists in a world of its own, distinct from the problem situation. It can be called upon, however, when a problem arises or threatens to arise. For example, the small child tells his mother, "I cannot reach the cupboard," and the mother offers the knowledge, "Stand on a chair." A man has a severe head cold and takes two aspirins and a cup of tea upon retiring. The motorist will decrease his speed upon entering a turn to reduce the effect of centrifugal force. The nurse will teach her patients how to cough preoperatively so that they will be able to cough postoperatively. The teacher will encourage the poor student rather than scold him.

It may be said that knowledge is the forerunner of problem-solving situations. That is, we can anticipate the answer to problems without solving them. Why? Because they have been solved previously. We need only to make the judgment that the problem can be classified as one of the same order of problems for which solutions previously have been obtained.

To anticipate the solution to a problem is a powerful weapon. The guesswork and the trial-and-error procedures are removed from problem-solving. The problem-solving process itself is reduced to a minimum because we can predict the proper answer or answers with reasonable certainty and concentrate on merely a few propositions. To predict, to know what to expect and perhaps what to do when presented with a series of obstacles provides man with considerable security. With knowledge we gain some control over our environment.

Knowledge reduces one's dependence upon chance. If a person is thrown unaided into the world, he is forced to act upon each situation by sheer trial and error. Tell him, however, what others have discovered in similar situations and he can direct his actions so that he is more certain what consequences they will have.[18]

Why accumulate knowledge? We only need to look at the world about us to answer the question. We only need to compare our world with that of a primitive society, with that of our parents, with that of the ignorant. Knowledge is the channel through which the secrets of yesterday become the realities of tomorrow. Knowledge is man's gift to man.

What Are the Attributes of Knowledge?

It may be recalled, in reference to the case of the head nurse and her problem (see p. 15), that more than one solution was considered. The head nurse thought initially that each of the practical nurses could be assigned to two of the critically ill patients. She concluded later that this proposal was inappropriate.

Knowledge has different attributes. What is appropriate for one situation may not be adequate for another. What are the attributes of knowledge? Upon what basis does a person select from one body of knowledge rather than another? Let us attempt to answer these questions by examining the various kinds of knowledge that are available and considering, hypothetically, how the head nurse could have made her selection.

Accessibility. One of the attributes of knowledge is accessibility. There are different sources of knowledge to which a practitioner may turn. Such practical considerations as time and effort may influence her choice. Knowledge that is more readily available, though less reliable or worthy, may be employed more frequently.

The first body of knowledge to which the head nurse may turn is contained within herself. Each of us is a reservoir of information, drawn from or influenced by our experiences, mental faculties and formal and informal education. This is common-sense knowledge, which is composed of many unrecorded solutions that have been accumulated from problems faced daily in the process of living. It is common-sense knowledge because we may not apply any particular abilities or technics to problem-solving other than those with which we are equipped at the time the problem arises. It is common-sense knowledge because the solutions may have been with us so long that we simply take them for granted. "How do you know that this is the best answer?" is asked. "Why common sense will tell you" is the reply.

Long before the beginnings of modern civilization, men acquired vast funds of information about their environment. They learned to recognize substances which nourished their bodies. They discovered the uses of fire and developed skills in transforming raw materials into shelters, clothing, and utensils. They invented arts of tilling the soil, communicating, and governing themselves. Some of them discovered that objects are moved more easily when placed on carts with wheels, that the sizes of the fields are more reliably compared when standard schemes of measurement are employed. . . . The acquisition of reliable knowledge concerning many aspects of the world certainly did not wait upon the advent of modern science and the self-conscious use of its methods.[19]

Common-sense knowledge may be considered to be an unorganized collection of solutions. It is unorganized because the solutions may not have been collected and recorded in their proper places in an organized body of knowledge. It is unorganized because man may not take the time, may not know how or may not feel the need to bind the solutions together in any deliberate or systematic fashion.

It may be extremely difficult, if not impossible, to separate the unorganized common-sense knowledge from the more systematically collected and organized knowledge. No sharp line separates beliefs that generally are subsumed under the familiar but vague term "common sense" from those cognitive claims that are recognized as "scientific." What is common sense today may become organized knowledge tomorrow. When Pasteur made his discoveries at about the middle of the nineteenth century, the idea of contagion as a cause of infection was centuries old.[20] But the cause was not known, nor was it investigated systematically. It was accepted simply as common-sense knowledge. Many explanations were offered, such as an influence in the air, a spontaneous generation of life, and the like. Nevertheless, the fact that contagion or contact caused the spread of some diseases was understood over two thousand years ago by the Hebrews who isolated lepers. The discovery of bacteria by Pasteur formalized this knowledge. A reason was provided. This contribution was placed within a framework consisting of other sources of knowledge.

Furthermore, what is organized knowledge today may be so well integrated by a society that it is accepted as common sense tomorrow. Knowledge regarding the transmission of contagious diseases has become common-sense knowledge. Today, people not only accept for themselves but demand that everyone else accept the social responsibility for voluntarily protecting the community from themselves when they have communicable diseases.

Common-sense knowledge has the important attribute of being readily accessible to the person when he needs it. The head nurse did not search through various source materials or seek authoritative advice from someone else when confronted with her task. She turned to herself, consulted her previous experiences, and chose what seemed to be the best solution. This is an extremely valuable time- and labor-saving device. We must call forth knowledge frequently during each day. Lacking common sense would place us at an extreme disadvantage.

Common-sense knowledge also has some limitations. Nagel differentiates common-sense knowledge (which he refers to as prescientific knowledge) from scientific knowledge in the following manner:[21]

1. Common-sense knowledge may be accurate within the margins of certain limitations. However, the information often is not presented with the facts that have been offered allegedly as support. On the other hand, the distinctive goal of science is the organization and the classification of knowledge on the basis of explanatory principles.

2. Although the claims of common-sense knowledge may be accurate, the boundaries signifying the extent to which it is valid and useful seldom are recognized. Thus it suffers from incompleteness.

3. Common-sense knowledge is preoccupied with what is considered to be immediate and observable. It is concerned with the effects that familiar things have upon matters that are valued by men; the relations of these events to each other are not explained or organized. Thus, there may be conflicts between judgments made in common-sense or everyday life. Science attempts to resolve such conflicts by introducing "a systematic explanation of facts, by ascertaining the conditions and consequences of events, by exhibiting the logical relations"[22] of each fact to every other fact. "Common-sense beliefs are not subjected, as a matter of established principle, to systematic scrutiny in the light of data secured for the sake of determining the accuracy of those beliefs and the range of their validity."[23]

4. In common-sense knowledge, terms are not used in precise and exact language; they generally are used in a broad and vague sense, and therefore do not offer a precise explanation

of an event or a phenomenon. Science, on the other hand, resolves the indeterminate character of everyday language by siphoning it through a more precise and exact definition and a thorough and critical testing by experience. Prescientific beliefs frequently are incapable of being put to definite and experiential tests in their original forms.

It may be said that common-sense knowledge contains a composite of reliable and unreliable information. The individual problem-solver must separate the two and evaluate each piece of knowledge accordingly. Since common-sense knowledge is based upon individual experiences and is enhanced by time, it may become highly resistant to change. This may be true even when very reliable information proves it to be wrong.

Referring once again to infection, cross-infection of patients in hospitals has become a serious problem since infection can be transmitted from one patient to another. Doctors and nurses know this. It has been proved also that a thorough hand-washing before attending each patient will aid materially in the reduction of infection. Yet frequently nurses and doctors will move from patient to patient without washing their hands.[24]

Common-sense knowledge, unorganized and unrecorded, is not accessible to everyone in the same degree. More intelligent, more experienced, better-educated people will have larger quantities than other people. Some will have more reliable knowledge than others. Therefore, common-sense knowledge will vary as much as the people who possess it. An individual who is rich in experience or exceedingly bright, or who has accumulated a large personal resource of knowledge, will have an abundance of common-sense solutions. Some of these may be well tested and exceedingly reliable. If he is lacking in these qualities, he may have a dearth of adequate common-sense knowledge.

These statements suggest another body of knowledge to which the head nurse might turn. That is, she may seek assistance from individuals who have accumulated a more comprehensive store of knowledge than she has, or from individuals who have accumulated abundant information with regard to the particular problem area in which she seeks knowledge.

Some people become more adept than others at solving particular problems. They accumulate and store within themselves large quantities of knowledge or solutions regarding a specific area of practice. They become our experts, the authorities, the people with whom we consult. The knowledge that they contain is organized and recorded. It has been organized and sorted as it has been experienced and recorded within the person. However, the knowledge may not exist outside the person.

In ancient days, these walking bodies of knowledge consisted of the tribe elders. They were the people who had lived the longest, had accumulated the greatest number of experiences and perhaps were the wisest in making judgments—sorting the appropriate from the inappropriate solutions. The world of today is considerably more complex and diverse. The wise men, although comparatively young, are highly specialized. They have accumulated considerable knowledge in particular fields. Some of them are available to provide service and offer knowledge, upon request.

If the head nurse had time and deemed it important, she could obtain the desired solution from one of these specialists. To whom would she turn? She might first approach other head nurses or her supervisors, who have had considerable experience in solving problems of this kind. If they could not provide adequate solutions and the situation warranted further efforts, she could address her problem to experts concerned with the management of personnel both in and outside the field of nursing practice.

This huge and diversified resource of knowledge has one very important attribute. Though not as readily accessible as the previous source, it is more reliable. It is more reliable because the expert has a greater abundance of solutions from which to choose and can exercise a wiser judgment in the selection process. It is more reliable also because his solutions have withstood the test of prolonged experience and have remained relatively unchanged.

The question remains as to the quality of this body of knowledge. In essence, it contains a wide variety of both good, well-tested, and poor, untested solutions. If, like the authors, one has little knowledge of motor mechanics, he consults with a specialist when his automobile breaks down. How does he know that the mechanic is providing the best possible service for his automobile? He really does not know; he simply relies upon the reputation that the mechanic has gained in solving his previous automobile problems. Since this information is recorded only within the person (consultant, mechanic, etc.) who has it, how can the individual practitioner (nurse, motorist, etc.) learn and understand the differences between the various solutions that are provided?

A third source of knowledge that is accessible to the head nurse is contained in the written record. This is knowledge contributed by the individual and shared openly by other individuals. In this regard, it differs from the other two sources. It is unlike them in still other respects. The amount of knowledge accumulated by any single individual is fixed and will die with him. Knowledge accumulated in written records does not have any such boundaries. It grows ceaselessly with time. It contains the contributions of many people—each building upon the works of their predecessors. It contains contributions in an endless number of areas. It can be dissected, evaluated, and employed in different ways.

Where can the head nurse find a written solution? She might begin by inspecting the hospital's records of previous assignments, including her own. She can examine the trade or professional journals for articles whose titles suggest that they cover problems similar to hers. She can consult texts on nursing service administration, hospital administration, or administration in general. There are many written records to which she can turn.

In what manner would the solution be displayed? Cronbach and others analyzed the various ways in which knowledge is presented in textbooks. They defined arbitrarily four categories that suggest how knowledge is transmitted: narration and description, prescription and directive, generalization, and theory.[25]

Narrations and descriptions portray a running account of an experience and a representation of the circumstance surrounding the event. They may make the reader feel that he actually is experiencing the event as it was experienced by the author. In this regard, the head nurse may attempt to seek out descriptive accounts of situations somewhat like her own, make a note of what was done, and contemplate whether or not that solution would satisfy the demands of her own situation. The various case-study materials presented in medical and nursing journals are typical of this kind of written report.

"Prescriptions and directives tell the reader what to do and how to do it."[26] This is exactly the kind of information that the head nurse would find to be the most desirable. It would tell her what to do when confronted with a situation like her own. Of course the question remains: Has anyone written any materials offering directives pertaining to this problem? Would the situation warrant a special set of directives?

Generalizations are solutions offered in abstract form that deal with the common properties of a whole class or group of situations. They do not concern the unique event or situation but may be applicable if the situation has the properties of the class or the group.[27] For example, examine the generalization—fewer nurses will be required to provide service when patients are grouped by common problems—and observe that it applies to a class of nurses and a class of patients. If the nurses and the patients of the problem situation have the same characteristics as those in the generalization, then the generalization may be applicable to the problem situation. The head nurse then will be provided with a valuable clue.

Theoretic knowledge is descriptive of the terms characterizing a body of knowledge that has been organized systematically. That is, this body does not accumulate an odd collection of solutions but, instead, organizes the solutions so that the relation of one to the other can be observed. In this way, other solutions can be derived. A theoretic construct depicts a relationship that cannot be observed or experienced by the senses. But we theorize logically on the basis of other facts, both observable and nonobservable, that it must be so. It may be possible to reconstruct in theoretic terms the situation that has become the case in point. This situation may be described, for example, in terms of a theory of group action or behavior that registers the advantages of a division of labor. Several possible solutions could be derived and made applicable to the nursing situation.

The reader will note from the above descriptions that knowledge secured from written records is perhaps the least accessible. The head nurse could search through many sources and still emerge without a definitive solution. The records, unfortunately, do not cry out and speak for themselves. The problem-solver will have to examine what is offered and make the required adjustments.

Knowledge displayed in this form is, perhaps, the most reliable. The reader has the opportunity to scrutinize the written report carefully. He can make comparisons with other reports and with his own or some authority's experience. He can observe the manner by which the data were collected. He can judge the degree to which the information is applicable to his own problems.

Summary. One of the attributes of knowledge is accessibility or the extent to which it is available to the consumer of knowledge. In this regard, common-sense knowledge, the expert consultant's knowledge, and knowledge contained within the written record were discussed. It was learned that some sources may be more accessible than others and that there may be a tendency for the more accessible to be less reliable.

Usefulness. Knowledge has a second attribute: it may be described by its usefulness. Some sources of knowledge have very limited application. Like narrations and descriptions, they may apply to unique situations. Sources such as generalizations have much broader applications.

The extent to which knowledge is used may be a result of

the manner in which it was derived initially. The authors already have categorized the subject matter of research into three types of problem situations: specific, common and underlying. These subject-matter areas or problem situations also may be considered as the springboard from which new sources of knowledge are derived. The utilization of the knowledge produced as a result of these undertakings may depend upon the type of problem that launched the enterprise.

The head nurse began her task with a specific problem. She required an on-the-spot solution. It did not matter at the time whether or not the derived solution would be applicable to other nursing situations or helpful to her on some future occasion. She needed a solution then and there and could not waste much time in obtaining it.

Common-sense knowledge would have been the most accessible and perhaps the most useful to her under these circumstances. The situation did not permit her to expend more energy or time on the matter. However, suppose that all of the more reliable source material was immediately available. Suppose, furthermore, that someone deliberately sorted the source material and discarded everything that was not highly pertinent. What would the probability be that a solution to her specific problem would remain?

There may be a slight chance of such an event. However, while on this occasion the solution would be useful to the head nurse, what future value would it have? How frequently could we expect situations to recur in the same way, even in the same place and to the same people? How useful is knowledge that is limited to a specific kind of problem?

Knowledge conceived and derived with regard to a very specific problem is limited in use to the specific problem itself. But, to the practitioner whose major concerns are the many specific problems encountered, this may be all that is required. She may rely principally upon her common-sense sources of supply. The action researcher suggests that she use more reliable methods. Until that time, however, she will remain essentially a common-sense problem-solver.

The head nurse could become a better common-sense problem-solver by increasing the quantity and the quality of her source of supply. She could seek continually new and better solutions to problem situations. These are obtained through experience, word of mouth, and the written record.

Nevertheless, we may ask: How could this person or any person acquire great quantities of knowledge and be prepared with the proper solution when the occasion arises? The probability is that she will be limited considerably. It is likely that she can acquire only a very small portion of this kind of knowledge during her lifetime. The process of acquiring knowledge is time-consuming for all and difficult for most.

However, the burden can be eased by another characteristic of knowledge: its generalizability. Knowledge need not be solely a unique answer to a unique problem. This would be satisfactory only momentarily, since the specific event could not be expected to occur again. Instead, the usefulness of knowledge increases when the solution can be transferred from the specific problem situation from which it was derived to a multitude of events. Then, with but a few potent pieces of knowledge, man can control, or at least understand, a large part of his environment. It is not the multiplicity of facts that stretches man's horizons but his ability to reach out and obtain those few items that span a multiplicity of situations. Indeed, the more useful solution may be conceived as the one with a wider applicability, and the search for knowledge continually takes this direction. Those who seek knowledge

are uninterested in single and completely unique events per se. Instead, their aim is to discover under the surface layer of diversity the thread of uniformity. Around a discovered uniformity a logical class is constructed; about the class and its observed pattern a descriptive generalization is formulated. (They) are alert to opportunities for combining comparable classes into a broader class and for formulating a wider and more abstract generalization to comprehend the discrete generalizations thereby embraced.[28]

Knowledge also may be timeless, for the solutions derived from yesterday's problems may be applicable to tomorrow's.

The problem may change its outer appearance; but if the solution is a useful one, it should hold true consistently.

In order to develop this kind of knowledge, the problem or the seeds from which it springs must be conceived initially in the broader frame of reference. But problems exist only in specific situations. For this purpose, the authors deliberately created two abstractions: the common problem and the underlying problem. Both these problems are figments of the authors' imaginations but gain meaning when represented in a series of common specific situations.

The *common problem* was defined previously as one that has properties shared by specific problems within a given area of practice. Perhaps there is a wide range of common problems. They may relate, for example, to the common problems that are shared by such persons as the head nurse, or by other persons like her (other head nurses), or by members of allied groups, such as teachers or social workers. The extent of the coverage will govern the applicability of the common problem.

The head nurse could conceive that her specific problem has properties that are shared commonly with other specific problems. Solutions pertaining to the latter might be useful in her own situation. She recognized, for example, that the problem dealt in part with the care of the critically ill. Someone else had been involved also in a situation of this kind and suggested that critically ill patients could be grouped together in a single unit, and intensive care could be given to them by a small number of professional nurses. Would this solution work in her case? It should if the patients and the nurses were of the same type as those in the similar situation.

We may consider that workers in the applied field of research are engaged to provide solutions for common problems. They are employed because the practitioners within a given field of activity recognize the need for better modes of practice, better solutions. The concern of the applied researcher is not the individual practitioner at work with a particular problem at a particular time. This is the job of the practitioner herself. Instead, the researcher centers his attention upon the needs of practitioners as a whole, and the problems they share in common. His concern is the solution or the knowledge to be derived and its degree of applicability to the field of practice that employs him.

Knowledge also may have application outside the realm of specific or common practice. The scope of application may transcend fields of practice—what is applicable to nursing may be applicable also to medicine, teaching, social work, industry and even the process of daily living; it also may transcend time and place. Knowledge exists that may apply anywhere, at any time, to anyone.

Underlying problem situations may be said to occur universally, and their solutions apply universally. They are shared by all men, but differ from the common problem in that they are not man-created. They are the problems that exist in nature, and the knowledge derived is from the solutions that nature has devised. In a sense, our most useful forms of knowledge are borrowed from nature and reflect nature's attempts at problem-solving.

Underlying basic or nature's knowledge has been grouped together in several bodies. These bodies have been classified into two major subdivisions: the sciences and pilosophy.[29] Each subdivision differs with regard to a third attribute: authenticity. This attribute, which is discussed on page 106, concerns the manner by which knowledge is secured. The sciences and philosophy also differ in their perception of knowledge or the type of knowledge developed by each.

Science is analytical description, philosophy is synthetic interpretation. Science wishes to resolve the whole into parts, the organism into organs, the obscure into the known. It does not inquire into the values and ideal possibilities of things, nor into their total and final significance; it is content to show their present actuality and operation, it narrows its gaze resolutely to the nature and process of things as they are. . . . But the philosopher is not content to describe the fact; he wishes to ascertain the relation to experience in general, and thereby to get at its meaning and its worth; he combines things in interpretive synthesis; he tries to put together, better than before, that great universe-watch which the inquisitive scientist has analytically taken apart. Science tells us how to heal and how to kill; it reduces the death rate in detail and then kills us wholesale in war; but only wisdom—desire co-ordinated in the light of all experience—can tell us when to heal and when to kill.[30]

Science and philosophy may use the same subject matter. For example, the acts, the powers and the habits of man are subject matter in both scientific and philosophic psychology. The differences arise mainly (though not solely) from the different standpoint or goal that characterizes each.

Science of psychology limits its analysis to acts, powers and habits —belonging to the phenomenal order of man's life. . . . Philosophy of psychology . . . advances its analysis beyond the facts of induction (to reach) some notion of the nature or substance of man.[31]

Scientific psychology is interested primarily in the laws of operation and their relationships; philosophic psychology is interested in the laws of being. Thus, they have the same subject matter, namely, the acts, the powers and the habits of man, but each approaches it from a different point of view and with a different goal.

Each discipline contributes a distinct kind of knowledge because its approach to problems is different. Therefore, the use of scientific or philosophic knowledge must be governed by the problem. The head nurse might find solutions from both the sciences and philosophy. If the question or the problem pertains to the scheduling of nursing personnel, she may find some solutions from an analysis of the scientific knowledge dealing with such topics as the division of labor or the organization of men. But if the problem is to decide which patient is entitled to the greatest amount of the available nursing care, a philosophic issue may arise.

The authors will consider, for reasons to be explained later, that research is more properly contained within the province of the sciences. The basic researcher thus is known more commonly as the scientist. He investigates nature at work. He is the pure researcher in the sense that he explores knowledge that is uncontaminated by man and his problems. It has been said that the basic researcher is impractical because he deals with problems outside the realm of practice. In reality, he is perhaps the most practical researcher of all, because the knowledge that he derives will be beneficial to the largest number of practitioners. It will be the most useful.

Summary. The derivation of knowledge can be envisioned as the series of concentric circles that form when a stone is thrown upon still waters. The ripples of water radiate, becoming larger and larger as they proceed from the point where the stone first made contact with the water. The initiating point can be denoted as the solution to the specific problem and is confined to the boundaries of the first circle. The area between this line and the outermost circle includes solutions to common problems whose applicability will vary over this entire range. The outermost circle contains the solution to the underlying problem and can be applied universally to everything that is included within its lines.

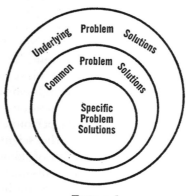

FIGURE 1

Authenticity. The third and final attribute of knowledge to be discussed here is authenticity. Is the solution correct? The information given to the head nurse may be most accessible and useful, but it also could be the wrong answer to her problem. In this event, it is not useful at all.

It has been said that one purpose of research is to seek the truth. In reality, when we seek the truth we search for the most authentic answer. When solutions are set aside in the reservoir of knowledge that is to be used upon the proper occasions, the judgment is made that the solutions befit the circumstances from which they are derived. Why is the contributor certain that this is the case? How does he know that it will work in other situations?

Two tests of authenticity or combinations thereof will be discussed: the test of empiricism and that of reason. Each order of knowledge will be related to the test of authenticity.

One of the most commonly used tests of authenticity is that of experience. "Seeing is believing" and "That's fine in principle, but does it really work?" are characteristic expressions of this mode of thinking. They imply that we must be able to experience the event for ourselves. It is an empiric test—that which can be sensed or observed.

Much of what is called common-sense knowledge is made up of solutions that have withstood the repeated tests of sense experience. The old-fashioned remedies persist because they appear to work, to work to a degree, or simply make us feel better. The head nurse may look for favorable reactions from her patients and staff, the presence or the absence of chaos, and other signs that seem to indicate that her choice was a good one.

Sometimes our experiences deceive us. The solution seems to work, but really does not. For example, did not man once consider that the world was flat and not round? Our common-sense experiences to this day will tell us that the world is flat. Yet other kinds of experiences will convince us that it is round.

Another test of authenticity is reason. The answer may seem to be logically correct. It was reasoned that if the world was flat, and a man sailed due west, he ultimately would fall off the earth. But man sailed west and did not fall off the earth. Therefore, the world must be more or less round.

The head nurse recalled an occasion when professional nurses provided care for critically ill patients. Her problem situation had characteristics in common with this previous occasion. She therefore reasoned that if the solution worked in the earlier situation it also should be appropriate in this one.

She reasoned further that two kinds of nurses—professional and nonprofessional—were available to give care to two kinds of patients—critically and not-so-critically ill. The nonprofessional nurse was qualified to perform many of the functions required for the latter group of patients and only a minimum of the functions required for the former. The professional nurse, on the other hand, was able to provide care at all levels. Perhaps it was more suitable, the head nurse reasoned, to utilize her limited resource of professional nurses to care for the critically ill and disperse her nonprofessionals among the not-so-critically ill.

The reasoning process implies that the problem-solver duplicates and re-enacts the situation on paper or in his thoughts. Then he is free to manipulate the events within the limits set by the rules of reasoning or logic and arrive at the best "paper" or hypothetic answer. The test of authenticity is that it must be logically correct. That is, the rules of logic must not be violated.

Reasoning, therefore, permits the problem-solver to make mistakes without any drastic penalty. All that is lost is time. However, he can reason incorrectly. He may do so by failing to reconstruct the events accurately or by violating the rules of logic.

The error made by man in describing the shape of the earth was partially an error of reasoning. In accordance with his observations at that time, the earth was flat. This was true no matter where he viewed it from. He therefore reasoned that it was flat all over.

The most appropriate test of authenticity may involve both reasoning and experience. It is questionable that, with his ability to conceptualize, man could do otherwise than apply both reasoning and experience. Where but from experience does the basis for his thoughts come? And where but from his thoughts can he select and evaluate the appropriate experience?

Sheer trial-and-error behavior or action without reason or thought is very rare. It is characteristic of the lowest organism or the newborn infant who has not had any previous experiences upon which to draw. But the human adult seldom encounters a situation that does not interrelate with some previous experience. What constitutes the event to be tried is something that was drawn by the process of reasoning from experience.

The ingredients for reasoning or problem-solving on paper are provided primarily by experience. We seldom can reason adequately without experience. The congenitally deaf, for example, who have never experienced sound, cannot conceptualize speaking. The young child's drawings reflect his limited experiences. Man, however, has found it possible to create or imagine events or things that he has never observed: an electric current, an atom. Nevertheless, even these in part reflect some previous experience.

The problem-solving process implies that a series of solutions are selected by reasoning and delimited by additional reasoning; the remaining solutions then are subjected to an empiric test that has been constructed deliberately for this purpose. We ultimately make the judgment or reason that the solution is authentic on the basis of the test. Thus, a series of tests, each interrelated and compensating for deficiencies in the others, generally composes the mark of authenticity.

There are some avenues of knowledge that do not lend themselves easily to empiric testing. Such very profound questions, as: What is knowledge? What is research? What is the purpose of research? are examples of problems that cannot be verified in a real situation. Findings of this type are developed and substantiated through the process of reasoning and simply cannot be subjected to empiric testing. For example, we cannot state conclusively that the definition of purpose that is being developed herein will represent the "final word." Instead, it can be offered only as a point of view.

Scientific and philosophic knowledge differ with regard to the attribute of authenticity, that is, in how they arrive at knowledge. The former is subject to both logical and empiric tests. Philosophic knowledge or solutions to such problems as those propounded above satisfy the test of reason, but not of empiricism.

The philosopher attempts to achieve understanding through reasoning.[32] He makes statements that are intended to be accurate and relies on argument to support his thinking or to refute the thoughts with which he does not agree. His statements are authentic to the degree that they unfold the deeper implications of reality; indeed, many of them cannot be rejected without denying reality itself.

The scientist, on the other hand, may limit his search to something less basic. In essence, he sacrifices the range of usefulness for authenticity or truth. He attempts to demonstrate in reality that, given certain conditions, certain events inevitably will follow. His method is a study of possibles; he employs precise methods for formulating and testing solutions. If his test is successful, he may feel more confident that his solution contains at least some element of truth.

There is not any clear line of demarcation between these two approaches to knowledge. In fact, there is considerable mutual interrelationship, and neither can be ignored. It was suggested previously that man tends toward both reason and empiric test. Parsons considered further that it is within the nature of a human being to strive for a rationally consistent account of all human experience that comes within his range.[33]

To restrict the body of knowledge to the scientific would simulate a house without walls or windows, or a novel without plot or theme. It would be crowded with the useful, the bare essentials, the "irreducible and stubborn facts." However, there would not be any wherewithal for binding the items together into a comprehensive and meaningful whole, for clarifying the vague, or for establishing new directions. Philosophy is the forerunner of science. It is not contained by empiric controls and, therefore, can deal with those broad questions that otherwise go unanswered.

All the world over and at all times there have been practical men, absorbed in "irreducible and stubborn facts": all the world over and at all times there have been men of philosophic temperament who have been absorbed in the weaving of general principles. It is this union of passionate interest in the detailed facts with equal devotion to abstract generalisation which forms the novelty in our present society. Previously it had appeared sporadically and as if by chance. This balance of mind has now become part of the tradition which infects cultivated thought. It is the salt which keeps life sweet. The main business of universities is to transmit this tradition as a widespread inheritance from generation to generation.[34]

All sciences rest upon presuppositions that are philosophic in nature. The principles of identity, generalizability, contradiction, causality, trustworthiness of the human intellect and the senses, and others, are philosophic, empirically unproven and unprovable.[35] We can reason that they are true, we can believe that they are true, but we cannot prove empirically that they are true. They represent problems of epistemology, a branch of philosophy. They deal with the validity of knowledge. They justify the foundations upon which science rests but which science is unable to justify by its own means and methods.

Philosophy, in turn, uses data from the sciences.

For though the philosopher as such need not use the affirmation of the special science to establish his own truths, he ought to make use of them (I) to illustrate aptly his principles, (II) to confirm his conclusions, (III) to interpret, throw light upon, and assimilate, the assured results of the sciences so far as questions of philosophy are involved. And finally he should use the affirmations of science (IV) to refute objections and errors which claim support from its results.[36]

There is another factor implicit in these statements about knowledge that is above and beyond reason and empiric test. There are some areas of knowledge that cannot be proved by reason or experience. We simply assume and accept their existence because of the principle of unity. The very foundation upon which the body of applied, scientific and philosophic knowledge is erected rests upon the fundamental faith that we live in an orderly world—that events do not happen by chance but occur in a consistent and logical manner. It is an inexpugnable belief that every detailed occurrence can be correlated with its antecedents in a perfectly definite manner, exemplifying general principles. Without this belief the incredible labors of scientists would be without hope. It is this instinctive conviction, vividly poised before the imagination, which is the motive power of research: that there is a secret, a secret which can be unveiled.[37]

The problem of gathering knowledge may be said to consist of discovering, eliciting and describing the details of an orderly system. We either have or do not have this belief about order in the universe. However, it would be rather difficult to acquire knowledge without it.

WHAT IS THE ROLE OF RESEARCH IN THE ACCUMULATION OF KNOWLEDGE?

The point of view was adopted in the first chapter that research is problem-solving. As such, it will incorporate the general steps of problem-solving, including the statement of the problem, the derivation of hypotheses through a process of reasoning, and the validation of hypotheses through empiric testing. We can observe, therefore, that the research process includes both reasoning and empiric testing.

It was intimated that research differs in purpose from general problem-solving activities. While the purpose of general problem-solving is to solve the problem at hand, it has been suggested that the purpose of research is to make a contribution or to add to a body of solutions or knowledge through problem-solving. A final question remains as to whether research contributes to all bodies of knowledge or to just a selective few.

Does research contribute to solutions of specific problems? If so, how does it differ from general problem-solving activities? If the intent is to provide a solution to a very specific problem, its usefulness is limited solely to the point of application. Common-sense knowledge, which also may be derived by the technics of general problem-solving, is more accessible. The authenticity of this type of knowledge, however, is questionable.

The proponents of action research have proposed that authenticity can be improved by utilizing the supposedly more rigorous methods of research. (There is no reason why we cannot and do not apply these technics in deriving common-sense knowledge.) Of course this procedure takes time. If the problem warrants such activity, the practitioner may pursue a more rigorous approach. What happens to the solution once the problem has been resolved is a point of controversy.

It has been suggested by some action researchers that the research practitioner looks beyond the needs of the specific problem situation and seeks to derive a solution that has meaning to the broad field of practice. In this regard, action research becomes akin to applied research. The interests of the researcher in the applied fields are directed toward the development of solutions for problems common to practitioners within the field. He employs the general problem-solving technics in the manner of the researcher to determine these solutions.

The knowledge contributed by applied research generally is considered to be more useful and accurate, though less accessible, than common-sense knowledge. It will have application to problem situations having properties common to the situation from which the knowledge was derived. However, it is not the most useful or authentic source of knowledge.

Knowledge determined from underlying problems is more useful and authentic. This knowledge consists of solutions provided by nature. It has universal application, transcending many fields of practice. Furthermore, it deals in solutions that have more basic origins. Applied knowledge, being more restrictive, may touch upon superficial solutions that work only within the context that is cast. Therefore, it tends to be less authentic.

Since the process of research implies both reasoning and empiric testing, it is concerned with that order of underlying knowledge that can be verified by experience. The term science often is restricted to this order, thus omitting philosophy, which verifies its conclusions by other means.* The latter rests upon reasoning. Scientific research entails philosophic principles, reasoning and empiric testing. Indeed, research often is called the method of science.

It may be concluded from this analysis that the role of research is elicited more clearly in projects pertaining to common or underlying problems. There is some question as to whether or not the researcher who deals solely with the specific problem is engaged in research activities. What differentiates general problem-solving activities from research activities is the question at hand. If it is merely a matter of technics, then all three activities might be construed properly as research. If it is a matter of purpose, then there is a sharp line of demarcation. The former two problem situations—common and underlying —are nonexistent in their pure forms, but describe a multitude of situations and have a bearing on problems to come. The latter problem situations—specific—are real, unique and limited in point of time and scope to problems as of the moment. The point of view expressed here is that the purpose of research is to contribute to a body of solutions or knowledge pertaining to problems to come.

THE GENERAL PURPOSE OF RESEARCH IN NURSING

The many diverse characteristics of nursing research were observed in reviewing the historical development. Different

---

* This book is devoted to the scientific method, with application to nursing. The authors have presented a few concepts regarding philosophy and its relationship to science in order to provide a broad frame of reference for these two orders of knowledge. The reader is referred to books on these subjects for further information. For example, see:

Martin, Oliver Wm.: The Order and Integration of Knowledge, Ann Arbor, Univ. Press, 1957; Nagel, Ernest: The Structure of Science: Problems in the Logic of Scientific Explanation, New York, Harcourt, 1961; Houde, R., and Mullally, J. P. (eds.): Philosophy of Knowledge: Selected Readings, Philadelphia, Lippincott, 1960; Feigl, H., and Brodbeck, H. (eds.): Readings in the Philosophy of Science, New York, Appleton-Century-Crofts, 1953; Koren, H. J. (C. S. Sp.) (ed.): Readings in the Philosophy of Nature, Westminster, Md., The Newman Press, 1958; Smith, Vincent: General Science of Nature, Milwaukee, Bruce, 1958.

kinds of people have been engaged in this practice in many areas of interest and perhaps for a multitude of reasons. Is the same underlying generating force beneath the myriad motivating conditions? Is there a general purpose of research in nursing?

The nurse—practitioner, educator, administrator, professional researcher; the sociologist; the psychologist; the statistician; the physician; and the industrial engineer have been participating in nursing research projects. Each may have been engaged in the same research activity, yet each could have embarked on the journey for reasons peculiar to himself. Also, they may have achieved satisfaction or settled upon goals miles apart. Why do people engage in nursing research?

Among the purposes extracted from the many nursing projects already reviewed were the following: to describe a state of affairs, to isolate problem areas, to determine solutions for problems, to analyze standards and guides for action, to determine cause and effect relationships, to predict. Each of these in turn was depicted in many ways. Sometimes the end-products appeared to relate, but more often they did not. Could we find a single unifying objective in the rapidly accelerating pool of research projects in nursing? Should there be a general purpose for research in nursing?

Nursing draws upon many resources of knowledge. Practically every science is represented. Many of the applied areas (including nursing) also have offered contributions. Nursing has borrowed to some extent from the more broadly displayed sources of philosophic knowledge. The area of coverage is quite extensive and there are numerous contributors. Then why does nursing itself engage in research?

WHY DO PEOPLE ENGAGE IN NURSING RESEARCH?

There are probably as many different reasons for engaging in nursing research as there are different types of practitioners. Lacking appropriate survey information, the authors would surmise the following to be among the most prominent reasons:

1. To satisfy some personal drive

2. To contribute to other pools of knowledge
3. To improve nursing practice.

As we have seen, nursing research was performed initially by a small body of women who constituted the founders of modern nursing. Judging from their publications, their intent was to reform the existing practices, to draw together the array of procedures that had been established, and to re-establish the general practice of what could be designated nursing upon a sounder footing. Why did they engage in nursing research? Personal motivations—the need to express their own ideas, disillusionment with the *status quo*—were no doubt among the propelling forces. These were the undeclared purposes. Their ultimate and stated aim, of course, was to improve and advance nursing practice.

During the second period, research was initiated by groups of people whose intentions were similar to those of the earlier body. Essentially, they desired to enhance nursing practice by improving leadership and education and defining the responsibilities of the profession. The projects themselves generally were farmed out to other nurses, who were assisted by statisticians. Why did these other nurses engage in nursing research? Personal motivations predominated, perhaps to a considerable extent. The conduct of research studies in nursing had become a principal occupation for them. We might suppose that this very small group of people became dissatisfield with their work as nurse practitioners and sought outlets in other areas of nursing. Some were chosen for and some drifted into the research activity. The job may have provided them with a new source of satisfaction.

The third period included a host of research practitioners for nursing, perhaps with a large variety of motivating conditions. The nursing leaders have made their presence felt, probably for the reasons already given. The supply of professional nurse researchers has grown as the demand for research services has increased. Nursing has made available for these people another channel through which drives left unsatisfied by nursing practice can be fulfilled. Lastly, the non-nurse professional researchers—the social scientist and the statistician—have made their contributions. Why?

Nursing, as we shall see, calls upon most of our primary sources of knowledge—the physical, the biologic, the social, the psychological and that of the humanities. Many definitions and interpretations of nursing (some broad and comprehensive, some narrow and largely technical) can be found in its literature. Assuming the comprehensive or broader concept of nursing for the purpose of our present discussion, we can see that its activities range from the very simple task of assisting a patient with his personal hygiene to the complex problem of establishing a therapeutic environment for the mentally ill. The following 21 nursing problems identified by Abdellah *et al.* are illustrative of this diversity in practice:[38]

1. To maintain good hygiene and physical comfort.
2. To promote optimal activity: exercise, rest, and sleep.
3. To promote safety through the prevention of accident, injury, or other trauma and through the prevention of the spread of infection.
4. To maintain good body mechanics and prevent and correct deformities.
5. To facilitate the maintenance of a supply of oxygen to all body cells.
6. To facilitate the maintenance of nutrition of all body cells.
7. To facilitate the maintenance of elimination.
8. To facilitate the maintenance of fluid and electrolyte balance.
9. To recognize the physiological responses of the body to disease conditions—pathological, physiological, and compensatory.
10. To facilitate the maintenance of regulatory mechanisms and functions.
11. To facilitate the maintenance of sensory function.
12. To identify and accept positive and negative expressions, feelings, and reactions.
13. To identify and accept the interrelatedness of emotions and organic illness.
14. To facilitate the maintenance of effective verbal and nonverbal communications.
15. To promote the development of productive interpersonal relationships.
16. To facilitate progress toward achievement of personal spiritual goals.

17. To create and/or maintain a therapeutic environment.

18. To facilitate awareness of self as an individual with varying physical, emotional, and developmental needs.

19. To accept the optimum possible goals in the light of limitations, physical and emotional.

20. To use community resources as an aid in resolving problems arising from illness.

21. To understand the role of social problems as influencing factors in the cause of illness.

The many-sided characteristics of nursing practice were inviting to a number of non-nurse researchers—especially to the social scientist. As a matter of fact, frequent references have suggested that much of the nursing research since 1950 has been conducted by these non-nurses. For example, a preliminary report of research sponsored by the American Nurses Foundation listed 17 professional nurses as project directors, codirectors or full-time research assistants, and 24 non-nurses (primarily social scientists) as project directors and codirectors.[39] To the social scientists whose subjects generally are the person in the school, the hospital or the community, nursing offered a unique laboratory. It was alive and could be semicontrolled; it presented a variety of experiences.

Although the studies in nursing performed by non-nurses were supported on the contention that they enhanced nursing practice (no doubt they did), these researchers were not as interested in nursing as they were in their major fields of endeavor. They primarily sought to contribute to their own pools of knowledge. And they also may have desired to do a job, to write a dissertation, to publish a paper. The enhancement of nursing practice may have resulted as a by-product. These feelings are summarized in a statement made by a social scientist in a discussion of this matter:

. . . basically we came to nursing research with an interest in some aspect of a problem which was not basically nursing, but . . . the nursing field did offer us a way of advancing our knowledge in this other field. . . . I would guess that non-nurses doing this research would have to approach it from a methodological interest, in which case the nursing area furnishes a vehicle for carrying out this more basic interest.[40]

An inescapable fact is that what has led many social scientists into nursing research is the available funds which have been set aside specifically in this area. A new set of relationships is developed, akin to the physician-patient relationship. The social scientist is more concerned in his role as practitioner and interpreter of certain "diseases" to his client, the nursing profession.[41]

SHOULD THERE BE A GENERAL PURPOSE FOR RESEARCH IN NURSING?

Since nursing is so diverse in practice, in the people practicing it, and in its research endeavors, should its research objectives be governed by a single underlying purpose? Since many private motivations prevail among the research contributors, can a single underlying purpose for research in nursing be developed?

The question or questions may pertain to the issue of whether nursing itself constitutes a special area for research or whether it is merely a vehicle through which other areas are served. That is, does nursing serve merely as the laboratory through which the principles of the related social and physical sciences are developed and tested? Or does nursing require special consideration for its own sake? Does it contain a resource of knowledge that is characteristically unique to the problems of nursing practitioners?

If nursing is merely a vehicle through which the research requirements of other technical groups are satisfied, it may not require a general purpose. The non-nurse researcher can be guided by the purpose of the society that is sponsoring his work. He makes his contribution to his own source of knowledge. Under these circumstances, nursing may be said to contribute to several sources of knowledge.

However, if this were the case, would not chaos result? Is it not possible that some of the cross-purposes would conflict with one another and perhaps with nursing practice itself? It was suggested, for example, that the nurse is educated to serve the patient now, utilizing the most appropriate knowledge available; the non-nurse, on the other hand, need not be concerned with this problem—he can withhold judgment or action until his hypothesis has been verified.[42] When the researcher requests the nurse to withhold certain nursing measures to attain long-term goals and to establish controls, an irreconcilable conflict may ensue.

Would it be possible to establish a single frame of reference for nursing research? Whose source of knowledge would be characterized? Who would undertake the development of such a framework? And, lacking this frame of reference or references, is nursing research destined to go on indefinitely without direction and without the capacity to interrelate the various contributions some day?

And what of the nurse researcher? To what does she contribute? Why are nurse researchers needed? Has this slowly evolving body been developing without a purpose? Should the so-called nurse researcher have been trained, instead, to practice in nursing research but to contribute to the parent science?

It is obvious that there are many answers to these questions. Underlying each, however, is the basic issue of whether or not nursing itself really should engage in research. The authors will seek to develop this issue and, in the course of the pursuit, to establish a point of view as to whether or not there should be an underlying purpose to research in nursing.

WHY SHOULD NURSING ENGAGE IN RESEARCH?

The previous discussion has emphasized the personal motivations of the researcher as some of the prime reasons for participating in nursing research. However, like "curiosity," these reasons may propel the individual rather than guide the group. They are, for nursing, the initiating causes—the reasons for getting started—rather than the final destination. In their attempt to derive the research needs of the profession, the authors therefore will consider the three other objectives:

1. To solve problems
2. To collect facts
3. To contribute to knowledge.

To Solve Problems

Is it the purpose of nursing research to solve problems? Almost every issue of the journals in nursing and related areas carry reports of studies that can be classified strictly as endeavors to solve problems. Here are some examples:

"The Hospital Is My Nursing Arts Laboratory."[43] The author considered the problem of finding the most appropriate setting in which to help students learn patient care. She described her experience at a school in which students were instructed only at the bedside. The procedure was detailed and the benefits derived were listed. She concluded that this was a worthy experience.

"A VNA Combats Staph Infection."[44] The authors described the manner in which their personnel and facilities were to deal with the problem of posthospitalization staph infections.

"Patients, Personnel and Therapy."[45] The author discussed the problem of upgrading the practice of patient care personnel. She described the effects of an in-service education program planned by her hospital in a small nursing unit.

These studies report the individual experiences of the various contributors. It is quite probable that many of the papers were not conceived initially as research problems, but were written up and circulated as afterthoughts. They may lack the attributes of knowledge derived through research, yet they may be received as the products of research. What actual purpose do they serve?

In reality, the results of these proposals may have satisfied the individual requirements of the contributors. However, would they be satisfactory again under different circumstances, in different situations, and for different people? They probably would not, because it was not the original purpose of the studies to be so. They were contrived around the specific problems encountered and in regard to the specific circumstances, situations and people involved.

It is quite possible that the projects could have been inaugurated with the same specific problems in mind, but planned and conducted in a manner more characteristic of research. This is what the proponents of "action research" would propose. The nursing profession, like the teaching profession, could recommend that their practitioners be trained to conduct studies of the specific action-research type. This type of activity would lend more credence to their problem-solving endeavors.

But is this to be the general purpose of nursing research? What end would these studies serve? The comments already made regarding action research are pertinent here. Studies of this type may yield few elements that can be transferred outside the circumstances in which they were developed. How many of the vast numbers of teaching practitioners actually practice action research also is questionable.

To Collect Facts

The nursing profession collects many facts. Most of the large nursing organizations periodically collect and publish facts. Many of these factual publications were mentioned in the first part of this chapter. In addition, almost every issue of the various nursing journals carries one or more articles that are concerned primarily with fact-collecting. We can judge the diversity of the fact-collecting activities from the titles of a sampling of these reports:

"Public Health Nursing Turnover"[46]
"The BLS Survey" (of salaries and working conditions of hospital nurses)[47]
"Mortality Among Former Student Nurses During the Last Decade"[48]
"The Patients' Reaction to Hospital Treatment"[49]
"A Study of the Professional Activities of the Faculty of the School of Nursing of Vanderbilt University, 1952-1953"[50]
"Staphylococcal Infections Among Hospital Personnel"[51]

What is the purpose of fact-collecting activities?

One of the authors formerly was responsible for co-ordinating the fact-collecting activities of a large nursing organization. This assignment had a long history, for the projects had been undertaken annually for many years. Since the various projects were quite time-consuming and expensive and involved numerous people, he inquired about their purpose: What end did these activities serve? Unfortunately, the person or persons who initiated the activities had passed from the scene long since. Others had some ideas, but not one actually could state a specific purpose. Like the snowball rolling down the hill, the projects simply had been started, had gathered momentum and had just continued to roll on.

The questionnaires that were employed to secure the necessary information tended to be lengthy. Since many of those surveyed did not care to respond to lengthy questionnaires, the author inquired the purpose of specific items. The response usually obtained was that the information "would be nice to have." And, more often than not, it was collected but not tabulated.

Of course, the examples cited are exceptional and are offered simply to illustrate that such conditions do exist. As we previously pointed out, fact-collecting has a purpose—to satisfy some other end—but it itself is not considered to be the ultimate objective of the research. Should this not be the case also with regard to nursing research?

To Contribute to Knowledge

The authors have expressed the point of view that the general purpose of research is to contribute to knowledge—specifically to formalized knowledge, derived and tested. Does nursing engage in research for this purpose? If so, what is nursing knowledge?

The task of describing nursing knowledge and setting its bounds is an arduous one. Nursing has many origins, not just one. Nursing is not a single practice but many practices. And nursing has not one, but many practitioners.

The Diverse Origins of Nursing. The noun nurse stems from the Latin *nutricia*, which implies care of or assistance for the infant or the very young child. It is implied further that this kind of nursing care is provided by a woman. The present concept of nursing was derived from the same origin—a mother caring for her babies, a woman caring for the infants or the older children of another person. While this concept of nursing has been formalized into such specializations as maternal and child care, it also exists today in its most primitive form in almost every home in the world.

There is a natural transition from the care of the very young to the care of the helpless or the infirm. As the infant and the older child require care or assistance, so do the ill, the poor, the invalids. With the rise of Christianity, with its emphasis upon service to our fellow men, organized societies for philanthropic purposes were formed. Religious nursing orders were developed to provide refuge for the travelers, the sick, the poor, the orphans. The hospitals of the Middle Ages were operated by these orders. They were assisted by the queen and her ladies of the court, wealthy widows who devoted their energies and time to the care of the sick.

The great wars of history that had such a devastating effect upon civilized society also served to implement the need for nursing. Wars created a large body of maimed victims who required care or assistance. Among the prime movers in this regard were the combined religio-military enterprises—the Crusades. This series of events, which covered an extensive period and involved long and hazardous journeys, established the need for hospitals and military nursing orders. The Hospitallers of St. John of Jerusalem were one such body, whose influence continued for over 500 years.[52] The impact of wars upon nursing in more recent times—the Crimean War, World Wars I and II— was such that new movements in the nursing profession followed each one of them, as the historical survey in Chapter 1 shows.

Lastly, the developments in the biologic sciences and in medical technology increased the requirements for nurses of a different type. Leeuwenhoek and his microscope, Pasteur and his germ theory of diseases, Koch and his development of modern laboratory methods, Lister and his developments in antiseptic and aseptic surgery, Simpson and Morton and their discoveries of chloroform and ether; and Holmes and Semmelweis and their emphasis on the communicability of puerperal fever laid the essential foundation stones for the development of modern medicine and surgery. In addition, each fostered the need for an assistant to the physician or the surgeon—someone skilled to care for the patient in the hospital, to administer complex medications and treatments and to assist in surgery.

The Many-Sided Practice of Nursing. Because of its diverse origins and the different factors that influenced its inception, modern nursing embodies a multitude of practices. The term comprehensive nursing care, for example, suggests that the nurse provides assistance that will help to satisfy the patient's physical, emotional and social needs. The 21 problems listed on page 119 illustrate this.[53] Nursing today also is concerned with the care of the healthy as well as of the sick—preventive as well as remedial and custodial care. Thus, nurses are expected to give physical care to patients, reassure them, administer treatments provided by the physician, teach patients and their families the essentials of health, participate in activities for the prevention of disease and the promotion of health, supervise other workers in the task of giving nursing care to patients, and co-operate and co-ordinate their services with those of such other health workers as the dietitian and the physical therapist.

The Many Different Practitioners of Nursing. As the practice of nursing has increased in complexity, the number of nurse specialists has increased. The term nurse may mean different kinds of people. We speak of the nurse in the hospital, the home, the community, the clinic, the school, the industrial plant. Within the hospital, we speak of the nurses who offer only custodial care, or the nurses who offer technical care, who offer professional services such as administering treatment and teaching patients, who counsel patients, or who do not minister nursing care directly but supervise others who administer care. Within the hospital, we speak of the nurse who cares only for pediatric or obstetric or surgical or medical patients. We also speak of the nurse who gives direct care to patients, or who teaches other nurses, or who offers consultation to other nurses. Although each calls herself a nurse, it is highly unlikely that they can interchange positions in all instances.

We realize from the above discussion that there is not a single body of nursing knowledge, but many bodies. There may exist a core area that defines a basic set of practices exemplifying all levels and specialties of nursing. Perhaps this core area can be described by the so-called general nursing curriculum. It is in a state of constant transition, however, as the respective fields of medical and nursing practice advance. There also may exist several special areas of nursing that define the practices of the smaller and more limited group of specialists. These areas often are described by the advanced curricula. They are more apt to reflect the changing practices in nursing.

What Is the Form of Knowledge in Nursing?

If knowledge in nursing is derived from many sources, how is each source made accessible to the nurse? That is, in what form or forms is knowledge in nursing presented? The three forms discussed in the previous section—common-sense, expert and written knowledge—will be considered.

Common-Sense Knowledge in Nursing

There is a large body of informal, common-sense knowledge in nursing. This consists of the knowledge that the beginning student brings with her to the school of nursing. It is synthesized in her educational program with the more formalized body of the curriculum. The combined resource of the formal and the informal then may be reshaped by experience into that body which ultimately serves the nurse in her everyday work assignments.

Considering again the derivation of nursing as the provision of care for children or the ill or those who simply cannot care for themselves, then there are very few places in the world where some type of nursing care is not practiced. That is, most people are exposed to some type of nursing care; furthermore, most people may administer some type of nursing care. In the course of these experiences, people will build up a body of informal practices that will serve them with varying degrees of success. Those who become more adept in solving problems of this type are quite often the people who are ultimately drawn into the more formalized nursing practice. And they bring with them the knowledge that they have acquired.

The student is exposed to a wider body of organized knowledge at the school of nursing. The sources of knowledge are generally the natural and the social sciences, the humanities and the formalized bodies of medical and nursing procedures. Learning the formalized nursing arts or procedures often is accomplished through an apprenticeship—the student attempts to practice the formalized procedures in an actual patient-nurse situation. Clinical learning, in reality, embodies a mixture of the formal and the informal—when left to her own resources, the student often must employ her common-sense or rule-of-thumb procedures. Thus, much of nursing education consists of synthesizing for the student the knowledge that she brings to nursing with that which is acquired in the organized classes and in her experiences in clinical situations.

Some of the student's common-sense knowledge will not serve her; it may even impede her progress in acquiring more formalized knowledge. Williams and Williams, for example, studied the socialization process of nursing students for a period of 6 years.[54] They found that many of the prenursing life experiences, such as intimate care of the body, care of the opposite sex, and problems of disfigurement, death, and odors actually conflicted with formalized nursing. Sometimes the conflicts were quite traumatic.

With successive years of experience, the nurse may blend her resources of knowledge to the point where they become indistinguishable. For example, she will not awaken and bathe her patient at 7 o'clock in the morning even though this procedure is routine hospital practice. She will postpone his bath and take care of another patient. She will place the bedside table in a position that is accessible to the patient. She will protect the patient from burns when applying heat. There are indistinguishable bits of formal and informal knowledge in each of these examples. However, for the nurse in the ward it may be all common-sense knowledge, for it is immediately accessible.

Expert Knowledge in Nursing

The expert nurse consultant has been employed extensively for a long period of time. The national nursing organizations have offered consultive services to schools, hospitals, public health agencies and communities. A wide variety of knowledge has been contributed.

Some of the more important services provided by the nurse consultant are:

1. To serve various health institutions and agencies as a source of technical knowledge in a specialized field such as maternal-child health nursing and cardiovascular nursing

2. To introduce and interpret new technics and procedures

3. To evaluate existing programs of service and education, identify their strengths and weaknesses, and plan programs for improvement

4. To serve as a source of general nursing knowledge for groups developing facilities for the provision of a nursing service, e.g., planning hospital construction

5. To serve nurses as a source of technical knowledge other than that of nursing, e.g., assisting state nursing organizations to conduct a survey of their nursing resources.

The nurse consultant is usually a nurse, but she also may be a specialist in some other field serving nursing, such as a social scientist, an educator, a dietitian or a statistician. The nurse who becomes a consultant is a person who has acquired extensive knowledge and experience in general nursing practices, specialized nursing practices, new technics in nursing, or practices and technics developed in fields other than nursing but employed in nursing.

The person who has acquired the status of a consultant also may have acquired the voice of authority. Authoritative evidence may be said to consist of formalized knowledge synthesized by years of experience. It is a composite, therefore, of both common-sense and formalized sources of knowledge. Many of the contributions made by the early research practitioners really were authoritative references blending the two sources. Much of the present-day research also is sprinkled with and in part supported by the voice of authority.

Written Knowledge in Nursing

Two major sources provide the written knowledge for nursing: books and professional periodicals. They cover a wide variety of topics, some quite specifically and others only indirectly. They generally are used *in toto* by the school as being representative of a thorough coverage of a given subject related to nursing.

The books can be classified under two major headings: textbooks and reference books. Textbooks are among the most widely employed sources of written knowledge in a school of nursing. They may contain extensive knowledge of nursing practices, as does the *Textbook of the Principles and Practices of Nursing* by Harmer and Henderson,[55] or the adaptation of other sources of knowledge to nursing, as does *Psychology and the Nurse*.[56] The reference books used by nurses are not always designed specifically for nurses but are employed in part because they contain some materials pertinent to nursing. Many reference books representing the related fields of biology, chemistry, physiology, medicine and pharmacology are used widely.

The nursing periodicals were initiated at the beginning of this century. They were established primarily as the organs of the various nursing organizations. As such, the journals initially contained reports of the organization to its membership. Gradually, authoritative papers on various topics of interest to the profession were included: new technics and developments within nursing, statistical reports, a variety of articles related to problems in nursing.

Since the advent of the *American Journal of Nursing,* numerous other periodicals have been published. These include *Nursing Outlook,* the *Canadian Nurse, The Catholic Nurse, Nursing*

World, Nursing Mirror, and *Nursing Research,* which is devoted exclusively to articles of a research nature.

The kinds of knowledge offered by books and periodicals can be reclassified in the manner suggested earlier in this chapter: narrations and descriptions, prescriptions and directives, generalizations, and theoretic knowledge. Most of the written materials in nursing are cast in the form of descriptions or prescriptions; very few materials containing generalizations or theoretic knowledge have been developed.

The journals are replete with narratives and descriptions. They range from case studies descriptive of care provided for a single patient to the nurse function studies that cover nursing behavior observed in a variety of situations over a period of time. The following are some typical examples of narrations and descriptions:

"The Nurse's Thursday in a Psychiatric Ward."[57] The nurse's behavior was observed and recorded, according to a prearranged classification, in consecutive intervals of 1 minute during several Thursdays. The nurse's actions were classified under 4 categories: care of patients, personnel matters, management and personal activities.

"Varying Images of the Professional Nurse: A Case Study."[58] Detailed descriptions were presented of graduates from an educational program that was radically different from the traditional program in basic nursing education. The authors depicted the graduate as seen by the dean, the faculty and the graduating seniors.

"The Role of the Infirmary in a Therapeutic Camp for Boys."[59] The nurse's role in a camp infirmary is described. The case of "Butch" and his use of the infirmary is depicted in detail.

Master's-degree students have tended to concentrate on the case-study approach in fulfilling their requirements for a degree. Among their contributions are the following:

"Descriptive Analysis of the Nursing Care of a Psychiatric Patient"[60]
"Nursing Needs of 4 Hospitalized Psychiatric Patients Receiving Thorazine"[61]
"Analysis of the Nursing Care of One Surgical Patient"[62]
"Study of Nursing Care: Orthopedic Patient With Fracture and Patient with Cerebrovascular Accident"[63]

Prescriptions and directives that tell the nurse what to do to whom, and when to do it, also abound in the nursing literature. The various nursing procedure books detailing the particular procedures used in the nursing care of patients can be found in most hospitals. The nursing organizations have produced several manuals on special nursing procedures: the use of tests, in-service education, student counseling, the curriculum guides, etc.

Many articles in periodicals contain directives to the reader. In addition, the journals often may carry columns that cater regularly to this need. For example, the *American Journal of Nursing* prints a monthly column, entitled "Trading Post," that frequently outlines different nursing procedures.

Generalizations and theoretic knowledge appearing in the nursing literature have been developed primarily as contributions from the allied sciences: anatomy, physiology, physics, chemistry and psychology. The nursing texts and reference books may specify applications to nursing of the principles or the generalizations. Articles that attempt to establish generalizations and theoretic knowledge within the specific context of nursing itself rarely have appeared. Peplau perhaps has developed a close approximation to knowledge of this type. She has prepared a miniature system from which several generalizations might be derived.[64]

The gross disparity in the literature between the first two and the last two types of written knowledge is quite obvious. Most nurses or nurse researchers tend to concentrate upon descriptive or prescriptive studies. The argument has been voiced that this type of study fulfills the need of the nurse to produce "firm, concrete, and, . . . useful findings."[65] It is risk-free because one is bound to succeed. But, on the other hand, the need to strike a balance also has been emphasized. "To the extent that research might serve to help elevate the nursing profession in the eyes of other health professions by providing it with a truly scientific underpinning, explanatory and hypotheses-testing research is badly needed."[66]

How Is Knowledge in Nursing Employed?

Why is knowledge in nursing gathered? It was suggested previously that, by definition, knowledge serves any area in reaching solutions to problems. What type of problems are served by nursing knowledge—specific, common, underlying? Does nursing knowledge satisfy past, present or future problems?

The largest consumers of nursing knowledge are staff nurses. There are so many of them. They deal in specifics. They are concerned with the present. The staff nurse has to solve the many problems that occur daily during her tour of service. Her patients depend upon her to have answers readily accessible.

The staff nurse lives in a practical world. She is called a nurse practitioner. She employs rather than develops or creates knowledge. Theories and even generalizations may be of only tangential interest. To her, practical knowledge that is readily applicable and readily available is the thing. To her, the purpose of knowledge in nursing is to solve specific problems.

The staff nurse's primary and most useful source of supply is her own pool of common-sense knowledge. It is accessible at all times. It is most applicable to specific problems. Her employing agency, a hospital or a public health agency, may provide her with a set of working rules or directives that pertain to the common problems that recur frequently within the institution. These are a source of knowledge or a series of mandatory solutions to be used when the occasion arises.

The staff nurse also may review periodically the written sources of knowledge. Her purpose is to keep abreast of the more recent developments in nursing that may be applicable to problems to come. The various articles and manuals on "how to do it" are perhaps the most appealing, especially if they can be applied in her situation. The articles on specific problem-solving, the narratives, the case studies also may be appealing to the extent that the staff nurse can empathize with the author. However, she often may find that the solutions offered will not quite satisfy the requirements of her situation.

The nurse supervisor's requirements for knowledge may be somewhat different. She may develop or enforce the procedures to be followed by the staff nurse. She must be available to act as the expert or authority to her staff when they are confronted with a difficult problem. At the same time, she has specific problems of a different order: those pertaining to the supervision of staff employees, to the administration of a department.

The nurse supervisor may be more common-problem oriented. Therefore, she must be less practical than her staff practitioner. She must center her attention upon knowledge applicable to problems to come. As in the case of the staff nurse, her greatest source of supply may be her own common-sense knowledge. Since she may have a more extensive and wider variety of experiences, her source of common-sense knowledge is more complete. She may have been selected as a supervisor on this basis. The nursing literature provides another effective source of supply. In this regard, articles referring to common problems may be more appealing. A head nurse of a pediatric ward, for example, may express considerable interest in "Problems encountered in different methods of limiting the separation of children from their parents during hospitalization."[67]

The author of this paper studied the effect of limiting the separation of children from their parents during hospitalization by (1) providing longer and more frequent visiting hours and (2) having one parent reside in the hospital. The problems encountered and their solutions in four hospitals were reported. The problems related to the attitudes of professional personnel and parents. The author recognized the need for staff preparation and the ability to understand parental problems.

The nurse supervisor's formal preparation (if any) and experiences will combine to produce a pool of common-sense knowledge in the area of administration and supervision. This will serve as her prime source. Expert assistance from the materials written by other nurses and non-nurse supervisors and administrators also may be of considerable value to her. It is questionable that this source of knowledge can be considered to be an integral part of nursing knowledge per se.

It is the primary concern of nurse educators to prepare people for the future practice of nursing. They must search out from the various sources of knowledge that which will be most useful to the nurse of tomorrow, and organize and disseminate the knowledge obtained in a comprehensible manner. Two kinds of problems also confront them: problems concerned with nursing itself, and problems concerned with disseminating nursing knowledge and educating the nursing student. The latter, like the problems of supervision, may be satisfied from pools of knowledge that have been compiled in and outside nursing.

The nurse educator deals with future nursing problems, with common, and perhaps underlying, rather than specific problems. She develops nurses who must practice in the future. She must train people to care for a variety of patients in a variety of situations, to perform skilled procedures that many practicing nurses may never have learned.

The nurse educator is more apt to employ written than common-sense sources of knowledge. The former generally are made available in bulk at the educational institutions. The latter are being developed within the student. Common problems replete with generalizations, rather than prescriptions and directives, will become the focus of her teaching, as in the following: The problem is to establish objectives for a curriculum, a course or a class, which can serve as guides in the selection of learning experiences (content and activities) that will lead to the attainment of the objectives. How to state these objectives in terms that will be helpful and not mere verbalizations is a common problem for educators at all levels. Instruction derived from such examples as the above is preferred by the nurse educator because the source of knowledge is not situation-oriented as are prescriptions and directives. The student who acquires this kind of knowledge can broaden her scope of experience more easily to include the care of patients in situations other than the one in which she was trained.

How useful a generalization is to the student will depend upon its scope—the number of nursing situations to which it can be made applicable. Generalizations or knowledge derived from underlying problems have a universal application. Nursing has borrowed generously from sources of knowledge pertaining to underlying problems. This is particularly true of the physical sciences, specifically anatomy and physiology, which make up a considerable portion of the general nursing curriculum. Many nurses become quite knowledgeable in these areas. Recently there has been an attempt to introduce the social sciences into the nursing curriculum. This source of knowledge is not as well organized as that of anatomy and physiology, nor are the applications to nursing as apparent. The struggle of social scientists to improve this state of affairs can be reflected perhaps by the great influx of these people into nursing research.

There has been some question as to whether or not nursing itself deals in underlying problems, as to whether or not nursing has a unique source of underlying knowledge. In other words, is there a science of nursing? Some investigators would say "yes." Johnson, for example, has attempted to isolate and identify an area unique to nursing and universal in scope.[68] In this regard, she has limited her search not to the supervisory and the managerial functions of the nurse, not to the study of the patient to whom she gives care, but to the area of nursing care itself, ministering to the needs of patients. Her feeling is that nursing knowledge can be systematized and a science of nursing can be formulated by studying the unique contribution of nursing to a patient with a particular pattern of response to stress.

Nursing care, which is provided to individuals or groups under stress of health-illness nature, has as its primary purpose to relieve tension and discomfort to the end of restoring or maintaining internal and interpersonal equilibrium.

Internal and interpersonal equilibrium . . . does not imply a state of health or well-being. It is rather a state in which opposing forces —biological, psychological, or social—are balanced momentarily . . . it can be conceived as a resting state. . . . It is a dynamic state, however, for it is fluid and transitional. . . . Nursing; requires therapeutic as well as supportive measures to assist the patient to achieve this state.

This goal is achieved through activities such as bathing, feeding, explaining, reassuring, and the like, which tend to reduce tension and to offer comfort, gratification, and assistance in relation to basic human needs (biological and psychosocial).[69]

If we hold to a rather rigid definition of a science (as the authors have proposed) as an embodiment of knowledge unique in function and universally applicable, then it is questionable that proposals such as the above constitute a science. Is the kind of knowledge described above unique to nursing? Is the kind of knowledge that is sought to be derived from and applied only to nursing problems?

Instead, this proposal appears to be an attempt to synthesize contributions from various sciences into a body of knowledge directed by a goal of nursing. The author herself suggests: "The major difference between the health professions does not appear to be sources of their bodies of knowledge, but their selection of concepts from those sources as pertinent to their respective specific social goals."[70]

The term science is construed here as the organization and the classification of knowledge rather than as a body of solutions to underlying problems. Does nursing have underlying problems that are unique unto itself? Or does it have a body of common problems to which the principles and the generalizations from the underlying sources can be applied?

The smallest consumers of nursing knowledge are the nurse researchers. There are very few of them. They deal in generalities. They are concerned with the future. The function of the nurse researcher is to solve the many problems that will occur tomorrow, 5, 10 and 15 years hence. The future staff nurse, the patients, the nurse supervisor, the administrator and the educator will depend upon her to have answers readily accessible.

The nurse researcher lives in a hypothetic world. Commonsense, practical knowledge related to the specific problems of caring for patients daily may be of only peripheral interest to her. She must take cognizance of the staff nurses' problems and seek, develop or create solutions that are useful to the greatest number. She provides theories and generalizations that may not be readily applicable or readily available. To her, the purpose of knowledge in nursing is to solve the common problems of the widest possible body of nurses and, perhaps, the underlying problems for which appropriate generalizations can be derived.

One of the nurse researcher's most useful sources of supply is the written material in and outside nursing. To isolate the many common problems that confront nursing, she may search through the various factual sources that are presented periodically. After she has gained some idea of the nature of the situations confronting her, she may search through the various descriptive and narrative reports of specific problem-solving in nursing and allied areas to develop appropriate solutions; she may examine the generalizations derived from the underlying sources of knowledge. To synthesize these solutions into an appropriate framework from which to derive additional knowledge, she may adopt the models suggested by Peplau,[64] Johnson,[70] or Kreuter and Kakosh.[71]

The written sources of knowledge may assist the researcher to isolate appropriate responses and to develop others. The ability to select from the appropriate source, to derive, apply and synthesize, and to create unique solutions is contained within the researcher herself. In this regard, she must rely upon her own comprehension of the nursing field and the related sciences. She also must be able to envision that which has yet to be derived. This is a unique characteristic, a unique source of knowledge that only researchers may have.

Since the nurse researcher cannot synthesize all knowledge, she may ally herself with the expert researchers from other fields: the physiologist, the social scientist, the engineer. Together they may pool their individual resources and bring to bear upon a problem the most extensive source of knowledge gained to date. This is a major contribution of interdisciplinary research.

How Is Knowledge in Nursing Obtained?

How trustworthy is the knowledge employed by the staff nurse, the nurse administrator, the educator, the researcher? The usefulness of the knowledge is limited to the extent to which it is the correct answer, to which it produces results: the staff nurse is able to aid the patient, the administrator is able to assist the staff nurse to aid the patient, the nurse educator can assist the student ultimately to aid the patient. This quality of nursing knowledge can be evaluated by examining the manner by which it is obtained.

Much of the so-called common-sense knowledge employed by the staff nurse is a curious blend of knowledge obtained by reasoning and trial-and-error experiences. Consider the following examples:

In accordance with a physiologic principle, it is necessary to balance the intake and the output of fluids to maintain the electrolyte balance in patients. The nurse knows that the electrolyte balance may be maintained by intravenous feedings. However, she may reason that it is more desirable to have the patient take the fluid orally, because this is the natural way of taking fluids into the body; it is pleasanter and more comfortable.

If the patient does not have any appetite or feels apathetic, the task of feeding him orally may be difficult. Therefore, the nurse may try different approaches before she obtains the patient's co-operation. In the course of her trial-and-error experiences, she may learn to enlist the support and the aid of one of the close members of his family to discover the patient's likes and dislikes, to supply the patient with special treats.

The nurse has learned that she can assist the restless patient to sleep by administering a hypodermic. However, she also knows that frequent use of a hypodermic may lead to a dependence on the drug and to narcotic addiction. Therefore, she may try a variety of measures until she finds the one that will help the individual patient to relax and fall asleep. She may give him an alcohol rub, a warm drink, emotional support, or adjust his bed.

The nurse who cares for a patient with empyema knows that anemia, malnutrition and avitaminosis commonly accompany the disorder. She recognizes, therefore, that the patient requires assistance to maintain a satisfactory state of nutrition. A high protein diet usually is ordered but frequently is rejected by the patient because of the "bad taste." The amount that the patient does eat often is dependent upon the nurse's actions. She may give small portions supplemented by in-between-meal feedings; she may try to arrange his tray in a more attractive manner. One patient who had been a poor eater became interested in his food when a certain spice was added to which he had been accustomed at home.

In each of the examples, the staff nurse had learned that certain knowledge, such as the need to maintain an electrolyte balance, is applicable to all patients without restriction. She also reasoned that some forms of knowledge will not be applicable in all instances. There was a need to create or adapt knowledge to the exceptional cases. In these instances, she obtained the appropriate solution by trying different things. The one that worked perhaps was regarded as the most trustworthy.

But is it really the most trustworthy, and will it work again? If the nurse does not understand why the solution offered was applicable, why it was relevant to the particular series of events, she may find that her source of derived knowledge is untrustworthy—it will not work again. The nurse may tell one patient that he has cancer and obtain a response of acceptance; she may relate the same information in exactly the same way to another and he will reject the fact. Knowledge obtained through sheer trial-and-error experiences may offer the nurse clues to further understanding but, without complete understanding, it may be useless, even disastrous.

The knowledge provided by authority figures in nursing— the nurse administrator, the educator, the expert consultant— is relied upon heavily. They deal with the common problems that span the field of nursing. They delve into the newer, untapped and, as yet, unexperienced activities.

The authority figures may deal in everyday problems. Typical of this are the functions, the standards and the qualifications of various aspects of nursing practice as set forth and amended periodically by a panel of experts.[72] Curriculum guides are other examples. These generally are based upon existing practices. The authority figures, particularly the nurse educators, also adopt newer practices, newer procedures. Abdellah *et al.*, for example, attempted to describe patient-centered approaches to curriculum development.[73] The experts may evolve a plan or a framework by which they can seek to understand current practices in nursing, and derive new practices, if possible. This was the approach of Kreuter and Kakosh,[71] Peplau[74] and Johnson.[75] Their purpose was to assist nurses to understand the nature of nursing practice.

How trustworthy is this source of knowledge? Consider the manner by which it is obtained. The hierarchic order of authority figures in nursing stems from the supervisor to the educator to the expert consultant. So, as the nurse ascends the order, she becomes further removed from practice. Therefore, as she ascends the order, her source of knowledge becomes less accessible to actual trial-and-error experiences. She may be required to develop solutions from past experiences or to construct future experiences as imagined and tested only by mental trial-and-error. In other words, she may reason the event.

How reliable are the functions, the standards and the qualifications specified by the American Nurses Association?[76] The curriculm guides? They were derived from a pool of past and current experiences of a panel of experts who have had many such experiences. They contain some factual information; they also contain material from opinionated authors. Will they work? They may look reasonably reliable, but no one ever has constructed an adequate test of their reliability.

How reliable are the conceptualizations of nursing practice? Each treatise represented a picture of nursing as it had been conceived and developed by the internal machinations of the authors. Some received additional assistance. Peplau, for example, drew heavily upon the works of Harry Stack Sullivan, which also represented the products of reasoning. Kreuter and Kakosh made extensive observations, but none of the models ever has been reconstructed in an actual setting and tested. None of the models has been subjected to a trial-and-error experience.

Theoretically, nurses should have considerable confidence in knowledge derived from research. We should expect the nurse researcher to develop her contribution through a process of reasoning and to subject her findings to the rigors of empiric testing. Unfortunately, we have learned that this generally has not been the case. For the most part, studies have evolved through a process of trial and error. Several examples have been cited in which the researcher simply has described a state of affairs. On the other hand, there have been a few instances, such as those discussed above, which have their roots in logical deduction. However, the authors have not been able to estab-lish concrete testing situations.

Perhaps this situation is a result of the current stage of de-velopment of nursing research. In the haste to produce results, the so-called empiric studies have abounded. The theorists have not had the opportunity, as yet, to complete the cycle. How-ever, the more complete contribution is beginning to emerge. The following are illustrations of studies that are moving in this direction:

The Nurse-Patient Relationship and The Healing Process.[77] The rationale of this study is based upon the "healing process" concept and its role in the development of nurse-patient relationships. The healing process is described as a complex involving the physiologic, the psychological and the sociologic functioning of human beings. It involves physical and chemical agents, the use of "people-self" and others in effecting various levels of human functioning. In gen-eral, the nurse has three broad areas of influence upon the healing process: she is involved in creating the environment or the milieu in which healing takes place; she manipulates physical agents used in the healing process; and she uses herself in relation to the patient as a psychological agent in the promotion of healing.

To date, the author of this report has been concerned with the development of an instrument that can be used in evaluating per-ceptions of the interpersonal relationship. Other studies have been planned to validate the instrument further and to test nurse-patient relationships in other settings.

Limit-Setting: An Aspect of the Therapeutic Nurse-Patient Rela-tionship With a Schizophrenic Patient.[78] Limit-setting was tested in this study as one aspect of the nurse-patient relationship to reduce anxiety in the schizophrenic patient. Limits were placed, beyond which the nurse's intervening in "out-of-control" behavior enabled the patient to re-establish himself on a more acceptable level. Concepts of limit-setting and some generalizations about it were presented for further study.

The Nurse: A Study in Social Perceptions.[79] This was a study of the role perception of nurses in relation to their perception of self and the institutional process affecting the nurse's role. It includes a quantitative assessment of self-image and role perception of "future" nurses, nursing students and graduate nurses, based upon Murray's conceptualization of needs.

The findings suggest the existence of significant areas in the needs-structure of nurses that differentiate them from a non-nurse control group. Areas of conformity and divergence are revealed.

The examples presented above have several features in common. Each was based upon empiric data and was cast in conceptual form through a process of reasoning. Each has suggested a series of relationships or generalizations that are to be or could be subjected to further empiric test. Therefore, they may be described as exploratory studies. The authors have just begun their quest for additional knowledge. In reality, they differ only in degree from the studies of Johnson,[80] Kreuter and Kakosh,[81] and Peplau.[82] Perhaps they have carried their assignments one step further.

The knowledge obtained is not wholly reliable. And years may transpire before it can be made more trustworthy. Furthermore, it is highly doubtful that the average staff nurse can comprehend the derived generalizations and translate them into action. They are written in the abstract language of the researcher, who must deal in generalities and abstractions. It will become incumbent upon the researchers to translate their findings into the more concrete terms of the applied situations and to test them accordingly. It will be the task of the staff nurse to relate the results to her specific problem. Considerable time and effort may be expended throughout the entire process. This is the price that nursing must pay to obtain knowledge through the medium of research.

THE PURPOSE OF RESEARCH IN NURSING—A SUMMARY

The authors have considered the point of view that nursing should engage in research to contribute to nursing knowledge. Two general questions were discussed:

1. What does nursing knowledge consist of?
2. How will research contribute to nursing knowledge?

Nursing knowledge is the embodiment of many resources of knowledge. These include the basic or the scientific and the applied. Nursing knowledge is concerned specifically with the application of the resources of knowledge to an understanding of nursing problems. Therefore, it is an applied body of knowledge.

Most of the problems arising in nursing are specific to the job, to the person, to the situation. These are operational problems. They concern the person on the job—essentially the staff nurse and, in some respects, the nurse administrator and the faculty member. The nurse researcher may contribute generalizations that perhaps are applicable to some of these problems. It is the task of the practitioner to determine whether or not the research findings are applicable. It is not the task of the researcher to solve the specific problems.

The practitioner may learn better problem-solving technics. This is a valuable tool under any circumstance. But does she also become a researcher? Does she have the ability? Does she have the time? Does she have the inclination?

The major task of the nurse administrator, educator, consultant or researcher is common-problem-solving. They must provide solutions that apply to a variety of jobs, persons and situations. In general, the nurse administrator, educator and consultant do not have the time or the capacity to apply the full treatment to problem-solving that is suggested by the research process. Therefore, they may employ their previous experiences, their accumulated knowledge, and/or their ability to reason in their problem-solving endeavors.

The nurse researcher should be able to develop and test generalizations applicable to common problems in nursing. Her major problem has been the inability to conceptualize and develop suitable hypotheses that can be subjected to empiric testing. Perhaps she has concentrated unduly upon descriptions of the ongoing job.

When the nurse researcher undertakes an underlying problem, she deals essentially with one or more of the sciences. The nursing situation serves as a point of departure, suggestive of the more underlying problem, and as an area in which the derived solution can be tested. The major problem of the nurse researcher in this regard has been her inability to move from the level of conceptualization to the level of reality. She has not been able to provide suitable situations to test the derived solutions.

REFERENCES

1. Hodgkinson, H. L.: Action research—a critique, J. Educational Sociology *31*:137-153, 1957.
2. Furfey, Paul: The Scope and Method of Sociology, p. 53, New Pork, Harper, 1953.
3. Hodgkinson, H. L.: *Op. cit.* (see Ref. 1), p. 143.
4. Shumsky, Abraham: The Action Research Way of Learning, p. 100, New York, Bureau of Publications, Teachers College, Columbia Univ., 1958.
5. U. S. Bureau of the Census: Seventeenth Census of the United States, 1950 Population, II.
6. U. S. Bureau of the Census: Labor Force, series 1959.
7. U. S. Public Health Service, Department of Health, Education and Welfare: Vital Statistics of the United States, 1959.
8. U. S. Education Office, Department of Health, Education and Welfare: Biennial Survey of Education in the United States, 1954-56.
9. U. S. Bureau of Labor, Bureau of Labor Statistics: Publishes studies on various aspects of labor annually.
10. U. S. Weather Bureau: Climactography of United States, 60, Climates of the States, Item 273-B.
11. Hardy, E. P., Jr., and Klein, S. S.: U. S. Atomic Energy Commission: Strontium Program Quarterly Summary Report, Nov. 19, 1958.
12. District of Columbia, Society of Professional Engineers, Yearbook, 1959. (Published annually)

13. American Medical Directory, Chicago, American Medical Association. (Published yearly)
14. Listing of hospitals, Hospitals *33*:15, August 1, 1959 (Part II).
15. Education for professional nursing—1958, prepared by Division of Nursing Education, National League for Nursing, Nurs. Outlook 7:448, 1959.
16. Teacher Supply and Demand in Universities, Colleges, and Junior Colleges, 1957-58 and 1958-59, Research Division, National Education Assn. of the United States, Washington, D. C., June, 1959.
17. Beers, C. W.: The Mind That Found Itself, Garden City, New York, Doubleday, 1935.
18. Cronbach, L. J., et al.: Text Materials in Modern Education, p. 29, Urbana, Univ. Illinois Press, 1955.
19. Nagel, Ernest: The Structure of Science, p. 1, New York, Harcourt, 1961.
20. Clegg, Hugh: Pasteur and the problems presented by bacteria *in* A Short History of Science, pp. 86-93, New York, Doubleday, 1959.
21. Nagel, Ernest: *Op. cit.* (see Ref. 19), pp. 1-14.
22. *Ibid.*, p. 6.
23. *Ibid.*, p. 12.
24. Geidt, W. R.: Clues to control of hospital infections, Mod. Hosp. *90*:88, 1958.
25. Cronbach, L. J., et al.: *Op. cit.* (see Ref. 18).
26. *Ibid.*, p. 32.
27. *Ibid.*, pp. 45-47.
28. Greenwood, E.: Social science and social work: a theory of their relationship, Social Service Rev. *29*:21, 1955.
29. Van Laer, H., and Koren, H. G.: Philosophy of Science, Part I, Science in General, pp. 46-47, Pittsburgh, Duquesne Univ. 1956.
30. Durant, Will: The Story of Philosophy, p. 3, New York, Simon & Schuster, Inc., 1926.
31. Brennan, R. E.: Thomistic Psychology, p. 52, New York, Macmillan, 1941.
32. Maritain, Jacques: Introduction to Philosophy, pp. 133-135, New York, Sheed and Ward, 1937.
33. Parsons, Talcott: The Structure of Social Action, p. 21, New York, McGraw-Hill, 1937.
34. Whitehead, A. N.: Science and the Modern World, pp. 3-4, New York, Macmillan, 1925.
35. Parsons, Talcott: *Op. cit.* (see Ref. 33), pp. 21-24.
36. Maritain, Jacques: *Op. cit.* (see Ref. 32), p. 122.
37. Whitehead, A. N.: *Op. cit.* (see Ref. 34), p. 18.

38. Abdellah, F. G., Martin, A., Beland, I. L., and Matheney, R. J.: Patient-Centered Approaches to Nursing, pp. 16-17, New York, Macmillan, 1960.
39. Nurses Invest in Patient Care, Preliminary Report on a 5-Year Program of Studies of Nursing Functions, New York, American Nurses Assn., 1956.
40. Nursing Research Conference, p. 8, Kansas City, Mo., Community Studies, Inc., 1957.
41. *Ibid.*, p. 8.
42. Hochbaum, G. M.: The nurse in research, Nurs. Outlook *8*:193, 1960.
43. Sullivan, Clare: The hospital is my nursing arts laboratory, Nurs. Outlook 7:521, 1959.
44. Pratt, M. K., *et al.*: A VNA combats staph infection, Nurs. Outlook *8*:310, 1960.
45. Walker, Virginia: Patients, personnel and therapy, Nurs. Outlook *8*:136, 1960.
46. Johnson, W. L.: Public health nursing turnover, Amer. J. Nurs. *57*:464, 1957.
47. Leopold, A. K., and Clague, E.: The BLS Survey, Amer. J. Nurs. *58*:1260, 1958.
48. Theodore, A., Berger, A. G., and Palmer, C. E.: Mortality among former student nurses during the last decade, Public Health Rep. *71*:914, 1956.
49. Calden, G.: The patients' reaction to hospital treatment, Public Health Rep. *71*:915, 1956.
50. A Study of the Professional Activities of the Faculty of the School of Nursing of Vanderbilt University 1952-1953, Final Report to the Tennessee State Nurses Assn., Nashville, 1955.
51. Taylor, C. H.: Staphylococcal infections among hospital personnel, Amer. J. Nurs. *58*:822, 1958.
52. Nutting, M. A., and Dock, L. L.: History of Nursing, Vol. I., New York, Putnam, 1907.
53. Abdellah, F., *et al.*: *Op. cit.* (see Ref. 38).
54. Williams, T. R., and Williams, M. M.: The socialization of the student nurse, Nurs. Res. *8*:18, 1957.
55. Harmer, Bertha, and Henderson, Virginia: Textbook of the Principles and Practices of Nursing (rev.), New York, Macmillan, 1955.
56. O'Hara, F. J.: Psychology and the Nurse, Philadelphia, Saunders, 1954.
57. Stevens, P. B., and Halpert, P. W.: The nurse's Thursday in a psychiatric ward, Nurs. Res. *6*:29, 1957.

58. MacAndrew, C., and Elliott, J. E.: Varying images of the professional nurse: a case study, Nurs. Res. *8*:33, 1959.
59. Godbout, R. A., and Hurvitz, I.: The role of the infirmary in a therapeutic camp for boys, Nurs. Res. *9*:23, 1960.
60. Sullivan, Sister M. Felicitas: Descriptive Analysis of the Nursing Care of a Psychiatric Patient, Master's Dissertation, Catholic Univ. America, Washington, D. C., 1956. (Unpublished)
61. Baer, Barbara: Nursing Needs of 4 Hospitalized Psychiatric Patients Receiving Thorazine, Master's Dissertation, Catholic Univ. America, Washington, D. C. (Unpublished)
62. Lee, Eugenia: Analysis of the Nursing Care of One Surgical Patient, Master's Dissertation, Univ. Texas, 1956; Abstract in Nurs. Res. *5*:130, 1957.
63. Guenther, Maria: Study of Nursing Care: Orthopedic Patient With Fracture and Patient With Cerebrovascular Accident, Master's Dissertation, Univ. Minnesota, 1955. (Unpublished)
64. Peplau, H. E.: Interpersonal Relations in Nursing, New York, Putnam, 1952.
65. Hochbaum, G.: *Op. cit.* (see Ref. 42), p. 193.
66. *Ibid.,* p. 194.
67. Dalzell, Irene: Problems Encountered in Different Methods of Limiting the Separation of Children From Their Parents During Hospitalization, Ed. D. Dissertation, New York, Teachers College, Columbia Univ., 1958; Abstract in Nurs. Res. *9*:97, 1960.
68. Johnson, Dorothy: The nature of a science of nursing, Nurs. Outlook 7:292, 1959.
69. *Ibid.,* p. 292.
70. *Ibid.,* p. 294.
71. Kreuter, Frances, and Kakosh, Marguerite: Quality of Nursing Care: A Report of A Field Study to Establish Criteria, New York, Teachers College, Columbia Univ., 1954. (Unpublished)
72. Past, Present and Future of FS&Q, A Guide for the Interpretation and Implementation of the Statements of Functions, Standards, and Qualifications for Practice, American Nurses Assn., 1957.
73. Abdellah, F., *et al.*: *Op. cit.* (see Ref. 38).
74. Peplau, H.: *Op. cit.* (see Ref. 64).
75. Johnson, Dorothy: *Op. cit.* (see Ref. 68).
76. Past, Present and Future of FS&Q: *Op. cit.* (see Ref. 72).
77. Whiting, F. J.: The Nurse-Patient Relationship and the Healing Process, Report to The American Nurses Association, Distributed by Veterans Administration Hosp., Pittsburgh, Pa., 1958.

78. Kachelske, Audrey: Limit-Setting: An Aspect of the Therapeutic Nurse-Patient Relationship With a Schizophrenic Patient, Paper Read at the National League for Nursing Convention, Miami Beach, 1959.
79. Mauksch, H. O.: The Nurse: A Study in Social Perceptions, Ph.D. Dissertation, Univ. Chicago, 1958.
80. Johnson, Dorothy: *Op. cit.* (see Ref. 68).
81. Kreuter, F., and Kakosh, M.: *Op. cit.* (see Ref. 71).
82. Peplau, H.: *Op. cit.* (see Ref. 64).

CHAPTER 3

The Climate and the Specific Purposes
of Research

It has been stated that the general purpose of research is to make a contribution to knowledge. However, these contributions do not appear suddenly or by chance. Usually they evolve through gradual stages of development. For example, we may note the different characteristics of knowledge appearing throughout each of the sciences: some of the reports are purely descriptive of a low order of concrete observations—the narrative; others are developed in highly abstract form to explain a wide variety of events—the generalization; some of the conclusions are offered as probable under certain circumstances; others are stated with the assurance of a law.

Some of the older sciences contain a large body of more fully developed knowledge. Researchers in these fields, therefore, may initiate their questioning at a more advanced stage. They can stand upon the shoulders of their predecessors. The newer and less tangible sciences are even labeled unscientific, at times. Nevertheless, any order of knowledge must begin somewhere, perhaps with the so-called unscientific.

A single contribution to knowledge, regardless of its character, does not constitute the be-all and the end-all. Usually it was derived from, and will in turn suggest, other knowledge. Items contained within a body of knowledge thus perform specific functions relative to other items within that body—one begets the other, one explains the other. It will be conceived here that knowledge is developed in sequential steps or stages, one unfolding into the other, each having special functions. If each step could be identified and its function recorded, more specific directions could be offered to the individual research worker. The research project then may be characterized by a specific aim or purpose specifying its function or contribution to the over-all body of knowledge.

Let us refer again to the trip analogy or the journey of research to identify the specific purpose of research. The general purpose was described as the final destination. The specific purposes may be conceived now as the interim stops along the way. These are the points through which the researcher must pass before he can attain his final destination. They usually are in sequential order. However, the traveler may plan a devious route that will circumvent some of these stops. He probably will soon recognize, nevertheless, that there are no shortcuts to knowledge and be forced to circle back to the original pathway.

Bearing these statements in mind, the authors will consider first the initiating cause or the reason for making the trip, and derive from this the specific purpose leading to the final destination. In this regard, three questions will be considered:

1. How do research projects get started?
2. What are the specific purposes of research?
3. How can the specific purpose of a research project be derived?

HOW DO RESEARCH PROJECTS GET STARTED?

A botanist studies the mating behavior of the tropical fruit fly. A virologist investigates the action of the colon bacilli upon the digestive organs of the monkey. A team of research chemists is concerned with the development of by-products from coal tar. A market research analyst prepares tables describing trends in the sales of railroad stocks. A psychologist constructs a battery of tests for the selection of insurance salesmen. A graduate student in nursing education conducts a study of the effects of instructor-staff nurse interaction upon student learning.

How did these projects get started? Was each motivated in the same way? Do they have the same underlying goal or purpose: to make a contribution to knowledge?

It is highly probable that these projects were not initiated in the same way. The botanist studying the fruit fly may have been moved by sheer intellectual curiosity. The virologist may have been on the threshold of an important breakthrough in this particular area of knowledge. The industrial projects could have emanated from someone or something other than the research workers themselves: a consumer demand, an executive order, expediency. The graduate student simply may have been trying to satisfy a requirement of her program.

Motives for engaging in research vary. Many industrial research projects, for example, originate from stimuli independent of the research worker or team. The demand of the society in which the researcher operates or is employed may have been the initiating force. However, many other projects may be the direct creation of individual researchers.

Motivating conditions also vary. Some, such as curiosity and the need to satisfy a requirement for a degree, frequently are extrinsic to the basic intent of research. These prevail upon the research worker to engage in his project. They do not seek a direct contribution to knowledge. The others may be fostered by a problem or a problem area of some type: How can the waste products of coal tar be employed? Should one invest in railroad stocks? How can insurance salesmen be selected? Knowledge is required to answer these "felt difficulties."

Thus, there are both extrinsic and intrinsic reasons for acquiring a program of research. Neither category is to be minimized, since each contributes to the launching forces. However, the discussion that follows will dwell upon the thought proposed by the previous chapter: the idea of moving toward a contribution to knowledge. It will be considered that research is started as an endeavor to fill the voids in an area of knowledge. The need for research signifies the need for knowledge.

The presence of a problem often is indicative of a gap in an area of knowledge. However, the character of this initiating problem may be quite distinct. The problem may be broad, narrow, specific, common or underlying. Since it must propel an inquiry, the problem generally will be a broad rather than a narrow one, a common or underlying problem rather than a specific one. Also, it will have been recognized by a society (usually a professional society) as a problem.

To avoid confusion, we might classify the so-called problem at this point as a general problem area. The intent of the researcher merely is to set the stage for an inquiry. It is *not* his purpose to state the exact problem. That comes later, since it is part of the actual problem-solving procedure. The distinguishing feature between research and general problem-solving is the intent of the researcher to contribute to knowledge rather than merely to solve problems. Therefore, he will examine the broader aspects of the problem area so as to extract the required contribution. If, in the course of this inquiry, he finds that a contribution has been made already, he may not pursue the problem area further.

A problem area that is defined in a narrow and highly specific manner will not permit the investigator to determine the actual requirements for the advancement of knowledge. If the head nurse, as a researcher, considers only the problem area of staffing her floor with the nurses available for the patients present, she immediately will narrow the scope of her investigation. She could address her problem only to the requirements of patients exactly like her own; to the capabilities of nurses exactly like her own; and to the layout of a floor facility exactly like her own. If, instead, she develops the more general problem area as the determination of staffing requirements for patients with varying degrees of illness, she can begin her pursuit of knowledge in one of several directions. It is true that she will not be able to solve her specific problem at this time but, as a researcher, this should not be her intent.

What would be the consequence of defining a problem area too broadly? It is possible to inquire: What is in the sky? or

What are the functions of education? However, it is readily apparent that any one researcher or any number of researchers could not begin to develop the complete solutions to these questions. In the course of his inquest, the investigator would be required to restrict the problem area to solutions within the grasp of man at that time. If he failed to do so, he merely would flutter about the sky with the rest of the objects.

Lastly, the researcher should be able to justify the actual existence of a problem area. Since research is a costly endeavor with comparatively large financial and energy expenditures, the researcher generally will begin with problem areas that are worthy of the efforts or the pursuit of knowledge. There are several ways to justify the existence of a problem area. Usually it will have been recognized as such by members of a professional society. The matter could have been the subject of previous research for which solutions were not complete —picture the current state of cancer research. The matter could have been unveiled as a result of a survey. Fact-finding information will uncover problem areas if the surveyor, like the diagnostician, is first made aware of the problem and its related symptoms. Lacking previous research or an actual survey, the matter could have been suggested as research by an authority or a group of authorities in the field. The weight of authority often is more persuasive than the other two sources of justification. However, since the voice of authority is based more upon opinion than fact, fact-finding information should bear more weight.

There are occasions when the need for research has not been recognized by a society or has been recognized only by a minority. The society may even voice antagonistic feelings toward a proposal. Consider, for example, the plight of Semmelweis when he advanced the need for asepsis. Sometimes the researcher must persevere without the assistance of others or even in the face of their disapproval. Some of mankind's greatest discoveries have been made in spite of such opposition. But these instances, while outstanding, probably are exceptions to the rule. If the researcher takes pains to justify the existence of a problem area, it is highly probable that the need also will be recognized by others.

Having acknowledged the problem area, it becomes the researcher's task to consider whether or not any knowledge already has been developed to answer the issue in question. The existence of a problem area does not necessarily imply a lack of acceptable answers. The state of knowledge in the world today has reached the point at which there remain very few unexplored areas. The researcher does not have to begin his search from nothingness. Instead, he must review first what has been learned already.

An exploration of the literature detailing previous research of the problem area may reveal that the question has been answered already. The head nurse had learned of a solution to her problem. Would further study be required? The researcher must consider at this point whether or not there is an actual need for additional research—whether or not the problem was solved adequately, whether or not the solution could be interpreted properly, whether or not the solution could be generalized extensively. He may decide at the completion of the review that there is no need for additional research. On the other hand, he may decide to pursue the matter further—to consider what additional research needs to be done.

Research often begets other research. Indeed, the fruitfulness of an individual study often is measured by the degree to which it generates other studies. Studies generally will arise from and build upon the creations of others. Note, for example, the following newspaper account of Dr. Albert Sabin's quest for an oral vaccine to combat poliomyelitis:

The first breakthrough . . . came in 1936 (when) . . . he established the fact that polio virus could be made to grow and multiply outside the body—on nervous tissues in test tubes.

The second big Sabin breakthrough came in 1939 . . . (when) he showed conclusively that paralytic polio viruses lived mainly in the intestinal tract of man.

It was not for 10 years that the next big breakthrough was made . . . a team of scientists at Harvard University . . . succeeded in developing a technique for breeding paralytic polio viruses on non-nervous monkey tissue outside the body.

The beginnings of final triumph came at the end of 1953. Dr. Sabin had found mutant particles of the paralytic viruses that produced no paralysis even when injected directly into the brains of monkeys or chimpanzees. The basic fact had been established—such mutants could be bred.[1]

The story continues until all are satisfied that the vaccine works. But it does not end, because other vaccines or discoveries of equal importance may be developed from this work.

The truly great accomplishments of our scientists may not be those recorded by history but, instead, may be measured by the new avenues of study that their research has unfolded. Claude Bernard, the eminent French physiologist, made the observation:

> Great men may be compared to torches shining at long intervals, to guide the advance of science. They light up their time, either by discovering unexpected and fertile phenomena which open up new paths and reveal unknown horizons, or by generalizing acquired scientific facts and disclosing truths which their predecessors had not perceived. If each great man makes the science which he vitalizes take a long step forward, he never presumes to fix its final boundaries and he is necessarily destined to be outdistanced and left behind by the progress of successive generations. Great men have been compared to giants upon whose shoulders pygmies have climbed, who nevertheless see further than they. This simply means that science makes progress subsequently to the appearance of great men, and precisely because of their influence. The result is that their successors know many more scientific facts than the great men themselves had in their day. But a great man is, none the less, still a great man, that is to say,—a giant.[2]

Surely Newton, among scores of others, learned from Galileo, and Einstein was fortunate enough to have succeeded both.

In seeking the need for additional research, it is probable also that the investigator is aware of a solution that has not been considered in the past. Let us surmise that much research is born from the germ of an idea whose seed is sown within the research worker or the potential research worker and perhaps is incubated over a long period of time. These "pet ideas" may occur almost anywhere, on or off the job. They are nourished and protected until they can be developed and tested. If the originator of the idea has any research talent or can be assisted in this regard, the idea may grow into an acutal research project and bear fruit of its own.

It was also Claude Bernard who developed "the germ of an idea" thesis. He conceived that research consists of "feeling," "reasoning," and "experiment." The idea itself arises only from the feeling. Not all individuals, Bernard stated, have the ability to perceive the idea. Nor is there a precise set of rules, as in the case of "reasoning" and "experiment," to which one may turn for this endeavor.

The idea is a seed; the method is the earth furnishing the conditions in which it may develop, flourish and give the best of fruit according to its nature. But as only what has been sown in the ground will ever grow in it, so nothing will be developed by the experimental method itself except the ideas submitted to it. The method itself gives birth to nothing. Certain philosophers have made the mistake of according too much power to method along these lines.[3]

At this point, the researcher may have narrowed his requirements for additional research to one or several areas of pursuit. He may decide to take up where someone else has left off for the lack of appropriate knowledge or for the inability to test his hypothesis. For example, some 30-odd years have passed and Einstein's theory of relativity has not yet been adequately tested. The researcher may decide to redo an entire study. He may concentrate merely upon the development of appropriate instrumentation for gathering data or testing a hypothesis. He may decide to take a new approach and develop a new idea. In any case, he should be ready to develop and state the specific purpose of his research.

WHAT ARE THE SPECIFIC PURPOSES OF RESEARCH?

Let us reflect briefly upon the criteria for knowledge derived through research and seek to establish the different stages of development. In accordance with the previous discussion, knowledge of this type consists of those attributes that enable man "to learn what to expect." That is, with this knowledge man becomes more aware of or alert to events to come: that X action leads to Y response; that a given set of conditions will provide for the development of a specific set of events.

Where do we secure the secrets of events to come? It was suggested, from time to time, that man could look to nature for the solutions of his problems. It is an orderly system that nature has provided for man and his cobearers upon this earth.

We need only to examine the inner workings of this system, matching problem for problem, to find the solutions to our own "felt difficulties." If we could observe nature in action in the unfolding of this system, we should "learn what to expect."

Since nature reveals itself at all times, why do we not just sit back, observe, and learn? The task is not that simple. We look but we do not see. Or events reveal themselves in different ways to different people. We may not agree that the same phenomena have been observed. Some events, like the splitting of the atom, are so obscure that they cannot be observed readily by the naked eye. Other characteristics, such as "hunger" or "pain," cannot be observed even with the most intricate of instruments.

Louis Pasteur served notice that great discoveries, the disclosure of some of nature's rarest secrets, do not occur by chance. It takes a prepared mind to make these observations. We have to know where, when and how to look and what to record. Above all, we must have a purpose for looking. Psychologists have suggested that observations often are colored by our needs, i.e., we see what we intend to see.[4] If we do not look for anything, the probability is that we will not see anything.

Therefore, man must be prepared before he begins his search. He should know in advance where to look and what he expects to find. This is possible if the system is an orderly one, as was assumed previously. If he can discover the order of events and the manner by which they were conceived, then he can learn to think along the lines of the system and anticipate what he expects to find.

"To know what to expect" implies also a bidirectional search. Before we can consider or think about what to expect, we must have a basis for our thinking. We must first be given a preliminary set of events, experiences or conditions, organized or disorganized. It then becomes our purpose to set these events in order or, at least, to seek to discover their order. At the opposite extreme, we must be satisfied that the expectations have been conceived properly—that they actually have a place or a niche within the order of events and fit consistently within this system. In this way, the expectations take on meaning and are considered with other expectations.

The research process, as was suggested, may thus be conceived as having functionally distinct phases. In this regard, it can be likened to the development of text material. Cronback *et al.* considered the functional requirements of texts and, as in this analysis, arrived at both general and specific purposes. The general purpose of the text, they say, is "to help the learner to interpret and respond to his own environment."[5] "If knowing what to expect" implies "knowing what to do," then this is simply another way of stating the same purpose.

We learned previously that this purpose may be served specifically by text materials in one of four ways: narrative-descriptive statements that present a running account of particular experiences; prescriptions and directives or "how-to-do-it" suggestions; generalizations or descriptions of a class of events; and theoretic statements that "communicate the precise meaning of concepts within systematically organized disciplines of knowledge."[6] We might determine that "prescriptions and directives" and "generalized statements" provide the necessary ingredients for learning what to expect. These, in turn, are fed and derived from the preliminary narrative-descriptive statements and gain meaning when cast into a theoretic framework.

It is possible then to think of three phases of the research process. Black reasoned in this way. He pictured the preliminary phase as the period for making observations, collecting data, *describing* experiences. In the second phase, the researcher may attempt to generalize about the observed or descriptive data and *predict* the unobserved. In essence, he would seek "to learn what to expect." The final phase considered those situations in which, for some reason, an exception to the predicted or the unobserved event did or might occur. In these cases, an explanation was needed, taking "the form of additional data and generalizations which, in conjunction with known data and theory, have the event to be explained as a consequence."[7]

We propose to consider that the research process falls into these three stages of development: the descriptive, the predictive, and the explanative. They generally will occur in sequence, in the order named. Each stage can be represented by a specific purpose: to describe, to predict, to explain. The research worker will ask himself, initially, "What is my intent? What do I expect to derive from this project—a description, a prediction or an explanation?"

To Describe

The first contraction period is apt to be short. After a wait of perhaps 20 minutes a longer and more intense hunger period arrives; then another and another. The infant's sleep becomes lighter. He is more easily awakened by external stimuli or by gastric discomfort. He is put to the breast, nurses vigorously, becomes fatigued or experiences satiety from distention and again goes to sleep.[8]

On March 18, 1937, Cat K (being hungry) was placed in the starting box and allowed to escape by an open exit door. This was done 3 times in order to establish a habit of leaving by the door. The door was then closed and the cat admitted to the box. On its first trial it struck the pole "accidentally" while turning in the box only 4 seconds after its admission. The same series of movements was repeated in the next two trials.[9]

(The) rat presented suddenly without sound. There was steady fixation, but no tendency at first to reach for it. The rat was then placed nearer, whereupon tentative reaching movements began with the right hand. When the rat nosed the infant's left hand the head was immediately withdrawn. He started to reach for the head of the animal with the forefinger of his left hand but withdrew it suddenly before contact.[10]

How can any of the preceding quotations be characterized? We will find that the search for words becomes confined to a limited few, each of which implies description. To state simply that they "describe" seems most fitting. Furthermore, they describe what is happening, what can be observed or sensed with little or no interpretation or value judgments. They seem to say, "This is what I saw."

Research begins and ends with description. In order to reach some of the more advanced stages of prediction and explanation, we must begin with description. Before we can turn our thoughts into action, some substance must be derived or observed to generate the process. We can only speculate now as to what lies on the opposite side of the moon, but countless theories will be developed when man has managed to catch a glimpse. At the other extreme, description is used to test the predictions or explanations that ultimately have been derived. The culminating generalizations must be scrutinized "in the face of indisputable facts."

The quotations above were reported from actual studies, which yielded a specific contribution to knowledge, in each case. The first quotation was taken from a study in which the author attempted to determine the infant's behavior pattern in response to the hunger drive. The second quotation is a partial description of an experiment that was designed to demonstrate the principle of association in learning. The third quotation pertained to a study that attempted to depict how the emotion "fear" is learned.

There are some who feel that all research is description— that the researcher can report only his observations and nothing more.

Since other people cannot sense my sense-data, or share my thoughts or feelings, they cannot verify the statements that I make about them; neither can I verify the corresponding statements that they make about their experiences. And if I cannot verify them, I cannot understand them either.[11]

This school of thought would argue that it is naïve to speculate about the underlying order of nature. There are too many exceptions to the rule to specify pure relationships. Instead, its adherents would be satisfied to state the probability that two events will occur together. The researcher who is so inclined, therefore, would not be interested in the order of events but simply would record the frequency with which two events occur together or the extent of their variation. He would utilize his observations to derive a statistical generalization that does not purport to ask why or how but states "what is."

On the other hand, the question is asked: "To describe" for what purpose? This point of view does not accept the relationship per se, but will inquire as to the order of the occurrence: which event led to another; how did they occur; and perhaps why. The adherents of this school of thought feel that the mere listing of correlated events is not enough. Is it not helpful to know, in addition, that certain events must be preceded by others? For example, is it not more useful for the physician to learn that a high temperature follows an infection than it is to be aware only that they tend to occur together? To be cognizant that an event can be attributed to another event (or events) is to be more knowledgeable than only to recognize that they vary in a particular direction. Is the nurse who recognizes that the action of a tranquilizing drug is to desensitize the autonomic nervous system not more informed than the one who observes simply that excitation or depression varies with the administration of the drug?

What is implied by this school is the notion of causality or a cause-and-effect relationship. A cause that yields a specific effect has been described as "any necessary antecedent or concomitant event or condition."[12] This definition infers that for each effect or event there is a specific cause or causes that occurred concurrently or in the past. Things do not happen by chance alone, but occur for a reason and can be related to that reason. The physician may attribute a patient's pain and discomfort to an infection. The nurse may recognize a hearty appetite as a sign that the infection has diminished and that more satisfying effects can be expected.

To describe, to observe the order of events and their relationship, may be conceived as a specific purpose for research. When we describe, we may be seeking out some measure of causality. Black cautions us, however, to be wary of cause-and-effect relationships. They are deceptive, nonspecific, multiple. He states that "cause sometimes means a condition (necessary or sufficient) which human beings can manipulate, while at other times it means a condition which for some reason is regarded as particularly interesting and important."[13]

Yet, at the same time, statements of probability also can be deceptive. It is possible to determine a statistical relationship, at one time or another, between any two orders of events. By chance alone, they will occur together to some degree. Sooner or later the question will arise: Why or how are these two events interrelated? Can two orders of events be singled out for observation unless considerable thought is given first to the propostion that they may be interrelated? It is not very comforting to live in an environment of probability. "I cannot believe," Einstein was quoted as saying, "that God plays dice with the world."[14] It is possible to make predictions on this basis. But how meaningful are they? How can we account for the exception to the prediction?

It will be suggested instead that this is an orderly world from which a system of relationships can be derived. But because of the many facets and intricate and devious pathways of cause-and-effect relationships, we may be unable to state with complete assurance that such relationships exist. We may have to be satisfied, as Black intimates, with statements like "most of the time" or "it seems highly probable" that A tends to be related to B or is the condition for B.

In accordance with these thoughts, what is described when we describe? Three orders of description will be considered. They will be differentiated by our level of conceptualization or thinking. That is, they will vary to the extent that we are able to depict relationship or sequence of occurrence. They will differ according to the extent of our knowledge in these areas.

At the lowest order of conceptualization, the researcher may be given two or more concrete observable events about which he may inquire: How does one relate to the other; or does one result as a consequence of the other? Are they both the conditions for or the effects of other events? It may be observed that certain mental patients become highly aggressive after visiting with their families. What is the relationship? Does the aggressive behavior result from the family visit? Or is it a symptom of some underlying condition that the visit has aggravated? At this stage of the investigation it becomes the purpose of the observer to describe the relationship between two events.

At the next level of thinking, we may be given an event (or events) and seek to inquire into the antecedent conditions. The researcher is presented in this case with an existing event and is asked to search the past for those events or conditions that must have preceded the given event. The physician examines his patient and observes a given set of symptoms or events from which he makes his diagnosis—he reasons that these symptoms should have arisen as a result of certain antecedent bodily states or conditions. At this level, we have sufficient knowledge to infer the order of events, i.e., that the given event resulted from other events. The purpose of the study is to describe those conditions that precede the given event.

The third order of conceptualization at the descriptive level evolves when we are presented with a set of conditions and are asked to determine the events that, of necessity, will follow. The physician makes his prognosis, which is that as a consequence of the patient's bodily condition such-and-such effects may be forthcoming. He prescribes a treatment that alters the conditions and produces other effects. In this study situation, the order of events is reversed from the past to the future. We are given antecedent conditions and seek to inquire as to the consequential events. The purpose is to describe those events that result as a consequence of the given conditions.

To Predict

It is sometimes stated that the aim of science is "to predict and control." To predict may be synonymous with "to learn what to expect"—to state that a relationship exists between two or more sets of events that occur in some type of order or sequence. Since the purpose of inquiry at the descriptive level is to uncover such relationships, the purpose at the predictive level is to determine whether or not this relationship actually enables us to learn what to expect. For example, if it were determined that the family visit was one of the predisposing factors to the onset of aggression in the mentally ill patient, then aggression would be expected after each visit.

A study at the predictive level actually may be considered to be a test of the relationship that could have been derived from a descriptive study. In a test of this type, only the events specified in the relationship are studied. All other events are deliberately held constant or out of the picture. Such a test is said to be controlled. Thus, the element of control infers that when a prediction is derived it will relate to specific events and to no others.

The validity of a test or the quality of a prediction depends upon the extent to which the factors under consideration can be controlled. Control itself is contingent upon the ability of the researcher at the descriptive level to identify and isolate all the relevant factors and specify their relationship or sequence of occurrence. Predictive studies, therefore, must wait upon and be served by descriptive studies.

One quality of prediction is accuracy. We desire to be reasonably certain that the prediction is correct, that the events will happen as expected. A prediction that is inaccurate may be detrimental because we sometimes plan as if the predicted events will occur.

It was noted previously that causal relationships are not easily contrived. Furthermore, they may involve a multitude of events, not all of which can be controlled at the same time. Accuracy in prediction might be described more aptly by the continuum or the line of probability. In other words, we learn to be satisfied with predictions of less than 100 per cent accuracy. The determination of the type and the size of the error of prediction may constitute a desirable objective of the researcher. It is more useful, perhaps, to have a large error and to be aware of it than to have a small error that has not been recognized as such. We will have learned what to expect.

Real life situations are not controlled, and events seldom occur a second time in exactly the same way. Then how useful is a prediction that is to be employed in different situations? How can we be reasonably certain that the predicted events will tend to recur?

The problem is overcome by another attribute of prediction: the quality of generalization or the ability to transfer solutions. This quality of generalization was described previously as a form of written knowledge. The researcher abstracts from the concrete or observable events those elements that probably would be present when the events occur upon a second occasion in an apparently different form. For example, the staff nurse may observe that patients become antagonistic and overdemanding when their expected visitors do not arrive. She may observe also that patients become overbearing when their food is cold or when they fail to recuperate as expected. The nurse, therefore, may develop the generalization that frustration (failure to have visitors, warm food, to recuperate) leads to aggression (becoming overdemanding, antagonistic). The prediction may not consider the specific events or situations observed, but abstractions from which the relationship actually is derived. The ability to identify these abstractions in other situations enables man to generalize or transfer solutions.

A prediction can be defined then as a generalization that is expected to occur at a certain level of probability. Perhaps the generalization is more descriptive of the relationship that occurs in a specific order of events than of the events themselves. At the predictive level, the researcher is given a relationship between two or more orders of consequent, antecedent, or both types of events. It then becomes his specific purpose to determine the probability that this relationship is true.

To Explain

To describe is faithfully to record events as they happen. A record of the past is provided and can be used to gain some insight into the future. Prediction is the channel by which the products of description are extended into the future. On the assumption that past events tend to recur, certain characteristics are abstracted and prescribed to entail the most probable descriptions of events as yet unobserved but to be expected. The level of description isolates and provides the ingredients for prediction. The ability to predict is a measure of environmental control.

We also can attain the level of prediction through the process of reasoning. It was stated previously that the predictor may generalize from the narrow and specific events observed to a much wider body of events to be observed. Generalizations that interrelate with other generalizations also might be developed. A network or system of interlocking generalizations can be formed from which it is possible to derive the very same generalizations or predictions secured from descriptive data.

It may be established, for example, that frustration also leads to regressive behavior, resignation or do-nothingness. That is, in response to frustration, some patients may become aggressive or more childlike, demanding excessive attention; others may engage in seemingly bizarre behavior such as asking the same question over and over again; and still others simply may lie in their beds for days, doing nothing, saying nothing. We may reason that these responses can be ranked in goal direction or in accordance with their respective abilities to overcome the source of frustration. Thus, aggression may be more adaptive in this respect than regression, fixation and resignation. It can be reasoned also that the patient may adopt each of the responses, in the order named, in accordance with the intensity of the frustration. Thus, as frustration is increased, his behavior may become less adaptive.

This process of conceptualization and system-development rests primarily upon deductive reasoning. To predict on this basis is to attain the level of explanation.

To reach the level of explanation is to surmount the apex of a body of knowledge derived through research. It is necessary to understand not only that events of the past tend to recur in the future, but how they occur and perhaps why. To explain is to overcome the limitations of description and prediction via description. To explain is to overcome some of the restrictions of control and to account for inevitable exceptions to the rule. To explain is to extend the powers of prediction beyond the narrow range of our senses.

There are some real limitations to the use of predictive data that are derived solely from descriptive analysis. Although it may be felt that this information has been derived from factual materials—that which can be sensed—the base may not be as reliable as it originally was thought to be. Our senses can deceive us. Our interpretation of what is sensed can be misleading.

"Let's get the facts." "Let the facts fall where they may," are statements of assurance that we can depend wholly upon this source of information. Research, as has been stated, will not accept into its order any statements of belief that have not been tested in the light of factual experience. Descriptive data that comprise statements of facts, however, can be deceptive or misleading. In this regard, it is not the facts that are at fault; they are there to be observed. But the observer can be misled, unintentionally or otherwise, in his attempt to obtain, describe and record his observations.

Black points out three areas of difficulty in the attempt to "observe the facts as they really are": the correction of personal biases, the inaccessibility of data and the perception of significant data.[15] On the one hand, the observer falls a victim to what he already knows; on the other hand, he is a prey to what he does not know.

Even with the best of intentions to remain objective, the observer may not be able to discard his previous experiences. This is especially the case, Black states, in relatively undeveloped fields of inquiry, where there is little agreement as to what is or is not an unbiased observation. The persons who made the initial observation become the experts of the time. Who is to state that their record is inaccurate?

This state of affairs also will hamper the researcher before he can make a single observation. He must inquire: Where do I look? What do I look for? How do I know I have obtained what I truly seek? The so-called miracle drugs that are employed today with great frequency and considerable success were not simply planted upon this earth during the past 30 years. But their discovery had to wait upon man's development and his readiness to perceive their existence.

Unfortunately, man does not make observations beforehand and he may not understand what he perceives. His observations, for lack of something better and because of the faith that is placed in the fact per se, may stand unrefuted for a long period of time. Until the Middle Ages, it was believed that the sun and the planets revolved around the earth.

A further complication is the recognition that many of the facts that we seek cannot be perceived by our sense organs. If we rely only upon what can be observed or sensed, then the descriptive statements may evolve only as partial facts. For instance, copper wires may be described, even by the most careful observer, as thin, hard, metal strands of varying widths and lengths. Does this description fit and account for the same copper wire through which an electric current is passed? We also may recall the experience of the six blind men of Indostan, which was limited to the sense of touch.* Each described the same elephant differently because each touched a different part of the elephant at the same time. Which one was correct? In a sense each was correct. But, in terms of what is already known about the elephant, would we dare to predict from any one of these descriptions?

Explanation helps to overcome some of these deficiencies. Instead of beginning the quest by looking for facts, the re-

* See page 338.

searcher will start with what is already known or assumed to be known. He will construct a model conceptualizing the system of which the facts to be evolved or made known are one part and not the only part. If he must construct the model with a small number of actual facts, his system may be incomplete. Therefore, he might borrow items from outside his specific field of knowledge, and/or invent facts. With each step, his system and its parts—the actual, the borrowed and the invented—are tested by the process of reasoning. If it is logically consistent, he will feel satisfied. If not, he will modify his system to make it so. As a further test, he may attempt to deduce from his system the facts that are already known. The ultimate test is to deduce the facts to be made known, and then to search them out empirically to determine that what has been deduced is actually so.

Numerous systems or models have been invented throughout the history of science. Some of them are confined to a very narrow body of events, and others may explain some of the burning issues of mankind. There is a system that describes the nature of the universe and, in one part, locates the earth and the other planets as bodies in space revolving about the sun. There is a system that can depict the characteristics of current electricity, describing its structure and movement with great accuracy even though the naked eye sees only a thin strand of wire. There are various systems—the circulatory, the respiratory, the digestive, the nervous, the endocrine—characterizing the inner workings of the physical organism. They may be treated independently or as interlocking to explain the action of each of the bodily organs in normal circumstances and in times of stress.

The goal of description and explanation is essentially the same: to provide a basis for prediction. However, each advances upon the goal from a different direction. Research initiated at the level of explanation can overcome some of the deficiencies of descriptive-level research. At the same time, one contributes to the other and is enhanced as the other is enhanced.

Personal bias as a source of error can be minimized at the level of explanation. Since the researcher derives first what is to be observed, he is made keenly aware of his biases. He then can take steps to set up or seek out a critical test situation in which to justify his derivations. The concern here is not that he believes that he knows the answer beforehand: he recognizes this and can testify on the soundness of his model that his hypothesis is reasonable. The system may substitute for the lack of qualified judges. The real concern is that he does not take sufficient steps to provide a critical test of his hypothesis. This source of bias is to be minimized or eliminated. In the case of descriptive analysis, the observer may not have been aware that his observations were biased. At the level of explanation, he is made aware of possible sources of personal bias beforehand and can do something about it, or at least account for it.

The data that are inaccessible to descriptive-level analysis do not constitute an immediate problem to explanative-level research. If the data cannot be observed but are called for in accordance with the demands of the model, they may be invented. That is, they may be developed in the mind of the model-builder and described in theoretic form. Hull defined them as intervening variables:

> Whenever an attempt is made to penetrate the invisible world of the molecular, scientists frequently and usefully employ logical constructs, intervening variables, or symbols to facilitate their thinking. These symbols or X's represent entities or processes which, if existent, would account for certain events in the observable molar world. Examples of such postulated entities in the field of the physical sciences are electrons, protons, positrons, etc. A closely parallel concept in the field of behavior familiar to everyone is that of *habit* as distinguished from habitual action.[16]

Hull suggests that these concepts can be used more fruitfully and less hazardously if they intervene between a set of observable events. That is, they can be tied down to and identified with concrete events that actually can be observed. While it is always more desirable to build on strictly observable events, these constructs serve a useful purpose until something better can be devised.

A model provides the additional advantage of casting the events to be observed in their proper perspective. The events may be derived from and regarded with respect to the model as a whole. Their role can be evaluated in this perspective. These same events may be cast alone, as often happens in the case of descriptive analysis. However, on what basis can it be stated that these are the significant events to be observed? The model, on the other hand, suggests what and where to observe and the meaning to be derived from the results of the observations.

Despite these advantages, explanation is still dependent upon description. It was indicated earlier that research begins and ends with description. There are very few, if any, theoretic models that are not based upon descriptive data, at least in part. The model ultimately must satisfy the test of empiricism. We have a circular condition in which descriptive analysis feeds the explanative models and is bettered as a result.

The elimination of bias waits upon the acquisition of reliable information; the acquisition of reliable information waits upon the elimination of bias. Without knowledge of generalizations, no significant observations; without significant observations, no generalizations.[17]

HOW CAN THE SPECIFIC PURPOSE OF A RESEARCH PROJECT BE DERIVED?

Let us summarize the foregoing and develop a procedure for deriving a specific purpose for a research project. What follows is not intended to be construed as a rigid format but should be regarded instead as furnishing some guidelines.

Initially, the researcher may inquire: *What is the general problem area?* This may be the reason for getting started. It can be "a felt difficulty," an initiating cause. He will wish to justify the existence of this general problem area by presenting documentary evidence of its actual existence and its importance. The evidence may take the form of previous research, fact-finding reports or authoritative judgments.

Having satisfied the initial requirement, the researcher then may ask: *What has been learned to date?* He will explore previous developments systematically to determine whether the problem has been solved wholly, partially, or not at all. He will investigate and list the pertinent sources of knowledge that already has been acquired. In this regard, he may inquire: Has a cause, an effect or a relationship been isolated? Have they been tested sufficiently? Are these just empiric relationships, or is there an understanding as to their exact nature? Has a system been established for deriving other relationships?

The researcher then may move to the opposite page of the ledger and consider: *What needs to be done?* That is, he will examine the information derived with regard to the previous question and determine the steps to be taken. It may be that the solution is at hand and that additional study is not required. His intended project may be concluded at this point. He may determine, on the other hand, that there are several steps to be taken and will list them in order of sequence.

The researcher should be ready to select from the list of needs the next step to be taken and to provide a *statement of the purpose of his study.* How can the purpose be stated? Table 2, below, may be of assistance. What has been learned to date is listed under "Given" at the three levels of investigation. What is "Needed" follows as a consequence. The purpose can be selected accordingly and stated in terms of one of the three levels of investigation:

1. To describe: to find an answer, or to discover, determine, identify, etc.

2. To predict: to know if it works, or to test

3. To explain: to know how it works, to understand, to derive further predictions.

The researcher may wish to justify the selection of his purpose. He may do so by stating how the results of his intended study will be helpful or what the contribution to the over-all area of difficulty will be.

TABLE 2. LEVELS OF INVESTIGATION

	TO DESCRIBE	TO PREDICT	TO EXPLAIN
Given:	1. A cause 2. An effect 3. Two events	A cause and an effect; a relationship	A series of relationships, unstructured or structured
Needed:	To determine the 1. Effect(s) 2. Cause(s) 3. Relationship(s)	To determine the probability that this is true	To determine the interrelationship of the various events; the derivation of other relationships

THE SPECIFIC PURPOSE OF RESEARCH IN NURSING

How do the concepts of the previous section apply to research in nursing? Let us center our attention upon a research project in nursing, utilize the concepts in a stepwise fashion and trace the development of the specific purpose. In this regard, the authors will attempt to describe the initiating conditions, isolate a problem area, justify the need for research, and determine the specific purpose or purposes as derived from several points of view.

Two factors, above all others, tend to influence the nurse researcher in her selection of a project: herself and the society in which she serves. Many projects emanate from the needs, the interests and the capabilities of the research person herself. The demands of the sponsoring agency also may be a prime determiner of who does what.

The nurse researcher often will engage in projects that are of particular interest to her. Thus, the psychiatric nurse will tend toward problems of mental health, the educator toward curriculum development, learning and evaluation, the specialist in maternal and child health toward obstetric nursing, and so forth. It is only natural that they should do so. The probability is that they were specialists in one of the subject-matter areas long before they had research affiliations. As a matter of fact, they may have selected or been selected to engage in a research project because of the subject matter rather than because of their expertness in research.

Accordingly, the type of project selected will be influenced also by the capability of the individual research worker. That is, she will tend to develop projects in a manner befitting the technics learned to date. She will limit the scope of her project in accordance with her ability to grasp or comprehend the total picture. She will pursue areas of knowledge with which she is familiar.

Unfortunately, many of the nurses engaged in research, either as students or as full-time or part-time researchers, are not equipped for the task. They may lack an understanding of some of the basic technics of research: experimental design, data gathering, statistical analysis, theory construction. They may even be deficient in the basic areas of knowledge upon which nursing must rely.

These deficiencies perhaps are exemplified by the character of the work that is produced. For lack of ability in theory construction, there has been an overemphasis upon descriptive studies. For want of technic, there has been a preponderance of specific technics: the questionnaire, the case-study approach, and some of the newly acquired but overused and misused technics such as Q-sort and critical incident. For lack of knowledge, there has been an overemphasis upon particular orders of studies such as the nurse function studies.

Projects often are initiated and supported by a sponsoring agency. Many of the large membership organizations, such as the National League for Nursing or the American Nurses Association or their state affiliates, the various governmental agencies, the smaller private organizations and foundations, including the universities and the hospitals, are among the groups issuing the call for projects. The student nurse researcher sometimes carries out the wishes of a faculty advisor who, in this case, assumes the role of a supportive agency.

The project can emanate from the agency in a number of ways. It may result from committee action. The committee itself may be drawn together to resolve a specific issue and perhaps may determine that it cannot do so without a detailed and controlled investigation. A committee may even be drawn together to specify avenues for research. The project could be initiated by a survey or sparked by a national event of an emergency nature, such as the spread of staphylococci among the hospitals.

In any event, the project is passed on to the nurse researcher from the sponsoring agency. The entire study may be spelled out in detail. Or it may be received by the nurse researcher as a recommendation for study, without further specifications. The nurse researcher, in essence, is presented with an assignment.

Let us assume that we have been presented with an assignment from such a committee: to investigate the problem area of nurse staffing. This committee was organized to specify some major problem areas in nursing, among the foremost of which was the one assigned. The committee did not limit the scope of the investigation in any way. It stated simply, "Here is the area to be investigated. Go to work."

Getting Organized

Nurse staffing! Do they mean nurse staffing in hospitals? Public health agencies? Clinics? Do they mean nurse staffing with regard to pediatric, obstetric, medical, surgical or psychiatric patients? The critically and the not-so-critically sick? Do they mean staffing with professional nurses, practical nurses, nurse's aides? Should the end-product be a series of nurse-patient ratios, or a body of relationships from which nurse-patient ratios can be derived?

During the initial stages of a research project, the researcher seems to stumble around in the dark. She has the problem, a very personal problem, of getting started. She may ask herself a number of questions similar to those just cited. She may have a flight of ideas, some of which seem fruitful, some of which are outlandish. But the ideas will wax and wane. At times, the researcher may be overwhelmed by the onslaught of questions and ideas. At other times, she may be completely devoid of any notion of how to go about solving the problem.

The crux of the researcher's personal problem is that she

must get organized. It may help considerably for her to ask herself: Where am I going? What am I trying to do? and then develop an outline or a plan of procedure. Although the researcher later may find the initial outline and even subsequent outlines to be inappropriate and subject to revision, this is the way to get started.

Our plan of procedure will begin as follows:

1. To examine the general problem area of nurse staffing
2. To determine the need for research in this area
3. To derive and state the specific purpose.

Although the topic to be investigated has been submitted as an assignment, the professional researcher should have the privilege of having certain questions answered before she attempts to make a detailed analysis. These questions pertain to the need for research. A professional researcher, just as a professional physician, must make a diagnosis before prescribing treatment.

The Problem Area

What is the general problem area? It may be the researcher's privilege also to establish a preliminary set of definitions. Committees sometimes express their demands in vague terms. The researcher may be required to restate the question more specifically. If the restatement does not satisfy the committee, it can always be altered.

The general problem area will be defined in this case as the need to establish a basis for making nurse assignments. We will not, at this time, specify the type of nurses to be assigned, where they will be employed, or for whom they will care. In this respect, the problem has not been severely curtailed and can be interpreted broadly.

How does one know that this need to determine nurse staffing requirements really exists? The committee apparently feels that this is the case. It has told us so. But is its judgment sufficient? Is it based upon opinions, the weight of authority? Or is it supported by factual evidence, the opinions of other authorities, or both? Factual evidence should have greater weight than opinion. A series of strongly supported opinions may have to suffice, however, when factual evidence is lacking.

What types of factual evidence may support the need for a study in this problem area? The following are samples of studies that were justified by the available facts.

Nursing Service and Patient Care: A Staffing Experiment.[18] This experiment on the effects of varying staffing patterns on the attitudes and the morale of patients and nursing personnel opened up some interesting questions. One question considered was: Are too many nurses worse than too few? It was found that nurses did not spend more time with patients when more nurses were introduced on the units; furthermore, they felt bored and restless with the extra time on their hands.

Twenty Thousand Nurses Tell Their Story.[19] Fifteen studies sponsored by the American Nurses Association on nursing functions were summarized and interpreted by the authors. These studies determined how nurses spend their time and who does what. The analysis of the results presented a very confusing picture in the area of staffing with regard to who does "what" tasks and the expectation of who should do "what" tasks. It would appear that the work of nurses has expanded. The number and the kinds of personnel who do the work also have grown. The question as to how the work should be divided remains unanswered.

A Study of Turnover and Its Costs.[20] The nursing department accounted for nearly half the total payroll and well over half the turnover costs of a large hospital. Costs involved in various phases of turnover—orientation, training, and reduction in job effectiveness—were determined. Costs were also found to influence staffing—the kind and the numbers of personnel and their utilization.

What kind of opinions may lend support? Here are some authoritative statements:

The American Nurses Association, in launching its program of studies of nursing functions, stated:

Studies of nursing functions for institutional nursing will make it possible to define specifically the duties and functions of the various workers on the nursing team. . . . Definitions of the duties of nurses and the establishment of patterns of team composition will serve as a basis for determining hospital staffing patterns—an increasingly important problem with the planned increase in hospital construction.[21]

The Director of the Department of Nursing Service Administration, National League for Nursing, expresses the philosophy of that department as follows:

The greatest need in administration of hospital nursing service today is for better prepared administrative nursing personnel. This has two aspects—more and better formally prepared administrative and supervisory personnel, and more and better on-the-job preparation for those unable to get formal preparation. Knowledge and skill in management techniques, and knowing how to put them into practice, are needed. Assistance also is needed in planning the nursing staff for hospitals. Related to this is the need for a better concept of nursing care around which to build the staff, in line with modern knowledge of the patient's needs.[22]

The problem of the shortage of nurses and the need for better utilization of nurse power is succinctly stated by one leader:

Clearly the time is here for a critical examination of the problem. Is there a shortage of *numbers* of nurses, or is the shortage more apparent than real? Is the shortage of nurse supply but a symptom of shortages that lie elsewhere? . . . Will we continue to focus attention on *numbers* of nurses without equal (if not more) attention to greater efficiency, and economy in their use, and better knowledge of where to use them?[23]

The researcher has developed an argument. The question is: Does the specified problem area exist? She will collect evidence to make a judgment. How much evidence should be collected? Enough to make an adequate judgment. She will conclude that the problem area is existent or nonexistent.

What is the role of the individual researcher in this regard? Does her opinion count? A strong need has developed throughout the history of research for objectivity—for the researcher to remain aloof from the argument. This seems to say that her opinion is not very important. But it is very difficult to stay objective, to remain aloof. The researcher's opinions and biases are contained in her selection of the topic and the supportive evidence, the organization of the materials and the development of the argument. There are many ways in which self enters into the argument; there are many ways in which self should or should not enter into the argument.

THE NEED FOR FURTHER RESEARCH

The existence of a problem area does not automatically justify the need for research. The researcher must determine what specifically is required—what voids in the body of nursing knowledge are to be filled.

The question of need may be examined by scrutinizing first what has been learned to date. The problem area may have been partially or completely answered or not answered at all. The researcher will wish to be aware of the present state of knowledge as applied to the question at hand.

She will scrutinize the resource of nursing knowledge again to determine what is already known about staffing. Have any of the variables associated with staffing been isolated? What are the causal factors? What are the effects? Have any relationships been determined? Is there sufficient evidence to establish their reliability? Can the relationships be explained?

After a diligent investigation of the pool of knowledge pertaining to staffing, a series of related factors may be determined. They may be listed and supported by appropriate references.

1. Staffing is apparently a function that is governed by the number of nurses available. That is, the nursing assignment is such that so many nurses will be required to fulfill the task. Furthermore, the number of nurses that can be assigned is dependent upon the number of nurses who actually are available for duty.

Nursing Service Staffing and Quality of Nursing Care.[24] The hypothesis was tested that the quality of the nursing care provided for selected groups of patients decreases when the numbers of patients assigned to the nurses increase. The study demonstrated that the work load of nursing personnel definitely was related to the quality of the nursing care provided for the patients.

Nursing Service Research.[25] Experimenting with the team assignment in medical and surgical units, the researcher found that a 1:2 proportion (nurse: nurse assistant) was optimal, and that it adequately and satisfactorily provided 2.2 hours of general nursing care per patient on the day shift in the selected hospital in which the experiment was conducted.

Nursing Service and Patient Care: A Staffing Experiment.[26] The problem of adequate staffing on hospital units led to the design of a study that would seek to answer the question: Is there an optimum nursing hours of care? For 9 weeks, nine different combinations of staffing were introduced with two variables: numbers of personnel and hours of nursing care per patient. The experimenters found a relationship between the numbers of nursing personnel, the staffing combinations, the types of activities engaged in, and patient and personnel satisfaction.

2. Staffing also appears to relate to the quality of the nursing care to be provided. Nursing personnel differ in ability, training and experience. Some perform functions that others cannot perform. Some provide service more skillfully than others. The nursing assignment, therefore, will be a function that is governed by the kinds of nurses available and the task to be done.

A Study of Nursing Functions in General Hospitals in the State of Minnesota.[27] The authors determined the distribution of nursing personnel in Minnesota hospitals and compared the on-job activities of licensed practical nurses, nurse-aides and professional nurses. They found that the assignment of a function to a member of a nursing team was dependent upon factors inherent in the local situation.

Institutional Nurses: Roles, Relationships and Attitudes in Three Alabama Hospitals.[28] The relationships among the nursing personnel in three hospitals were found to be affected by the roles that the nurses were required or expected to assume because of the existing situation regarding the number of personnel available and how they were used in each hospital. Where the functions were more clearly defined, the work loads more evenly distributed and the lines of communication clearly defined, there was less disharmony and misunderstanding among the various levels of nursing personnel, and consequently more qualitative care.

A Study of Nursing Functions in 12 Hospitals in the State of New York.[29] To determine the nursing activities presently carried on by nursing, observations were made of the personnel for a 24-hour period on each of 2 days. It was found that professional nurses were functioning at a professional level approximately 50 per cent of the time, at a nonprofessional level 25 per cent of the time, and at a non-nursing level 25 per cent of the time. Practical nurses functioned at a professional level (as defined in this study) 20 per cent of the time, at a nonprofessional level 50 per cent of the time and at a non-nursing level $33\frac{1}{3}$ per cent of the time. It was concluded that neither professional nor practical nurses were performing at the level of function for which they were prepared.

3. Staffing is a function that is governed by the types of patients to be cared for. Some patients require more care than others. Patients also require different kinds of care. The number and the kind of nursing personnel to be assigned will be dependent, therefore, upon the amount and the kind of care that is required by the patients.

Concepts of Progressive Patient Care.[30] The authors point out that the nurse staffing pattern for various progressive patient care units will depend on the type of patients being cared for. For example, one nurse per patient per tour of duty may be required in an intensive care unit housing patients who have had open heart surgery. On the other hand, one professional nurse and one practical nurse or one nurse-aide per unit of 5 or 6 patients per tour of duty might be sufficient in a hospital with less specialized services.

A Preliminary Study and Analysis of Nursing Requirements in Neurological and Neurosurgical Nursing.[31] A time study of the nursing care provided for approximately 5,000 patients in a neurologic hospital was conducted for a 3-year period. The experienced and highly specialized nurses spent as much time with the very ill patients on busy days as on slack days. Hence, the burden of the care of the moderately ill was left to untrained auxiliary personnel.

4. Staffing is a function of the nursing facility. That is, the physical layout of the nursing unit either will hamper or enhance the performance of the nurse. Some facilities are more conducive to nursing service than others. Accordingly, fewer nurses may be required.

Hospital Design, Function and Finance by Research in Hospital Planning.[32] This is the report of an interdisciplinary team that investigated factors relating to hospital design. Among the factors considered were the function of the nurse, the pattern of nurses' movements, and functional planning.

New Ideas in Hospital Design Fit New Ideas in Patient Care.[33] Three designs for hospitals planned to incorporate new ideas of patient care are presented by three graduate students of architecture. The designs consider the type and the degree of care required by various groups of patients.

5. The effect of certain staffing configurations also has been considered by a number of studies. Knowledge is available relating staffing to patient and personnel satisfaction.

Effect of Nurse Staffing on Satisfactions With Nursing Care.[34] The study was designed to test the extent to which feelings about the inadequacy of nursing service in general hospitals are related to the daily average number of hours of nursing care available per patient. Feelings about the inadequacy were found to be associated with the amount of care provided. Patient satisfaction was related directly to the amount of professional nursing service available.

Nurse-Patient Relationships in a Hospital Maternity Service.[35] Patients felt that, while their physical requirements were satisfied, their emotional needs were not. One of the main barriers to patient and nurse satisfaction arose from institutional practices that created a segmented assembly-line care.

6. The researcher will learn soon that, in addition to the many diverse and independent studies on nurse staffing, some attempts have been made to link the various elements together. These studies range from the empiric approach to the more rational analysis of the various roles of the nurse.

Patterns of Patient Care.[36] A basic staffing pattern for patient care based upon five studies of nursing service was developed. The studies combined the approach of management engineers and nurses toward the solution of nursing problems, determining better ways of performing many tasks, and improving the physical layout of ward space.

Education of the Nursing Technician.[37] The author diagrammed the concept of nursing function on a continuum. This continuum began with simple functions based on common knowledge, led to intermediate functions requiring skill and some judgment, and culminated in complex functions requiring expert skill and judgment.

We can observe from the studies cited that there is an abundant resource of knowledge on nurse staffing. The studies listed pertain only to the nursing literature. In addition, there is available perhaps a much wider body of related knowledge outside the nursing literature.

But the mere listing of knowledge secured to date will not be sufficient. The researcher must organize and evaluate her resource to consider: Is the knowledge adequate to fulfill the requirements of the assignment? If it is, she may complete her assignment at this point. If it is not, she may ask: What is lacking; what additional knowledge is required?

The researcher will establish a 3-column record from which to specify the need for further research and derive a specific purpose. Knowledge learned to date will be listed in the first column. The middle sector will evaluate these contributions. The requirements for additional study or knowledge will be listed in the third column.

The researcher has learned that there are many causal factors of which nurse staffing is a function: the numbers of nursing personnel, the quality of nursing personnel, the type of patient to be cared for, and the physical facility. These factors were isolated from a series of empiric, descriptive-type studies of an exploratory nature. Does the researcher feel satisfied that there are true functional relationships between the factors and staffing? Are there any more relationships to be explored?

She has learned that some of the effects of particular patterns of nurse staffing configurations also have been isolated: the effect upon patient satisfaction, upon nurse satisfaction. These, too, were derived from empiric, descriptive-type studies. Have these relationships been tested adequately? What of the other effects, especially of the patient's condition? Can a relationship be derived between each of the factors specified above and each of the effects? Can the derived relationships be tested?

She may question the meaning of these empirically derived relationships. The knowledge was secured generally from observations of the practices in existing situations. For example, the nurse-patient ratios cited simply reflect the staffing arrangement on the day or the days when the observations were made. They indicate that so many nurses were serving so many patients. They do not indicate how the ratios were derived, how they relate to the number and the kinds of nurses available, and, above all, how they relate to the requirements for care of the patients. Therefore, it may be best to approach the assignment from the explanative level. That is, the researcher might attempt to develop a frame of reference in which each of the causal factors and their related effects can be merged with the suggested conceptual patterns. The interaction of one set of variables with the other then can be studied in a more meaningful way.

STATEMENT OF PURPOSE

There are perhaps many requirements for additional knowledge in this area. It becomes obvious immediately that the committee's assignments cannot be answered in one fell swoop. Perhaps several studies may be proposed at the descriptive and the predictive levels. The researcher may even decide to investigate the problem area at the explanative level..

It also becomes obvious that the individual investigator cannot provide all the necessary answers in a single study. Nor should she attempt to do so. Only one factor at a time can be isolated and studied. Thus, the nurse researcher can study the effect of the numbers of nurses independently of the quality of the nursing care, or the kind of patient to be cared for, or the type of facility. The true effect of any factor will remain undetected as long as it is treated in combination with the other factors.

Knowledge gained through research in nursing, as in other areas of endeavor, is to be accumulated over the course of time. While one investigator may make several contributions, several investigators will contribute the bulk of the knowledge. A coordinated effort is essential. Unnecessary duplication should be avoided and studies should occur in sequence. The revelation of new knowledge often is dependent upon the awareness of some previous knowledge. Concentrated efforts should be made in the areas of greatest need.

But how can a diversified group of independent researchers co-ordinate their efforts? The source of written knowledge is perhaps the most useful medium of exchange in this regard. If the individual researcher can scrutinize this resource carefully and derive the next contribution to be made, she will assume her role among the team of researchers.

Essentially, the procedure that we have followed leads in this direction. The remaining question is: What is the next contribution to be made? What purpose can be derived as our specific contribution to the area of knowledge concerning nurse staffing?

The ultimate requirement is to provide some predictive statements, formulae or directives that can be applied by the nurse supervisor when she makes her nursing assignments. She desires a recipe suggesting that so many nurses are to be blended with so many patients to produce a cake of effective patient care. The problem perhaps is that we are not aware of all the ingredients to be blended; we do not know the rules for mixing the components; we may not even know what the end-product, effective patient care, may be like. The researcher may decide, therefore, that she is not ready to perform predictive-level research in this area.

Nevertheless, the researcher is aware that predictive-level research is fed by the products of descriptive and/or explanative-level research. In what direction should she concentrate her effort?

In scrutinizing and evaluating the large array of previous knowledge, the researcher may decide that the most crucial area of need is to describe adequately the end-product, the effects of nursing care. She may determine that the primary measure of effectiveness currently employed is patient satisfaction: the expressed feelings of the patient about the type of care received. Is this a sufficient criterion, or are more appropriate criteria required? Before she can truly evaluate the knowledge relevant to nurse staffing accumulated to date, and develop predictive statements, the effects of nursing care should be identified and described.

On the other hand, the researcher may determine that the nursing literature is saturated with an avalanche of unrelated descriptive-level studies. There has been accumulated a series of independent descriptive studies on numbers of nurses, nursing functions, patients' satisfaction, nurses' satisfaction and nursing facilities. Each has proceeded along relatively independent lines. There has been little or no attempt to interrelate the various components of nursing care. It may be difficult at this time even to describe the concept of nursing care, much less its effects.

The researcher, therefore, may seek to develop a model interrelating nursing care and its component parts. She may decide that we have sufficient descriptive-level knowledge upon which to construct an effective framework. However, it is necessary to provide some channel for understanding, to link together the *various* elements and allow future observations to be more meaningful. The model will serve to integrate the previous research and suggest not one but many additional requirements for further study.

The development of a miniature model follows. It has been expressed in outline form. The presentation may serve to demonstrate how the vast number of independent studies in nursing can be ordered properly and the requirements for future projects established.

The Development of a Model

The model to be constructed is intended to yield an understanding of the requirements for staffing.* When completed, it should produce a set of underlying components or constructs from which nurse staffing configurations can be derived logically. It is based upon the premise that the various nurse staffing patterns did not arise by chance but constituted responses to the demands of certain antecedent conditions. Knowledge of these preliminary conditions or events, however, was not recorded and became lost in the maze of developments following the establishment of the particular staffing configuration. The patterns remained, but without a foundation. If we could retrace and re-establish these anticipatory situations in nursing, a basis for nurse staffing also could be redetermined. It is the purpose of this model to stimulate the array of underlying circumstances on paper and to reconstruct these events.

A Reconstruction of the Past

There were probably many instances in the course of early history when the incapacitated man was abandoned and suc-

---

* Preliminary work done by one of the authors (Meyer) in a research study in this area. (See Abdellah, F. G., *et al.*, Patient-Centered Approaches to Nursing, p. 51, New York, Macmillan, 1960.)

cumbed to the elements. On some occasions, however, he was assisted and even may have managed to survive. Perhaps he was merely comforted; he may have been fed; and no doubt there were times when crude attempts were made to correct whatever incapacitated him. When that situation arose in which he was first assisted, whatever the circumstance, the practice of patient care began.

The practice grew with the passage of time. More people were assisted; more people were comforted and sustained and had their impairments corrected. In the course of this development, learning took place. On the one hand, people learned to seek assistance when in need. On the other hand, something was learned of the mechanics of giving care: comforting, sustaining and correcting. Something was learned also about the human organism, why it became incapacitated and in what ways it could be assisted. Technics were developed and a body of knowledge was accumulated.

As the body of knowledge grew and was disseminated, more people became aware of the art and the practice of giving care. Some began to practice patient care more frequently and more skillfully than others. Some became more adept at comforting, sustaining or correcting. They even may have been called upon or directed specifically to perform their acquired skills. The art of patient care flourished and a group of specialists came into being.

The practitioners also learned that they were not without assistance in their art. They discovered potions that had curative values. They developed and utilized equipment to compensate for their own limitations. They found it better to house their patients and equipment and to conduct their practice in special facilities. Thus, there also was accumulated a storage of specially devised equipment and facilities.

It may be supposed that, in the process of being assisted, the patient or the recipient of care would have acquired a special type of feeling or source of satisfaction. This feeling may have been such that, when future states of impairment arose, an urgent need would be felt for the assistance that was received formerly. He actually may have been urged or forced to seek the assistance. Upon each occasion when assistance was given and satisfaction was derived, the need for care would have been strengthened. Thus, perhaps a special order of need was acquired. It was man-made and initiated on special occasions. In time, it became accepted almost universally. However, we might consider also what happened upon those occasions when the assistance offered was not satisfying. Three alternatives may be conjectured: the patient remained incapacitated and perhaps even failed to survive: he sought the assistance of another practitioner; or both the patient and the practitioner persisted until the kind of assistance or care was developed that was satisfying to the patient. It was perhaps as a result of the latter state of affairs that the body of practices grew and were augmented. Thus, the specific needs for care may have fostered the growth and the development of practice and become the basis for specific types of practice.

An Underlying Assumption

The model is based upon the assumption that nursing is composed of an accumulation of activities created and shaped by man to satisfy the requirements of the human being for assistance. Therefore, all nursing functions should be derived from a study of the normal human being and of the patient and his requirements for care or assistance as administered by a nurse. Nursing would cease to exist if people had no need for care.

A Concept of the Whole

In accordance with the underlying assumption, the researcher must initiate her study of nursing with the patient. The requirements for nursing personnel can be derived ultimately from a study of this person. The total framework can be cast in the form of a triangle at whose apex lies the patient, radiating a series of requirements for nursing personnel. The patient can be described by his needs for nursing care, which yield a picture of those nursing services required to satisfy his needs. Since the services are to be performed by nurses, they can be translated accordingly into numbers and kinds of nursing personnel.

The single triangle may describe the requirements of the single patient. However, several patients may be grouped into the various combinations to produce a variety of nurse staffing patterns. Thus, while the requirements for nursing personnel are initiated from a study of the patient, the requirements for staffing may be derived when patients are treated as a group.

A Concept of the Parts

1. **The Patient.** A patient will be described as a person who requires care. This person may be portrayed in many ways. It is the purpose here to limit the description to those characteristics of the person that may necessitate the services of a nurse. Certain terms have been invented to assist in this regard. They pertain only to the meanings assigned in the discussions to follow.

Three characteristics of the person may interplay to produce a need for nursing care. They will be termed: personal need, self-help ability and an impaired state.

A. *Personal Need.* When a person is deprived of one of the essentials for optimal living, a state of need may be said to exist. The need may be primary, if it is unlearned and basic to the survival of the individual. It may be acquired or learned, if it is not basic to survival: through learning it has acquired characteristics of primary needs.

B. *Self-Help Ability.* An important attribute of the person is his ability to help himself and provide for the satisfaction of his personal needs. Every individual is endowed to some extent with self-help ability. Persons will vary in this regard as a function of their innate physical emotions, capacities, levels of maturation and learning, type of environment and available resources.

C. *Impairment State.* An impairment of the body or the person may reduce self-help ability to a condition limiting the individual's ability to satisfy his personal needs. The impaired state may result from injury, disease, malfunction or maldevelopment.

2. **Need for Nursing Care.** The three characteristics of the patient may be conceived as interacting and creating a condition requiring nursing care. An impaired state may lower self-help ability to such a degree that the patient, of his own accord, cannot satisfy some of his personal needs. He may require a nurse to assist him. It may be desirable, in addition, to strengthen the self-help ability in anticipation of an impending or a threatening impaired state. The nurse also may assist the patient to attain this strengthened ability.

Thus, two general requirements for nursing care can be derived: one to compensate for a lowered self-help ability, and the other to enhance self-help ability. The former will be designated as the need for impairment care and the latter as the need for preventive care.

A. *Need for Impairment Care.* This need will be occasioned by an impaired state. Care directed toward this end may serve three functions: to sustain the individual and assist him to satisfy his personal needs; to treat, correct or reduce the impairment; and to restore the self-help ability to its normal state.

B. *Need for Preventive Care.* This need may arise to ward off or prevent an impaired state. The aim of preventive care is to raise self-help ability from a normal to a plus condition.

3. **Nursing Services.** The kinds of assistance to be provided by the nurse to fulfill the patient's needs for care can be described in the form of nursing services. These services are to be directed toward the specific objectives just discussed. They may be characterized in terms of the kind and the amount of care required.

A. *Kind of Care.* The kind of care required by the patient can be described by a series of activities to be performed by the nurse. The activities may be exercised directly by the nurse or indirectly when she is called upon to assist some other member of the medical or the nursing staff.

The activities, of course, should relate directly to and be derived from the patient's requirements for nursing care. Impairment care, for example, will be composed of a series of sustenal, remedial and restorative activities. Sustenal activities will consume an array of functions to assist the patient to satisfy his personal needs, e.g., eating, bathing, eliminating bodily wastes. Remedial activities, such as administering medication, will be directed toward the reduction of an impairment. Restorative activities will entail a set of teaching functions to assist the patient or some member of his family to perform sustenal care activities independently of the nurse. Preventive care also will involve a variety of activities. They may vary from administering a vaccine to a number of teaching functions such as assisting a diabetic patient to exercise proper foot care.

A series of peripheral activities also may be identified that are to be performed by nurses in support of the more direct care activities. These activities stem from the need to plan and evaluate periodically a program of patient care.

B. *Amount of Care.* The amount of care required by the patient can be measured by its intensity and duration. Some nursing activities may involve an extensive amount of nursing participation upon a single occasion; other activities may necessitate minimal participation. The activities may vary also in duration. That is, they may be administered over a short or a long period of time, on only one occasion or periodically.

4. **Nursing Personnel.** Nursing services are functions to be performed by nurses. The component parts of this category can be transcribed and summated to yield the kinds and the numbers of nursing personnel required to satisfy the derived requirements for nursing services. That is, the kind of care or activities should suggest a set of skills possessed or acquired by nursing personnel of a particular quality. The amount of care may be translated into some quantitative function indicative of the numbers of the various categories of required nursing personnel.

A. *Level of Skill.* The activities may vary in complexity. Some may involve little or no judgment and can be performed by nurses with minimal skill, experience and training. Another group of activities can be classified in accordance with the amount of highly specialized technical knowledge required.

These activities may be planned and performed under supervision, but their performance requires a person who has developed sufficient technical ability. Lastly, there remains a category of activities that suggest requirements for independent action. In this regard, the nurse must have sufficient understanding of the situation to be aware of the consequences of one course rather than another course of action.

B. *Numbers of Nurses.* The level-of-skill category suggests three classifications of nurses. An estimate of the amount of care required for nursing activity (as measured by intensity and duration) may be derived from a study of the single patient care plan. This estimate should be translatable into the numbers of each classification of nurses required per tour of duty. The accumulation of the several patient care plans of a nursing unit should suggest the numbers of each classification of nurses required per tour of duty for the entire nursing unit.

The model has been summarized in Figures 2 and 3. They may provide the reader with a feeling for the total configuration as well as for the interrelations among the parts.

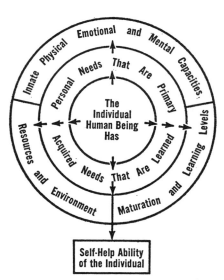

Fɪɢ. 2. The personal needs and the self-help ability of the individual human being.

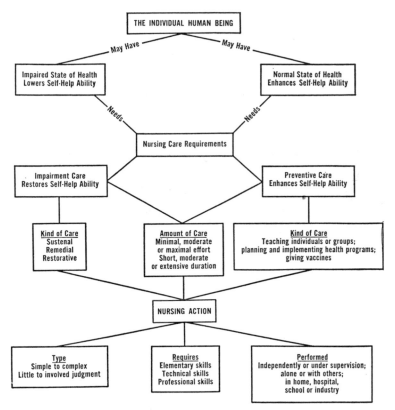

Fig. 3. A model for deriving nursing care requirements and action from the needs of individual patients.

An Application of the Model

This model represents a structure by which the researcher can bind together the various studies in nursing. It can be considered as a rough classification system of nursing knowledge pertaining to staffing. That is, it suggests a means for interrelating the rather large accumulation of independent knowledge in this area and determining how each study may impinge upon the desired outcome—the derivation of nurse staffing patterns. Above all, the model will suggest the requirements for further study.

This structure has several limitations. The model rests upon an assumption that, if unfounded, could upset the total framework. Also, it has been developed about certain concepts that require stringent definitions and that must be anchored securely to observable, concrete events. The model is far from complete. There are other factors to be answered that also impinge upon staffing, such as the facility, the team concept, the supervision. The model should allow for the introduction of these factors. Lastly, there are huge gaps within the framework that are devoid of knowledge.

However, these limitations may be twisted about to represent the model's most useful application: the derivation of not one but many requirements for interrelated study. The researcher can examine the gaps within the structure and attempt to piece together the missing parts. She will employ existing knowledge first. Whatever remains will compose a hierarchy of research projects.

It may be surmised at this point that many worthy projects can be derived at each level of inquiry. Below is a sampling of what can be done.

Descriptive Level of Inquiry

Among the first steps to be taken is to fulfill the requirements to isolate, identify and describe the various components of the model. It also is necessary to describe some unit of measurement that can be employed to manipulate and evaluate the interaction of the different components. Then an attempt can be made to depict and isolate a series of empiric relationships.

1. **To Identify the Components.** The model suggests that nursing care can be conceived to stem from an actual or an impending impairment state. A system is required to classify, describe and list the various impairment states. The researcher may then proceed to isolate the components of the model as a function of each classification of the impairment states. For example, if we assume that she starts with Impairment State X, her tasks may include the following:

To identify self-help ability minus conditions resulting as a function of Impairment State X

To identify personal needs to be sustained as a function of Impairment State X

To describe sustenal (remedial or restorative) requirements for nursing care as a function of Impairment State X

To identify the nursing activities needed to satisfy the sustenal (remedial or restorative) care requirements as a function of Impairment State X

To determine the intensity (or duration) needed to perform Nursing Care Activity A to satisfy sustenal (remedial or restorative) care requirements as a function of Impairment State X

To determine the effect of Nursing Care Activity A given at I Intensity for D Duration upon the sustenal (remedial or restorative) care requirements as a function of Impairment State X.

2. **To Describe the Unit of Measurement.** A companion sequence of studies concerns the need to devise functional units of measurement descriptive of each component. The components displayed in the sequence of studies are constructs that should be tied concretely to observable events. For example, the researcher should devise technics to measure and describe impairment states, self-help ability, personal needs, care requirements, intensity, duration and levels of skill. This series of studies will permit the researcher to deal more constructively

with the problem that has plagued the nurse researcher for a long time: how to determine and measure the effects of nursing care.

Explanative Level of Inquiry

There are many relationships eluding the researcher at the descriptive level of inquiry that would become apparent at the explanative level. The value of the model in construct form enables the researcher to manipulate the components of care and derive these otherwise elusive relationships. Here are some examples:

With the current shortage of nurses, it is fairly common practice to concentrate skilled professional nursing services among the more intensely ill patients. There is also the feeling that the comparatively well patient requires little or no nursing care.[38] In accordance with the model, however, this state of affairs may not be the case. The seriously ill patient may require a series of highly technical services to assist in the reduction of the impairment state and some relatively low-level sustenal services to satisfy personal needs. On the other hand, the recuperating patient may require some intense and highly professional services of long duration to restore self-help ability and enable him to become independent of the nurse. Accordingly, the following relationship may be derived: as the need for remedial service diminishes, the requirement for restorative service may rise.

People do not seek out preventive care as they would impairment care. Why? The model will explain that impairment care results when an actual impairment state produces a situation in which a person is unable to satisfy some personal needs. This will force him into the care situation. However, preventive care is given in response to an anticipated impairment state. The intrinsic requirement to satisfy personal need is lacking. Accordingly, the following relationship may be derived: the need for preventive care will be a function of some extrinsic form of motivation such as fear, the desire to please someone, and the like.

The researcher can proceed to derive countless studies in this one area of nursing. Each project can be expressed by a specific purpose suggesting another contribution to the body of knowledge organized within the model. The framework will serve as a standard by which knowledge is put in order and evaluated. When the specific contributions are placed in their proper positions within the framework, the researcher can determine more accurately the next step to be taken.

REFERENCES

1. New York Times Magazine, p. 42, Sept. 6, 1959.
2. Bernard, Claude: An Introduction to the Study of Experimental Medicine, pp. 41-42, New York, Dover, 1865; Eng. Trans., 1927.
3. *Ibid.,* p. 34.
4. Morse, W. C., and Wingo, G. M.: Psychology and Teaching, pp. 462-464, New York, Scott, Foresman, 1955.
5. Cronbach, L. J., *et al.*: Text Materials in Modern Education, p. 31, Urbana, Ill., Univ. Illinois Press, 1955.
6. *Ibid.,* p. 32.
7. Black, Max: Critical Thinking, An Introduction to Logic and Scientific Method, pp. 362-363, Englewood, Prentice-Hall, Inc., 1946.
8. Taylor, R.: Hunger in the infant, Amer. J. Dis. Child. *14*:233-256, 1917.
9. Guthrie, E. R.: Conditioning, a Theory of Learning in Terms of Stimulus, Response, and Association in the Psychology of Learning, p. 39, National Society for the Study of Education, Forty-first Yearbook, 1942.
10. Watson, J. B.: Psychology from the Standpoint of a Behaviorist, p. 232, Philadelphia, Lippincott, 1924.
11. Ayer, A. J.: Logical Positivism, p. 18, Glencoe, Ill., Free Press, 1959.
12. Ingle, D. J.: Principles of Research in Biology and Medicine, p. 24, Philadelphia, Lippincott, 1958.
13. Black, Max: *Op. cit.* (see Ref. 7), p. 296.
14. Lincoln, Barnett: The Universe and Dr. Einstein, p. 29, 2nd rev. ed., New York, Sloane, 1957.
15. Black, Max: *Op. cit.* (see Ref. 7), pp. 336-339.
16. Hull, C. L.: Principles of Behavior, p. 21, New York, Appleton-Century-Crofts, 1946.
17. Black, Max: *Op. cit.* (see Ref. 7), pp. 336-337.
18. New, P. K., Nite, G., and Callahan, J.: Nursing Service and Patient Care: A Staffing Experiment, Kansas City, Mo., Community Studies, Inc., 1959.
19. Hughes, Everett, *et al.*: Twenty Thousand Nurses Tell Their Story, Philadelphia, Lippincott, 1958.
20. A study of turnover and its costs, Hospitals *29*:59, 1955.

21. Research and ANA program for studies of nursing functions, Amer. J. Nurs. *50*:770, 1950.
22. Miller, M. A.: Institutional nursing *in* Cowan, C. (ed.): The Yearbook of Modern Nursing, p. 197, New York, Putnam, 1957-1958.
23. Geister, J.: The trouble is not lack of nurses, it's lack of sense in using them, Mod. Hosp. *89* (No. 2):63, 1957.
24. Stafford, B. J., and Scholtfeldt, R. M.: Nursing Service Staffing and Quality of Nursing Care, Nurs. Res. *9*:149-154, 1960.
25. Bredenberg, Viola: Nursing Service Research, Philadelphia, Lippincott, 1951.
26. New, P., *et al.*: *Op. cit.* (see Ref. 18).
27. Hanson, H. C., and Stecklein, J. E.: A Study of Nursing Functions in General Hospitals in the State of Minnesota, St. Paul, Minnesota Nurses Assn., 1955.
28. Ford, T. R., and Stephenson, D. D.: Institutional Nurses: Roles, Relationships and Attitudes in Three Alabama Hospitals, Univ. Alabama Press, 1954.
29. A Study of Nursing Functions in 12 Hospitals in the State of New York, New York Univ., 1952.
30. Halderman, J. C., and Abdellah, F. G.: Concepts of Progressive Patient Care, Reprinted from Hospitals (May 16 and June 1, 1959) by U. S. Dept. of Health, Education and Welfare.
31. Flanagan, E. C., and Herdan, I. M.: A preliminary study and analysis of nursing requirements in neurological and neurosurgical nursing, Canad. Nurse *51*:855, 1955.
32. Heyward, Jean: Hospital design, function and finance by research in hospital planning, Nurs. Times *53*:346, 1957.
33. New ideas in hospital design fit new ideas in patient care, Mod. Hosp. *93*:73, 1959.
34. Abdellah, F. G., and Levine, E.: Effect of Nurse Staffing on Satisfactions With Nursing Care, Hospital Monograph Series No. 4, Chicago, Ill., American Hospital Assn.
35. Lesser, M. S., and Keane, V. R.: Nurse-Patient Relationships in a Hospital Maternity Service, New York, Mosby, 1956.
36. George, F. L., and Kuehn, R. P.: Patterns of Patient Care, New York, Macmillan, 1955.
37. Montag, Mildred: Education of the Nursing Technician, New York, Putnam, 1951.
38. Halderman, C., and Abdellah, F. G.: *Op. cit.* (see Ref. 30).

CHAPTER 4

The Statement of the Problem

It was suggested previously that research is a form of problem-solving—for a very special purpose, and performed in a carefully defined manner. Once the specific purpose of a research project has been stated, the researcher can begin the problem-solving. His first task is to state the problem. What is it? How does it differ from purpose? What are the various types of problems? How is it derived? How is it stated? This chapter will present a detailed discussion of the matter of a problem.

WHAT IS A PROBLEM?

The term problem often is misunderstood. It was described in the first chapter as a "felt difficulty." The terms general problem area and underlying, common and specific problems also have been mentioned. We shall speak soon of a procedural problem. Purpose and problem often are confused and used interchangeably. What is the meaning of each of these terms? How do they interrelate?

A "felt difficulty" is an obstacle to a goal. For example, a motorist may enter a strange community for a predetermined appointment. Lacking a map and being unfamiliar with the town's layout, he may be unable to locate the place of his appointment and thus will be blocked from keeping the appointment. It may be conceived also as a question requiring an answer or, as Burton *et al.* have suggested, "a situation involving doubt" or a "puzzle."[1]

The attribute of "blockage" or "doubt" does not fully substantiate the existence of a problem. Burton *et al.* have indicated that the problem should be correlated with the problem-solving process or with a problem-solving situation.[2] The latter formerly was defined as a situation "in which an answer is required to a question in the absence of reliable information concerning the appropriate procedures to be adopted."[3] These authors would contend, therefore, that a queston for which there is an answer does not constitute a true problem. For instance, if the slightly bewildered motorist stopped at a service station and secured complete and detailed directions, he may not truly have had a problem. On the other hand, Burton *et al.* would contend that a true problem must be capable of being solved in a rational manner.[4] That is, the problem-solver should not be so completely bewildered that he does not know how to proceed, or proceeds blindly. If the motorist simply is instructed to proceed to town X to keep an appointment, without being told with whom and exactly where the appointment is to be kept, he may be in such a state of bewilderment. This situation does not lend itself to the problem-solving process.

We may piece together these considerations and arrive at a preliminary definition of "problem." It contains an obstacle or a blockage to a goal. It may be conceived as a question about the way in which the obstacle can be overcome or circumvented. It lacks an available and known answer but can be submitted to the process of problem-solving. Lastly, it is perceived by the problem-solver as a "felt difficulty."

The terms "general problem area," "underlying," "common," "specific" and "procedural" problems are used here to pinpoint the meaning of the term "problem." Each has its own unique meaning, which is stated in this chapter.

General Problem Area

The general problem area may be the reason for getting started. It is the motivating factor that sets the stage for an inquiry. It is the situation for which a company seeks an answer, which the professional society recommends as an area for research, for which the government will contribute funds, and about which the individual researcher is curious.

The general problem area may have some but not necessarily all of the attributes of a problem. The very fact that it was selected is an index of a "felt difficulty." It is generally a puzzle, a source of bewilderment, an area of doubt or an obstacle to a goal. It may be phrased as a question: What is the cause of cancer? How can buyer resistance be overcome? Should capital punishment be abolished? But it may not satisfy some of the other criteria. For example, answers to each of these problems may exist. The researcher need only cite the appropriate source. On the other hand, the problem area may not be amenable to the problem-solving process; e.g.: How many stars are in the sky?

The researcher should employ the general problem area as a point of departure. That is, it may serve as his reason for getting started. Then he may attempt to isolate the true problems, depicting what is already known and what is to be made known. A specific purpose for his particular project can be derived from this analysis.

PROBLEM AND PURPOSE

The terms problem and purpose often have been confused. A purpose is not a problem, nor is a problem a purpose. A purpose has been defined here as an aim or a goal: to describe, predict or explain a solution to a situation. It is a task to be accomplished. "A task," as Burton *et al.* describe it, "is a job-to-be-done, and not a problem to-be-solved."[5] The problem is the situation or the circumstance for which the solution is to be described, predicted or explained. Thus the problem is associated with the specific purpose of the research project. It is not the purpose itself.

However, the problem should be related directly to the specific purpose. If it is not, then the intent of the research project, as exemplified by the specific purpose, is not being pursued.

For example, if the specific purpose is to describe a cause, then the problem should be: What is the cause?—and not: What is the effect? or What is the relationship? The purpose states the aim of the project. The problem-solving process is intended to carry out the aim or the purpose. A problem is stated as the first step of the problem-solving process. Therefore, it should be derived directly from the specific purpose.

Underlying, Common or Specific Problems

An underlying, common or specific problem, as distinct from the general problem area, should display all the attributes of a problem. Each differs with regard to the level at which the problem is conceived. One is more abstract than the other. One can be derived from the other.

A mother observes that her 2-year-old child clings to an old blanket. She will not leave the house without the blanket. How to assist the child to do without this article has become a very *specific* problem for this mother.

It may be observed that other parents have similar problems. Their 2-, 3-, 4- and 5-year-old children cling to old blankets, rag dolls or articles of clothing. Some of the children must have the object at all times; others simply desire it on particular occasions, such as at bedtime. Each parent has a specific problem with her child. Yet the parents share a common problem. A solution derived from this *common* problem may relate to each of the specific problems.

It may be observed that adults themselves create similar problems. A psychiatric patient rejects the hospital garb and clings to the clothing she wore when she entered the hospital. We also tend to revert to old habits in times of stress. In other words, there may be a relationship between "identity with the familiar" and the need to be secure. A problem of this type may occur at any time, at any place, for or with anyone. It seems to *underlie* each of the other problems.

The underlying problem is the most abstract. It underlies the common and the specific problems, which, in turn, can be derived from an underlying problem. The specific problem is the most concrete and relates to a unique situation. It can be derived from a common as well as from an underlying problem.

Each of the problems may be expressed also in relation to the specific purpose. If it is the intent or the specific purpose of the researcher to isolate knowledge that has universal application and underlies all situations, then he will state an underlying problem. This is usually the assignment of a basic researcher. The applied researcher usually will pursue knowledge related to common situations within a given field of endeavor, or he may seek to apply underlying knowledge to common situations within a given field of endeavor. In either case, he will state a common problem. Lastly, the action researcher, whose concern is the answer to a unique situation, will state a specific problem.

A specific problem must be derived ultimately, no matter what the original statement of the problem was. The research process requires an empiric test of the solution derived or to be derived. That is, the researcher must locate or concoct a real situation, reconstruct his problem and test his proposed solution. Underlying and common problems, however, are abstractions. "Identity with the familiar" and "the need to be secure" are merely concepts or words. They may describe a series of specific situations that seem to have these factors in common. But they do not exist in reality. Therefore, the researcher must derive the specific problem situation depicted by the underlying or common problem situation under investigation.

He also must consider how he will test his derived solution. This is his procedural problem. Often undue and premature emphasis is placed upon a procedural problem. The researcher may concentrate upon how he will collect data or facts before he actually has determined the reason for collecting the facts. The procedural problem of "how to test" should wait upon and be derived from the specific problem of "what to test."

HOW IS THE PROBLEM STATED?

The statement of the problem is a focal point in the development of a research project. It will link the specific purpose to the derivation of the solution. How it is stated will be affected directly by the derivation and the statement of the specific purpose. How it is stated will affect the derivation of the solution.

Let us look back to the derivation of the specific purpose and consider its effect upon the statement of the problem. What has been done? We started with a broadly stated general problem area and delimited its scope to something that requires an answer and can be subjected to the problem-solving process. We may have segmentalized the general problem area into an orderly series of specific problems and selected the most urgent requirement as the specific purpose. Therefore, the statement of the specific purpose has determined the problem, limited its scope, and specified the level of investigation as underlying, common or specific.

The task ahead is to find a solution to the stated problem. The solution will be derived through a process of reasoning and will be subjected to an empiric test. The rational solution is essentially a paper solution or one that is contrived and established in the thoughts of the researcher and set down on paper. The researcher, like the architect, will construct a model on paper as the solution to his problem. Then he will erect his model in a realistic setting to determine whether or not it actually works. In order to do this properly he must know the kind of solution that is required and the ingredients that will compose his solution. Analogously, the architect cannot develop his blueprints until he knows the kind of house to be built and its make-up. The kind of solution to be expected and the necessary ingredients are to be established in the statement of the problem.

Therefore, two cardinal rules in stating the problem will be cited and discussed:

1. To state a problem adequately is to know the kind of answer that is needed.

This rule is actually a restatement of a statement made by Black.[6] It implies first that the researcher knows what he is looking for—whether it is a cause, an effect, a relationship, a prediction or an explanation. This should be specified in the purpose. It also should be exhibited in the problem.

The researcher may ask: If I know the kind of answer that is needed, do I really have a problem to be solved? or If I know the kind of answer that is needed, am I not biasing my results? To know the kind of answer that is needed does not imply that the investigator knows the answer. To inquire What is the cause? does not imply that the investigator knows the cause. It simply restricts the scope of the investigation to the determination of a cause. This is the intent of the investigation.

To know the kind of answer that is needed also will limit the subject matter of the investigation. The researcher will inquire: The cause of what subject matter?—and will specify the subject matter accordingly. This rule, in essence, instructs the researcher to restrict the range of his study to something highly specific. It will not permit him to seek out "what is in the sky."

2. To state a problem adequately is to know of what it consists.

This rule relates to the first in that it specifies the subject matter, and does so definitively. It requests the researcher to select the terms of his problem and to define them. The enactment of this rule actually will set the stage for problem-solving.

The terms of the problem are the ingredients with which he will construct his model. They may be described, as the authors have implied, as a cause, an effect, a cause-and-effect relationship, a prediction or an explanation. They will be exhibited in accordance with the first rule: to determine the kind of answer that is needed.

Let us erect a series of models to describe the problems cited by the above example. The problems will be displayed symbolically, using the following symbols:

A = A 2-year-old child
B = Carrying an old blanket
C = Contentment
D = A cause-and-effect relationship
E = Being in the presence of the mother
f = function

G = Sucking the thumb

1. *Given:*   *To Determine:*

The function $\boxed{B}$ upon $\boxed{A}$ = $\boxed{C}$

Problem: What is the effect (C) of B (carrying an old blanket) upon A (a 2-year-old child)? The unknown, or the kind of answer that is needed (to be determined) is C (an effect). The terms to be defined are what is given or known—A (a 2-year-old child) and B (carrying an old blanket).

2. *Given:*   *To Determine:*

$\boxed{C}$ of $\boxed{A}$ = a function of $\boxed{B}$

Problem: What is the cause (B) of C (contentment) of A (2-year-old child)? The unknown or the kind of answer that is needed (to be determined) is B (a cause). The terms to be defined are what is given or known—C (contentment) and A (a 2-year-old child).

3. *Given:*   *To Determine:*

The function $\boxed{B}$ and $\boxed{C}$ = $\boxed{D}$

Problem: What is the relationship (D) of B (carrying an old blanket) and C (contentment)? The unknown or the kind of answer that is needed (to be determined) is D (a relationship). The terms to be defined are what is given or known—B (carrying an old blanket) and C (contentment).

4. *Given:*   *To Predict:*

a. f $\boxed{B}$ upon $\boxed{A}$ = $\boxed{C}$ f $\boxed{B}$ upon $\boxed{A}$ = $\boxed{C}$

b. $\boxed{C}$ of $\boxed{A}$ = f $\boxed{B}$ $\boxed{C}$ of $\boxed{A}$ = f $\boxed{B}$

c. f $\boxed{B}$ and $\boxed{C}$ = $\boxed{D}$ f $\boxed{B}$ and $\boxed{C}$ = $\boxed{D}$

Problems: a. Does B (carrying an old blanket) have the effect C (contentment) upon A (a 2-year-old child)?

b. Is the effect C (contentment) upon A (a 2-year-old child) the result of B (carrying an old blanket)?

c. Is there a D relationship (cause-and-effect) between B (carrying an old blanket) and C (contentment)?

The unknown(s) or the kind of answer(s) needed (to be predicted) is that the total proposition(s) will hold true. The terms (wherever applicable) to be defined are each term in the proposition(s)—A (2-year-old child), B (carrying an old blanket) C (contentment), and D (the relationship between carrying an old blanket and contentment).

5. *Given:*   *To Explain:*

a. $f\boxed{B}$ upon $\boxed{A} = \boxed{C}$ $f\boxed{B} = f\boxed{E} = f\boxed{G}$

(B will cause C effect upon A)

and

b. $\boxed{C}$ of $\boxed{A} = f\boxed{E}$

(E will cause C effect upon A)

and

c. $f\boxed{G}$ and $\boxed{C} = \boxed{D}$

[G (cause) and C (effect) constitute a cause-and-effect relationship]

Problem: Does B (carrying an old blanket) and E (being in the presence of the mother) and G (sucking the thumb) have the same effect (C) (contentment) upon A (a 2-year-old child)? The unknown or the kind of answer that is needed (to be explained) is that the function of B is the same as the function of E and the function of G. The terms to be defined are A (a 2-year-old child), B (carrying an old blanket), C (contentment), D (a relationship between sucking the thumb and contentment), E (being in the presence of the mother), and G (sucking the thumb).

This series of models exemplifies conditions at the descriptive, the predictive and the explanative levels of research. The purpose of each is implied and the derived problem is stated. The terms and the kinds of answers that are needed are also cited. Two or more terms may be selected for definition. The number and the kind of terms to be defined are a function in each case of the kind of answer that is needed. That is, the terms are the ingredients required to produce the kind of answer that is needed.

The mere selection and designation of terms will not suffice in themselves to produce an appropriate solution. They also must be adequately defined or described. The definitions serve a very useful and necessary function. They will influence the progress of the researcher in his problem-solving efforts. They will specify the direction that he will pursue. They will limit the available resources of past knowledge. Lastly, they will affect the manner by which he ultimately will test his solutions. Therefore, the definitions should be formulated carefully.

The progress of the researcher may be advanced or deterred by the manner in which he defines his terms. The terms are merely words, and words are abstractions that may or may not be descriptive of a specific concrete event. The terms also describe the thoughts of the researcher as he attempts to relate them to himself and to others. If he fails to communicate these thoughts adequately to himself, then he cannot establish a sequence of logical operations that will link the terms and produce the kind of answer that is required. If he communicates the wrong meaning to himself, then he may produce erroneous answers. If he fails to communicate adequately to his readers, then his research project and the knowledge contributed will have meaning only to himself. These difficulties of communication tend to accelerate as the researcher moves in the direction of the underlying problem and toward the level of explanation.

The direction to be pursued by the researcher will be influenced also by the definition of terms. If he defines his terms in the language of the specific situation, he must solve only the specific problem. He cannot produce a solution that will be applicable to other situations. Furthermore, he will restrict the fund of past knowledge to that which relates only to the terms of his problem.

Consider the examples. If the definitions pertain to a very particular 2-year-old boy, a very particular act of carrying an old blanket, and a very particular kind of contentment, then the investigator will search for knowledge and derive solutions that are akin to his definitions. Since the situation described by these very particular definitions may not recur frequently, it is unlikely that additional knowledge applicable to this very particular situation can be located. If, on the other hand, the definitions are broadened to include young children, familiar objects and general contentment, a larger fund of knowledge may be available in the child-development literature. Furthermore, if the definitions are broadened to relate to the concepts of identity with the familiar and the need to be secure, then a much larger fund of knowledge will be available in the general psychological literature. Indeed, it will be difficult to solve the problem at the level of explanation unless the more abstract definitions are employed.

Nevertheless, the researcher must conceive the specific problem situation in which the solution to be derived will be tested. It is possible that the definition of terms will be so abstract and so general that a highly abstract and general solution will be derived. If this is the case, it may be difficult to define a test situation at the level of reality. The process of moving from the specific to the abstract and back again to the specific is an arduous one. The researcher can first develop the concept "identity with the familiar" from a term such as "carrying an old blanket," and later construe it to mean something entirely different, such as "knowing how to read." Unless a linkage is maintained from one level of abstraction to another, meanings become altered or distorted. The two specific definitions on the ends may become opposite and even contradictory.

Operationalism is the practice of linking the specific to the abstract. An operational definition of terms is one in which "a concept can be defined only in terms of the set of operations that has been assigned to assess it."[7] This statement implies that the results of a research project gain meaning only with respect to the operations that were performed to test them. Just as our system of weights and measures relates only to the standards upon which it is based, so the generalizations derived from a research study relate only to the operations designed and performed to test them.

The researcher may therefore plan a 2-fold definition of terms. He may conceive of the terms in their abstract or generalized form. He may also link or anchor the concepts to one or more specific situations by describing the specific processes or operations implied by each concept. The term contentment, for example, may be described abstractly as a general state of relaxation following need satisfaction and, more concretely, by the behavior of the person, e.g., the child sits quietly, he smiles, his body is not tense, etc. Thus, a series of operational definitions also may be employed.

We can gather from this discussion that the definition of terms should be developed carefully. If the architect does not list exact measurements in his blueprints, the builder will determine soon that the joints of the house may not meet. So it is with the research project. If the terms are defined loosely, the researcher may find that he has been led astray, that he has derived a solution that does not pertain to the problem, that he has become too abstract, that he has become too specific.

The definition of terms relates strictly to the problem under study. It should be performed to facilitate the derivation of an adequate solution. Webster's definitions will not suffice. They were derived for an entirely different purpose. It is incumbent upon the researcher to make the definitions fit the problem.

HOW IS THE PROBLEM DERIVED?

The steps followed in the derivation and the statement of the problem are depicted in Table 3. The relationship of the various problem levels to the various purpose levels is shown. The derivation of the problem from the specific purpose is summarized briefly.

A problem stated at the underlying level is purely hypothetic and exists only on paper. The objective in stating a problem at this level is to derive a solution at the descriptive or the explanative level. Examples are presented of some specific purposes and their related problem statements.

TABLE 3. DERIVATION AND STATEMENT OF A PROBLEM

PROBLEM LEVEL	PURPOSE LEVEL	STATEMENT OF PURPOSE	STATEMENT OF PROBLEM
Underlying (hypothetic: exists only on paper)	To derive a solution a. Describe b. Explain	Given: An effect Purpose. To determine cause Given: A cause Purpose: To determine effect Given: Two events Purpose: To determine a relationship	What is the cause of A from B? What is the effect of A upon B? What is the relationship?
Common (hypothetic: exists only on paper)	1. To derive a solution (see above) 2. To apply a solution (to predict)	(See above) Given: A cause-and-effect relationship Purpose: To determine that the cause leads to the effect	(See above) Does the cause lead to the effect?
Specific (actual)	1. To derive a solution (see above) 2. To apply a solution (see above) 3. To test a hypothesis	(See above) (See above)	(See above) (See above) What are the operations described by the hypothesis?
Procedural (actual)	To test a hypothesis		How can the hypothesis be tested?

A common problem also is hypothetic. It may be derived, however, from the more general or abstract underlying problem. If the common problem is depicted independently of the underlying problem, again it will be the purpose of the researcher to derive a solution. If the common problem relates to the underlying problem, the purpose may be to apply a solution or a generalization derived at the underlying level. The specific purpose and the related problem statement are to determine if the generalization is applicable to the common problem situation.

A specific problem actually exists. It may be derived from an underlying or a common problem or may exist independently (at least for the researcher) of either the underlying or the common problem. If this is the case, then it may be the researcher's purpose to apply a solution or to test a hypothesis (which is actually the application of a solution). All problems depicted initially at the underlying or common-problem level must be derived and tested at the specific-problem level. The problem, in this case, is to determine *what* is to be tested: What are the operations described by the hypothesis? Therefore, it can be stated only after a hypothesis has been derived.

A procedural problem is also a realistic one. It is derived from the specific problem. The objective in stating the procedural problem is to test a hypothesis. In this case, the researcher questions: How can the hypothesis be tested? It, too, can be stated only after a hypothesis has been derived and the specific problem descriptive of this hypothesis has been stated.

THE PLACE OF THE PROBLEM IN NURSING RESEARCH

Observe and compare the following studies in nursing:

1. A Study of Clinic Nursing Service[8]

The purpose of this study was to examine the objectives, policies, organizational pattern, and nursing practices in the University of Illinois Clinics in the light of current trends and generally accepted principles of nursing practice, and to propose recommendations based upon the findings.

Summary of Findings. There was considerable disparity of opinion among the nursing staff about the purposes of the clinics and about the way in which nursing service contributed to meeting these purposes. . . .

The nurses were then asked in what ways they believed nursing service contributed to meeting the objectives of the clinic. Each of the 20 respondents gave more than one answer. All of them felt a responsibility for "keeping the clinic running"; 3 said that this was their primary responsibility. Another named as her chief responsibility assisting in the teaching of medical students. . . .

There was also evidence that lines of authority to the medical and nursing administrative staff needed clarification. The nurse in charge of a given clinic has a dual responsibility: (1) to the department head of the particular clinical specialty . . . ; and (2) to the associate director of nursing. . . . Of the 20 nurses interviewed, 9 recognized this dual responsibility; 11 believed that they were responsible only to the medical group. . . .

The results of time studies for staff and supervising nurses revealed that the responsibilities which they assumed in actual practice were not consistent with the responsibilities outlined in their respective job descriptions. . . .

The level of responsibility for a group of nurses classified as "clinic nurses" was found to need clarification. . . .

An analysis of the time studies revealed that there was a need for studying ways to make a greater amount of nursing time available for the care and teaching of patients. . . .

The amount of nursing time which was diverted into nonprofessional activities indicated the need for making additional auxiliary personnel available.

2. An Evaluation of Nursing Care on an Obstetric Service[9]

(The following statement apparently is the purpose.) This study was undertaken to obtain a qualitative and quantitative comparison of the nursing care given in a well-established Rooming-in program with that given in a traditional maternity ward and nursery.

(The following were listed as conclusions.)

Concerning Nursing Service Hours and Quality of Care. A comparatively inexperienced nursing staff in R5 was observed to provide significantly better care for mothers and babies than was provided by a more experienced staff in T4, in 0.9 hours of nursing service per mother and baby day less than was used in T4. . . . (R5 refers to a Rooming-in ward and T4 a standard maternity ward and nursery.)

Concerning Nursing Education and General Health Education. The frequencies of possible learning opportunities in specific topics of conversation indicated that Rooming-in was a particularly valuable experience for nurses and especially for those who planned to do public health work, since it gave the nurses much more practice in working with families as a unit than did ward and nursery care. . . .

Concerning Nursing Administration. The Rooming-in mothers, on their 1st to 3rd postpartal days, were found to give better care to their babies than nurses and aides gave to ward babies in the nursery. When this was found to be the case, it was realized that fluctuations in census and the general dearth of nursing personnel in the past decade had frequently been responsible for heavy assignments in the nursery. . . .

Concerning the Future of Obstetric Nursing. On the basis of the above findings, the Rooming-in program must be recognized as offering a more professional type of obstetric care to the families, and greater educational opportunity to both student and graduate nurses. However, the real challenge which confronts the nursing profession today in all services, including obstetrics, pivots around the development of team nursing.

3. The Study of Student Anxiety in a Tuberculosis Nursing Situation[10]

. . . the aims of this study were to determine the extent of fear relating to tuberculosis in the student group (nursing students); to develop a tool which might objectively measure this anxiety; and to determine whether anxiety would influence the level of achievement attained by the student.

The Problem. Previous research suggests that the presence of fear or anxiety may impede both learning and the development of positive attitudes. If this is the case, certain important questions must be addressed whenever students are faced with learning experiences that arouse anxiety. In the present study, answers were sought to the following questions:

1. What degree of anxiety is experienced by nursing students who come to the tuberculosis teaching unit?

2. Does the anxiety level change during the tuberculosis nursing experience?

3. What influence does previous experience in communicable disease or tuberculosis nursing have on student anxiety?

4. Is anxiety related to student achievement and performance in the tuberculosis nursing situation?

Conclusions:

1. Nursing students evidenced some anxiety regarding tuberculosis, but this anxiety should not be considered extreme.

2. Anxiety toward the disease decreases slightly during the first 2

weeks of experience, then remains relatively constant for the rest of the experience.

3. Degree program students with previous experience (including previous contact with tuberculosis patients) were significantly less anxious with regard to tuberculosis than were degree program students without previous experience. The same trend was found for diploma program students, but the differences were not statistically significant.

4. No significant relationship was found between a student's performance and achievement and her level of anxiety.

4. Nurse-Doctor Relations and Attitudes Toward the Patient[11]

Purpose. The present study hoped to shed some light on the factors influencing the kinds of interpersonal relations which doctors and nurses establish with each other . . . to investigate the nature of some attitudinal differences of doctors and nurses and the degree to which these influence the quality of the relationships established by the two groups.

Problem. In particular, it (this study) raised two questions:

1. What are some differences in the attitudes doctors and nurses have about the patient?

2. Are these differences related to poor interpersonal relationships between doctors and nurses?

Results. The evidence in Table 1 supports the hypothesis that doctors and nurses differ in their esteem for their typical patient. . . . In summary, then, the doctors and nurses differed in their perceptions of the typical patient mainly with respect to his intellectual ability, his emotional stability and maturity, and his surgency. However, even where differences were not significant, there was a general tendency for the nurses to esteem the patient more than the doctors did. . . .

Thus, the results clearly support the second hypothesis . . . (which concerned the relation between differences in attitude and the interpersonal relations established by doctors and nurses. . . .) The nurses, as a group, held different attitudes toward the patient than did the doctors. Nurses who had those attitudes most strongly were seen as inferior by the doctors. In turn, doctors who differed most from the nurse group were considered inferior by the nurses.

Discussion. The findings indicated definite differences in the attitudes of the doctors and nurses toward the patient, and suggested that these differences influenced the kinds of interpersonal relationships which members of the two groups had with each other. . . .

The first two studies may be characterized perhaps as nonspecific, general and indecisive. The authors apparently had established broad guideposts. They did not confine themselves to a narrow range of subjects. As a consequence, their studies produced broadly stated results that touched upon many topics without satisfying one conclusively.

On the other hand, note how succinctly the second pair of studies can be summarized. The statements of purpose yield clear-cut statements of problem, which, in turn, are answered directly. The results are intended to satisfy the purpose and pertain only to the problem as stated. Thus, they are somewhat more definitive.

The quality of indecisiveness pervades much of the nursing-research literature. Many factors may contribute to this characteristic, such as the absence of a complete and carefully compiled body of nursing knowledge or the desire of the researcher to accomplish too much with the single study. The authors will suggest and explore a third factor—the lack of a direct and positive approach to problem-solving—as a deterrent to the production of more fruitful results.

A discussion in Chapter I indicated that there may not exist a truly direct approach to problem-solving. A certain amount of floundering in the dark, running back and forth mentally, is involved before an adequate solution can be forthcoming. This may be particularly characteristic of problem-solving in research, especially research that touches upon the frontiers of knowledge.

The discussion suggested, however, that some general rules could be prescribed to ease the task of the problem-solver. Among the rules was listed the need for an adequate and clear-cut statement of the problem. While observance of this rule may not lessen the requirements for "running back and forth mentally," it should focus the attention of the problem-solver upon a particular problem and request solutions only in answer to the problem as stated.

The examples cited above were selected to illustrate the need for a clear-cut statement of problem. The so-called "indecisive" studies have not focused upon precisely stated problems. Therefore, they lack the straightforward character of the other two studies, wherein the presence of concise problem statements is evident.

The authors contend that this rule, which specifies the requirement for an adequate statement of the problem, has not been observed carefully by researchers in nursing. The lack of directiveness and its product, indecisiveness, may have resulted as a consequence. The place of the problem in nursing research has not been firmly established as yet.

What is the place of the problem in nursing research? A survey of past and current research activities would not pinpoint the position of this term. It apparently has acquired different meanings and has been employed in different ways. Accordingly, it may be considered that the problem has had not one but several places in nursing research.

A number of questions arise. There is a question of what the problem actually is. There is also a question of when or whether it should be employed. Lastly, there is a question of how meaningfully it should be stated.

THE PROBLEM—WHAT IS IT?

The problem has been utilized in a variety of ways by researchers in nursing. A survey of any issue of any nursing journal will reveal obvious differences. Some researchers never state the problem. Other researchers state the problem, but in different forms and apparently for different reasons.

The following statements were extracted from studies of what were purported to be problems in nursing:

(The) Problem. While incontinence and untidiness were in themselves a serious problem, they also contributed to social problems, since it was difficult to take the patients out of their environment due to their extraordinary need for physical care. It was thought that if some method or methods could be found to induce the patients to take greater responsibility for their physical care, they might be able to participate in a wider range of activities previously unavailable to them.[12]

Statement of the Problem. The purpose of this study is to construct an instrument for investigating some of the ways head nurses and staff nurses feel about the use of authority in ward nursing service.[13]

Statement of the Problem. The problem of this study is to investigate the attitudes that may influence the progress of each student in nursing. The areas of home and family relationships, personal relationships, nursing activities, and future plans and aspirations have been selected as being particularly important in the student nurses' progress.[14]

The Problem. . . . The Problem for study was predicated upon three statements: (1) there are differences of opinion concerning who should teach the patient; (2) there are differences of opinion regarding how the patient should be taught; and (3) there are differences in practices of teaching patients.

From these predications two questions arose: First, are there differences in patients who have been the subjects of these different ideas and practices? Second, if there are differences, what type of practice seems to offer patients the most favorable situation for the conduct of their long cure?[15]

Which of the above statements actually describes a problem? If, as the authors maintain, each is a problem, then the term problem is employed differently. How would you describe a problem based upon these examples—as a general problem area, a purpose, a question, or a series of questions?

A Problem Area

The first statement seems to be more indicative of a problem area. It specifies a "felt difficulty" and points out an area of need. A problem is inferred perhaps, yet not stated definitively.

Examine the so-called problems below. They, too, appear to reflect the presence of a general problem area rather than a specific one.

The Problem. . . . Limited experience with the clinical technician group at another Army hospital had pointed up the fact that this group of workers were not being used at their highest potential. The high quality of their training required that they function at a somewhat higher level if they were to be kept from becoming frustrated in their jobs. . . . Previous studies have demonstrated that the hours of professional nursing service required by patients is in direct relationship to their nursing needs, taking into consideration the degree and intensity of: (1) their nursing procedural requirements; (2) their physical restrictions; (3) their emotional disturbances; and (4) their instructional and rehabilitation needs.

Thus, it can be seen that the readiness factor, a basic principle of learning, was present for this project. The situation was ready; the clinical technicians were ready. There was much interest in such a study. The only unknown factor was the degree of functioning that could be permitted the clinical technicians.[16]

The Problem. During recent years a definite trend toward collegiate education for nurses has been apparent in the increasing number of schools offering degree programs and in the proportion of total student nurse population enrolled in these programs. The proponents of this trend emphasize the professional nurse's need for a broader educational background if she is to meet successfully the challenge of increasing responsibilities. Nevertheless, there are members of the nursing and allied professions and laymen who question the practicability and even the desirability of college preparation for the professional nurse. But both proponents and opponents would probably agree that the acquisition of clinical knowledge and nursing skills is fundamental in all nursing education programs. Evaluation of achievement in these areas of nursing should, therefore, be acceptable as one index of a program's proficiency.[17]

Statement of the Problem. Psychologists have established that there are many motivating factors in human life. These have been categorized by Carroll as (1) the need for emotional security; (2) the need for achievement or mastery; (3) the need for recognition or status; and (4) the need for physical satisfaction. It is logical to assume that in his vocational pursuits the worker's psychological needs operate to create satisfactions or dissatisfactions with his employment. An examination of workers' complaints in business and industry supports this assumption.

Science Research Associates reports that workers' chief complaints fall into the following categories: (1) supervisor-employee interpersonal relations. . . .

It seems reasonable to assume that nurses' complaints may be similar to the complaints of other workers.[18]

How do these statements of problem assist the researcher? They do not reflect specifically the kind of answer that is needed or even suggest the known terms. Instead, they appear to recommend an area or a subject for further study. They may be considered as the introductory reason for "getting started." Is this what a statement of problem should do?

Problems or Purposes

Two of the statements given before (Refs. 13 and 14) tend to confuse the terms problem and purpose. They are stated more specifically than the "general problem area" statements just given. Yet they convey an objective or a goal rather than a question or an area of doubt. Let us scrutinize some additional statements of this kind:

Statement of the Problem. The specific purposes of this study were as follows: (1) To identify and analyze the on-the-job problems and responsibilities as perceived by a selected group of nurses serving public school children. (2) To determine to what extent, if at all, differences in perception are related to specific aspects of professional education, professional experience, or the present work situation. (3) To analyze the significance of such data in relation to the development of preservice and inservice curricula for school nurses.[19]

The Problem. The purpose of this study was to determine, on the basis of nursing observations, the amount of formula that premature infants of a given weight and age will tolerate and at the same time maintain a satisfactory weight record.[20]

Statement of the Problem. The purpose of this study is to construct an instrument for investigating some of the ways head nurses and staff nurses feel about the use of authority in ward nursing service. This instrument would provide a method by which head nurses and staff nurses might examine objectively their own feelings and attitudes about the way authority is used in the ward nursing situations.[21]

Although each author has indicated that his is a statement of a problem, the statements begin with "the purpose(s) of this study is (are)" and proceed to state a purpose. Should the term problem be stated synonymously with the term purpose? Do they actually have the same meaning? Are they to be used in the same way? If so, why employ one rather than the other?

Problem or Procedure

Another source of confusion arises when the procedure or what is to be done is stated as the problem. Here are some examples:

Statement of the Problem. It was the purpose of this study: (1) to make an operational definition of what psychiatric patients perceive as therapeutic interaction among themselves in their daily life on a psychiatric ward, (2) to get some general experience with the research tools being used, (3) to plan to continue this study in the future on a larger scale, and (4) to attempt to apply any concepts formulated to the development of a more therapeutic environment for the psychiatric patient.[22]

The Problem. The purposes of this study were:

1. To determine some opinions and plans of a selected group of graduate nurses with regard to graduate nurse education.
2. To determine whether certain factors may be associated with the opinions and plans of nurses regarding graduate nurse education.
3. To consider the implications of the information for the Division of Nursing Education, School of Education, Indiana University, which offers programs in graduate nurse education.[23]

There is a real need to consider how subjects and materials will be selected and how data will be collected and analyzed. The answers to these questions will compose the means by which the researcher will obtain and test the knowledge to be derived. But do these problems pertain directly to the end itself: the acquisition of additional nursing knowledge? Should not the statement of the problem inquire what knowledge is to be obtained rather than how the knowledge will be obtained?

The nurse researcher has thus tended to employ the term problem in different ways. Should this be the case? If the term is employed differently, then it has acquired varied meanings in the eyes of the different researchers, such as a purpose, a question, a procedural problem. Although researchers are wont to interpret terms differently, there is a real need for consistency. This is exemplified in the conflicting utilization of terms in studies that actually were reported by the same journal. The problem of communicating knowledge through written sources is sufficiently difficult. It need not be exaggerated by the imposition of ambiguous terms.

If there is a place in nursing research for each of several different kinds of statements of problem, the nurse researcher should recognize the meaning of each and categorize them accordingly. Then the various terms may become meaningful rather than confusing to the individual researcher. She should employ them to direct her problem-solving endeavors rather than blindly to strew the pathways to a solution with additional, but noncontributory, requirements.

THE PROBLEM—MUST IT BE STATED?

Is there actually a need for a problem statement? Some researchers may state either a purpose or a problem, but not both. Other researchers may state both a purpose and a problem, but in an apparently unrelated manner. That is, while the purpose may suggest the determination of a solution to problem X as the study's objective, the question stated may be problem Y. Thus, these studies may be directed by the purpose or the problem, but not by both. If either term fails to assist the researcher, could one or the other be omitted?

The authors recognize the differences inherent in each term and recommend stating a purpose and a problem. They agree that one—the problem—is often a restatement of the other—the purpose. Yet they also feel that each has a distinct place within the research project and serves specific ends.

The authors have reiterated that purpose and problem should be closely interrelated. The area of knowledge suggested by the statement of purpose can be construed as the kind of solution fitting the situation stated by the problem. One, the purpose, poses the kind of solution to be determined, while the other, the problem, suggests the question. Perhaps the confusion between purpose and problem can be attributed to this relationship.

This interpretation of the purpose and the problem also can be illustrated by examples of studies in nursing:

Purpose. To test the validity of a speculation often heard in the nursing profession; namely, that increases in the amount or the quality of nursing care will produce improvements in patient welfare.

Problem. Is there a relationship between increases in the amount or quality of nursing care and patient welfare?[24]

Purpose. . . . to identify, in that system (social system of a modern hospital), the social and organizational factors significantly related to efficiency and job-satisfaction of nurses.

Problem. Four questions to which the research would seek answers were indicated:

1. What is the place of the nurse in the formal and informal organizational structure of the modern hospital's social system?

2. What social and organizational factors in the social system of the hospital are significantly related to the efficiency of nurses and nurse teams?

3. What social and organizational factors in the social system of the hospital are significantly related to the job-satisfaction of nurses?

4. What relationships exist between job-satisfaction, nursing team morale, and efficiency?[25]

Observe the interrelationship between purpose and problem in each case. Several can be denoted. Each purpose specifies what the researcher intends to determine. The problem states specifically what he is looking for. Each statement of problem relates directly to the purpose and follows the statement of purpose. Each statement of problem, furthermore, is presented in the form of a question inquiring what is to be made known. The researcher is ready to begin problem-solving. The reader may have a clearer understanding of the action to be taken.

There are places for the purpose and the problem in nursing research. The purpose can serve as the concluding statement summarizing the requirements for study in the light of previous investigations. The problem can be made the focal point between the derivation of the purpose and the problem-solving process.

An adequate derivation of purpose will assist the researcher to state the problem as well as the purpose. In the course of this development, the researcher should become acquainted with the body of previous research in the area of concern and isolate the requirements for additional study. She should be able to distinguish between the real problem under study and the problem area. (This feature may be lacking in the two indecisive studies already presented.) Furthermore, she should be able to distinguish between what is already known or given and what is to be made known.

The problem, as a focal point, should link previous knowledge (as stated by what is known or given) with knowledge to be acquired by the ensuing project (implied by what is to be made known, and stated by the purpose). If the problem is stated adequately, the products or the results of problem-solving should augment what has been contributed in the past.

The purpose and the problem statements can assist the nurse researcher by directing her efforts along more confined and appropriate channels. The purpose should specify the goal of problem-solving. The problem should initiate the problem-solving process by clearly defining the situation for which a solution is required.

The Problem—Is It Meaningful?

The goal of problem-solving is to make known the unknown. A key to problem-solving is to link what is already known with what is to be made known. In other words, our best estimate of what is unknown often is contained in the past and has been made known. The intent of problem-solving, therefore, is to explore and/or manipulate what is given or known to produce the unknown.

The terms of the problem may be described by what is given or known. A major task of the researcher is to isolate and describe what is given from a rather concise statement of the problem. The success of the problem-solving efforts to follow will depend in large measure upon the researcher's ability to communicate these terms to herself.

Faulty communication in this regard has contributed perhaps to the indecisive quality that is characteristic of some studies in nursing. The nurse researcher sometimes may state the problem and yet fail to describe what is known about the characteristics of the situation in question. She may experience difficulty in isolating and selecting the terms of her problem. She may fail to convey the appropriate meaning of the isolated terms.

Definition of Terms

Two difficulties in particular have hampered the nurse researcher's effort to isolate terms. First, there has been a tendency to select words or the parts of terms rather than the whole term. Second, the nurse researcher may have failed to isolate and define each of the pertinent terms. Let us refer again to the nursing literature and illustrate the difficulty by an example.

The investigation was undertaken in order to test the hypotheses: (1) that nurses fear tuberculosis and associate themselves with the disease; (2) that fear produces certain attitudes in the nurse which make her reluctant to accept assignments to a tuberculosis service as readily as to other types of service; (3) that some nurses have changed their attitude through education.

Definition of Terms. The following terms are defined in the sense in which they are used in this study. . . . (Other words defined similarly included nursing, nurse turnover, social adjustment, tuberculosis service and environment.)

Attitude is a tendency to act toward or against something in the environment which becomes thereby a positive or a negative value. An attitude has meaning only in relation to some value. Attitudes are the subjective counterparts of objective phenomena. The distinguishing evidence of attitude is behavior. . . .

Fear complex is an unreasonable and persistent fear of some object or situation and an attempt to avoid it. This fear may be concerned with what may happen to one, or with what one might do to another person.

Job situation, when used or referred to in this study, means the total sum of factors that affect positions the nurse holds.[26]

We may surmise from the hypotheses (a problem statement was not given) that the author wishes to ascertain relationships among several terms—"fear of tuberculosis" and "identification with the disease," "fear of tuberculosis" and the "nurse's attitudes also, making her reluctant to accept assignments." Instead of describing these terms, the author delineated and defined the parts composing them. These separate definitions of the parts do not necessarily describe or even imply the meaning of the whole. Furthermore, some of the defined words are not even pertinent.

Statement of Problem. The problem may be stated as a study of some of the psychological effects of early ambulation in the adult surgical patient.

Definitions. The majority of terms used in this study have a common meaning and need no further interpretation here. Some variation of the term "early ambulation," however, is revealed in the literature. Early ambulation in this study is based on Webster's definition, with further consideration of the time element lapsing between surgery and the ambulation of the patient. From her study Faller found that early ambulation usually meant continuation of body activity, including walking, self-care in matters of toilet, dressing and feeding. For the purpose of this study, early ambulation connotes ambulation from 8 to 72 hours postoperatively.[27]

The author sought to determine (1) the psychological effects of (2) early ambulation in the adult surgical patient. She defined only "early ambulation." It was suggested that the definition of the term "psychological effects" was understood. Does it really have "common meaning"? Would not problem-solving have been made easier by an actual, stated definition of this term?

Once the terms have been isolated, they should be defined appropriately. Definition here does not have the same meaning that it does in a dictionary, which serves a broad and diversified public. Its definitions refer more generally to common word usage. They are tersely stated. The illustration that follows, for example, may comprise good dictionary definitions.

Environment is "the aggregate of all influences and external conditions which bear upon the individual's development."

Nursing is defined in its broadest sense "as an art and a science which involves the whole patient—body, mind and spirit; promotes his spiritual, mental and physical health by teaching and by example; stresses health education and health preservation as well as ministration to the sick; involves the care of the patient's environment—social and spiritual as well as physical; and gives health service to the family and community as well as to the individual."[28]

The question remains, however, whether these definitions are useful to the researcher. They tend to cover the universe.

They talk of many things. Could the researcher actually study the concept nursing, as implied here, in a single project?

A more useful definition might narrow the frame of reference to that which can be manipulated by the problem-solving process. Consider the following examples:

The construct "nursing effectiveness" as used in this study denotes those proficiencies of the graduate professional staff nurse which are most crucial in that they have been responsible for outstanding performance of the nurse engaged in her job. In operational terms, nursing effectiveness may be defined as the kind of behavior which a clinical instructor might cite in the classroom to exemplify nursing skill, or the kind of behavior which might evoke favorable pronouncement by doctors, head nurses or patients.[29]

A *covert nursing problem* is a *concealed* or hidden condition faced by the patient or family which the nurse can assist him or them to meet through the performance of her professional functions. (E.g., a patient with a tracheotomy tube is unable to sleep because of his anxiety of being alone and unable to get help should the tube become plugged with mucus. The covert nursing problem is the patient's anxiety, which the nurse must find ways of relieving. The solution to the covert problem will solve the overt nursing problem —the patient's inability to sleep.)[30]

These examples deal with single terms that may be associated with other comparable situations within nursing. They provide a link to the past. The nurse researcher of the first illustration thus may employ knowledge gained from other studies on "nursing effectiveness" (as defined here) to enhance her own problem-solving efforts. She could have made the definition more abstract to gain access to studies outside the nursing literature. Each term also can be identified with and observed in a specific situation. Lines of communication have been established, therefore, with the concrete and actual situation.

The definition of terms, as well as the problem statement, will exercise a large measure of control over problem-solving. The nurse researcher's approach will be straightforward in accordance with her ability to pinpoint and convey the meaning intended by the terms of her problem. She will be able to make use of available knowledge only to the extent that she can communicate with the literature. Eventually, she will be able to isolate observable situations to the extent that she can identify the elements to be observed.

Stating the Problem

Let us select one of the specific purposes used as an example in Chapter 3 and consider what must be done to effect an appropriate problem statement. This exercise may enable us to summarize, by illustration, the major points of the preliminary discussions.

Purpose: To determine the sustenal requirements for nursing care as a function of Impairment State X.

Prior to stating the problem, the researcher may plot a mental picture of the purpose, listing exactly what is given and what is to be determined.

Given: *To Determine:*

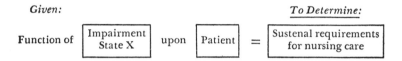

Function of | Impairment State X | upon | Patient | = | Sustenal requirements for nursing care

This model implies that what is given is already known. That is, a fund of knowledge is available by which to describe the function of Impairment State X upon the patient. (This assumption will be made throughout the remainder of this exercise.) The problem is to relate what is given to what is to be determined; the latter will depict the unknown or the kind of answer that is needed.

Problem: What sustenal requirements for nursing care can result for the patient as a function of Impairment State X?

Unknown Term or Kind of Answer That Is Needed: Effects, namely, the sustenal requirements for nursing care that may be anticipated as a function of Impairment State X.

Known Terms: 1. Impairment State X
2. Patient

The need to define the terms remains. The known terms should be described explicitly so that they can be interrelated. It also will be necessary to focus upon the unknown terms and to limit the direction and the scope of the problem. That is, the researcher will desire to consider Impairment State X as it affects those characteristics of the patient to produce the unknown, sustenal (not remedial or restorative) requirements for nursing care.

Definition of Terms

1. Impairment State X. The broad or general connotation of impairment state, as described in Chapter 3, should compose part of the definition of this term. Thus, any generalization derived with regard to impairment state should be applicable here.

An impairment state has been described previously (see Chapter 3, p. 189) as an impairment to the body or mind that hampers the individual's ability to satisfy his personal needs. It can be conceived to arise when the person reacts with an unfavorable environment, which may be:

A. External to the individual, e.g., a puncture, an infection, a blow on the head;

B. Internal to the individual, e.g., excessive strain, a malgrowth such as cancer;

C. A combination of external and internal forces, e.g., anxiety. The unfavorable environment may be characterized then by injury, disease, malformation or maldevelopment.

The term also should be depicted by the more specific X factor. An actual term would be substituted for the X term in an actual study. X was employed here deliberately to illustrate the obvious need to make the meaning of the term known. This requirement is not so obvious in other studies that substitute words for X's even though the words may be meaningless.

Specific impairment states might be classified in terms of what happens to the person. In this regard, it may be conceived further to cover such structural defects as an opening, an obstruction, a fracture, a strain or an amputation and/or as accelerated or depressed bodily malfunctions. A category of malfunctions that may not have a physical base, such as misunderstandings and feelings of insecurity, etc., also can be developed.

Impairment State X may be classified accordingly. It should be described specifically with regard to the source from which it arose and its effects upon the body structure (if any) and function. This state also should be depicted by the symptoms that enable the observer to be aware of its presence. In other words, the description should link the concept to something more tangible and observable, such as signs and symptoms.

2. Patient. A patient may be defined as a person in need of assistance or care.

There are many ways to describe this person. It will be our purpose, however, to limit the description to those characteristics of the person that cast him in the role of a patient. The model suggested two characteristics of this order: personal need and self-help ability.

A. Personal Need. The following description is a variation of a definition of a state of need developed by Hull.[31]

A considerable variety of optimal conditions is required for survival: air, water, food, temperature, intactness of body tissue. When any of these necessary conditions departs from the optimum, a state of need may be said to exist. Deviation from the optimum may result when the person lacks or is deprived of one of the essentials—air, water, food—or when the body is injured or discomfited by the presence of an irritating agent.

Needs may be described in two ways:

1. Primary. When the need is unlearned and basic to the survival of the individual—the need for food, oxygen, elimination, relief from pain—it may be said to be primary.

2. Acquired or Learned. When the need is not basic to the survival of the individual but has acquired certain characteristics of primary needs through the process of learning, it may be said to be acquired or learned. The need for nursing care, for example, may be conceived as acquired or learned. When the patient himself cannot satisfy his primary need for food and is assisted by the nurse, he may acquire a secondary need for nursing assistance.

Needs classified under this category may relate to physical as well as nonphysical requirements of the person. Social and psychological motives (believed by some psychologists to be related to biologic needs and by others to be learned) influence our behavior. The needs for affection, for a feeling of personal worth, for social approval or respect provide direction for most of our striving.[32]

B. Self-Help Ability. An important attribute of the person is the ability to provide for the satisfaction of his personal needs. Every individual is endowed with this ability, to some extent. It is quite probable that most people can provide for the satisfaction of their primary needs.

Self-help ability is governed and may be measured by the physical and mental capacities of the person and the degree to which they have been developed. Individuals will vary, therefore, in self-help ability in accordance with their physical and mental capacities and their stage of development. Self-help ability also will vary for the same individual. For example, it will be minimal during the infantile stages of life before the bodily organs have developed fully, maximal at maturity, and diminishing in the later years when the bodily organs may function less adequately.

Self-help ability may be described by its normal state, which is the one most typical of the individual at any one developmental level. It may be described also by a minus state, which is lower than that which is normal for the person. This state may arise when the body or the person is impaired and the person's ability to provide for the satisfaction of his personal needs is hampered. The extent of the limitation will be a function of the degree of impairment.

A patient may be described now as a person with a minus self-help ability who, as a result, cannot satisfy some of his personal needs. He may require the assistance of some other person to supplement his self-help ability and provide for the satisfaction of these needs.

These general descriptions will permit the researcher to manipulate the constructs in abstract form. Thus, she can deal with more underlying problems and derive solutions with more universal applicability. They also will enable her to employ other systems of construct manipulation such as the learning theory.

However, a person is composed of a variety of abilities that relate to many personal needs. It would be difficult to isolate and describe each of these conditions and impossible to study them at any one time. Therefore, descriptions should be restricted to the patient rather than to the person state. Self-help ability will then be described as it may be limited by Impairment State X. The researcher may also list and describe those personal needs that remain unsatisfied as a result. The behavioral changes taking place in the person at this time may provide the researcher with observable descriptions of the patient.

3. Sustenal Requirements for Nursing Care. Since this is the unknown term, it is assumed that our knowledge is limited in this regard. The description of the term is to be derived as a function of what is known or given. However, a few words may be offered to limit and define the scope of the study.

Care might be defined in its abstract form as some form of assistance to perform functions that is rendered to one person by another person when the former lacks the ability to perform these functions independently.

Sustenal care refers to a particular kind of assistance that is rendered to compensate for the individual's inability to satisfy his personal needs. It is directed toward the satisfaction of these needs.

A nurse is a person who has learned to render care. She has acquired knowledge and developed a set of skills and may be able to perform certain functions commensurate with and satisfying the requirements of the situation for care. Sustenal nursing care will pertain to those functions that the nurse can or may be able to perform to satisfy and sustain the personal needs of the patient. Sustenal requirements for nursing care will concern the secondary needs that the patient has acquired for this type of assistance when he is unable to provide for himself.

The definition should limit and direct the problem-solving process to solve for this unknown and for no other.

This exercise has uncovered a number of requirements for defining the problem in nursing research:

A. There may be a need to elicit a picture of all the other pertinent terms—what is given and what is to be made known. Some of these terms may be implied but not stated in the purpose. They should at least be incorporated in appropriate sequence in a statement of the problem.

B. There may be a need to develop an adequate system for describing the known terms. The descriptions may be invented or borrowed. They may relate to the abstract as well as to the specific. They should interrelate with one another.

C. There may be a need to define the unknown term to the extent that the researcher can limit its scope and direct the problem-solving process more specifically.

REFERENCES

1. Burton, W. H., Kimball, R. B., and Wing, R. L.: Education for Effective Thinking, p. 21, New York, Appleton-Century-Crofts, 1960.
2. *Ibid.,* pp. 21-25.
3. Black, Max: Critical Thinking, An Introduction to Logic and Scientific Method, pp. 247-248, New York, Prentice-Hall, Inc., 1946.
4. Burton, W. H., *et al.: Op. cit.* (see Ref. 1), p. 22.
5. *Ibid.,* p. 22.
6. Black, Max: *Op. cit.* (see Ref. 3), p. 249.
7. Ingles, D. J.: Principles of Research in Biology and Medicine, p. 80, Philadelphia, Lippincott, 1958.
8. Osgood, G. A.: Study of clinic nursing service, Nurs. Res. 7: 33-35, 1958.
9. Holman, B. L.: An evaluation of nursing care on an obstetric service, Nurs. Res. 9:125-128, 1960.
10. Heinemann, E., Hill, R. J., and Birkbeck, L.: The study of student anxiety in a tuberculosis nursing situation, Nurs. Res. 8:155-159, 1959.
11. Dodge, J. S.: Nurse-doctor relations and attitudes toward the patient, Nurs. Res. 9:32-36, 1960.
12. Carpenter, H. A., and Simon, R.: The effect of several methods of training on long-term, incontinent, behaviorally regressed hospitalized psychiatric patients, Nurs. Res. 9:17, 1960.
13. Copeland, M., Derryberry, J., Eaton, D., and Harper, M.: A projective technique for investigating how nurses feel about the use of authority, Nurs. Res. 4:79, 1955.

14. Ingmire, A. E.: Attitudes of student nurses at the University of California, Nurs. Res. *1* (No. 2):36, 1952.

15. Wandelt, M. A.: Planned versus incidental instruction for patients in tuberculosis therapy, Nurs. Res. *3*:52, 1954.

16. Bredenberg, V. C., and Hincker, E. A.: Utilization of clinical technicians, Nurs. Res. *3*:33, 1954.

17. Jessee, R. W.: A comparative study of fully accredited basic nursing programs, Nurs. Res. *7*:100, 1958.

18. Grivest, M. T.: A personnel inventory of supervisors, head nurses, and staff nurses in selected hospitals, Nurs. Res. *7*:77, 1958.

19. Grossman, J.: The school nurse's perception of problems and responsibilities, Nurs. Res. *5*:18, 1956.

20. Iffrig, Sister Mary Charitas: Nursing observations of 100 premature infants and their feeding programs, Nurs. Res. *5*:71, 1956.

21. Copeland, M.: *et al.: Op. cit.* (see Ref. 13).

22. Carter, F. M.: The critical incident technique in the identification of patients' perception of therapeutic patient-patient interaction on a psychiatric ward, Nurs. Res. *8*:207, 1959.

23. Allen, Dotaline E.: Opinions and plans of a group of graduate nurses in relation to graduate nurse education, Nurs. Res. *5*:121, 1957.

24. An Investigation of the Relation Between Nursing Activity and Patient Welfare, Nurse Utilization Project Staff, p. 1, Ames, Iowa, State Univ. Iowa, 1960.

25. Bullock, R. P.: Position, function, and job satisfaction of nurses in the social system of a modern hospital, Nurs. Res. *2*:4, 1953.

26. Wago, Helen: An analysis of expressed attitudes of registered professional nurses toward tuberculosis nursing and the implications of these attitudes, Nurs. Res. *3*:114, 1955.

27. Stanford, E. G.: A Study of the Psychological Effects of Early Ambulation on the Adult Surgical Patient, Master's Dissertation, Washington, D. C., Catholic Univ., 1952. (Unpublished)

28. Wago, Helen: *Op. cit.* (see Ref. 26).

29. Bailey, J. T.: The critical incident technique in identifying behavioral criteria of professional nursing effectiveness, Nurs. Res. *5*:52, 1956.

30. Abdellah, F. G.: Methods of identifying covert aspects of nursing problems, Nurs. Res. *6*:4, 1957.

31. Hull, C. L.: Principles of Behavior, New York, Appleton-Century-Crofts, 1946.

32. Morse, W. C., and Wingo, G. M.: Psychology and Teaching, p. 430, New York, Scott, Foresman, 1955.

CHAPTER 5

Formulating the Hypothesis

THE GENERAL CASE

After the problem has been stated, then what? Naturally, the next step is to find the answer. This purpose—to develop a given piece of knowledge conceived as a solution to a problem —has been proposed for a specific research project. The problem statement will depict the particular situation or condition necessitating a solution. The remaining task is to determine the solution.

How does the researcher determine the solution to his problem? Three very normal modes of response are: to ask the expert, to peruse the literature, and to observe situations wherein the solution may be located. Each process presupposes the presence and the availability of ready answers. Each step seemingly vaults the thinking phase, logically deducing the answer. Let us examine the three processes and consider their pitfalls.

ASK THE EXPERT

Expert knowledge has been discussed previously as an important resource for general problem-solving activities. Some of the advantages and disadvantages were considered. This form of knowledge has been employed also in so-called research matters. It has not been unusual to consult with the subject-matter specialist or a team of authorities in the field in question.

Different methods have been employed to secure experts' solutions. The researcher has solicited the brief responses of large groups of experts upon single occasions. He also has secured some rather detailed and extensive responses from a small number of specialists.

The opinionaire has been established as an instrument to obtain the reactions of many respondents at one time. This technic asks the specialist to respond to a set of predetermined questions or issues. The number of items may be small or large and vary in diversity. The respondent may be restricted to a limited set of alternative responses or encouraged to react freely to open-end questions.

The election ballot is a good illustration of an opinionaire. Here the voting public constitutes the population of experts. The candidates represent a set of alternative responses to the question of who is best fitted to hold office. Actually, many issues are embodied.

It may be judged, however, that this example is not representative of research. The issues may be stated too broadly. The sample of experts may be questionable. On the other hand, studies based on the opinionaire, not too dissimilar to the election ballot, have been called research. They are used frequently and pertain to a large variety of subjects, e.g., buyers' needs, TV listeners' interests, stock market forecasts, curriculum matters. The items may be phrased more rigidly and the populations defined in a more restrictive manner than on the election ballot, but the general process of seeking opinions—expert judgment—is the same. What is or is not termed research may be merely a question of degree.

The expert or experts also may be requested to respond to a single problem or to a small number of problems in a more detailed fashion. In this case, only one expert or a small group of experts may be interrogated. The person or persons chosen for this undertaking may represent a more selective segment of the so-called expert population than the larger groups mentioned in the previous examples. They may be classified as subject-matter specialists in a well-defined and limited area of knowledge. They may be expected to issue a report listing an analysis of alternative proposals and recommended solutions for the problem.

Consider the case of the medical specialist such as the surgeon or the cardiologist who is called upon for consultation. He is presented with the problem of a patient who has been observed by another physician, who may not be certain that he has diagnosed the problem correctly and/or prescribed the proper treatment. The medical specialist may be requested to confirm the diagnosis or prognosis or to prescribe other treatment. His report may be long or short. It may be written or oral.

Another example pertains to the panel of experts who are brought together to resolve a major problem. The Supreme Court of the United States of America constitutes such a panel. This group is required to resolve legal issues that may not have right or wrong answers. A question of judgment is involved. The group may concur as a whole and issue a decision. The members also may differ and present two sets of judgments, with the majority opinion becoming the accepted interpretation.

It is highly unlikely that either example would be considered to be research. Nevertheless, they represent variations of practices that sometimes are termed research. It has not been unusual to call upon a private consultant or a panel of experts to consider some major community, industrial or governmental problem. Questions pertaining to health, national security, education and the economy have been resolved in this manner in recent years. The end-products have been issued sometimes as research reports. What is or is not termed research in these cases may be a question of subject matter.

Is problem-solving by expert judgment really research? Let us consider the process and observe the limitations.

There is a question as to who the expert is. Is the expert one who knows the answer? If so, the problem (as it has been defined in Chap. 4) really may not be a research problem. If the answer is known, only a question is necessary to elicit it. If the expert does not know the answer, how is it determined?

He may resort to his fund of accumulated knowledge and deduce the answer.

This process does not eliminate the thinking phase of problem-solving but is the thinking phase. As a matter of fact, it may never move beyond this phase. Herein lies the difference. The solutions are not tested empirically. They are accepted because the expert says so. They carry the weight of authority and are accepted solely on this basis. But authorities have been known to be wrong.

What is the role of the researcher? Is he merely a statistical clerk who surveys the population of experts, summarizes their thoughts and issues a report? Or is he also a subject-matter expert? Has he not fortified his resources of pertinent knowledge to develop an appropriate purpose and state the problem? Can he not also advance the project through problem-solving and deduce the answer or answers? Who should be more familiar with the very specific matter in question than the researcher?

The researcher also may be more alert to the problem of securing an appropriate test of the solution that is deduced. It has been the authors' point of view that the problem-solving process is incomplete unless an empiric test of this kind is exacted. If problem-solving by expert judgment is to be labeled research, this limitation should be observed.

PERUSE THE LITERATURE

The researcher may turn to the written record for a solution to his problem. This method of problem-solving, sometimes called library research, utilizes a variety of records: opinions, observations, reasoning processes. The researcher will isolate, evaluate and pool the available literature systematically and then make his own judgment as to the best possible solution or solutions.

Legal problems tend to be resolved in this manner. The lawyer often will define his problem and search the legal literature for similar cases or precedents. Judgements and/or interpretations made in previous situations and recorded in the literature serve as precedents for future judgments. Therefore, he may cite them as arguments in support of his case.

The historian often may not have any resource available except the written record. The problem situation may not be observed directly. All actual eyewitnesses of the problem situation may have passed from the scene long since. This may be true also of secondary and tertiary sources of information. Only written observations, if any exist, may contain the solution to some questions of the past.

The historian, therefore, may have little choice in the matter. He either will employ the written record or fail to find an appropriate solution to his problem. But what of the researcher in current-day problems? Should he employ the written record exclusively?

Using written records exclusively results in the same limitations as using experts exclusively. If a worthy solution to the problem appears in the literature, then the problem again was not really a problem but a matter of inquiry. The researcher would have made this determination in the process of deriving his purpose, and would not have proceeded to the stage of problem-solving.

If the answer is not stated definitively in the literature, it may be surmised by a compilation from a variety of sources. However, this process also is questionable. The individual source materials may be open to question. For example, the ancient record-keeper upon whom the historian relies may have been extremely biased and selective of the observations that he recorded. The modern-day record-keeper is not necessarily immune to this ailment. On the other hand, the historical review also may be incomplete. The literature available on certain current problems is so extensive that it has become extremely difficult for the researcher to be aware of, much less review, all the source materials. What is selected and what is omitted certainly will influence the judgment of the researcher. He may not even be aware of the existence or the extent of this form of bias.

Therefore, the researcher may not actually find the answer in the literature but may deduce it in a give-and-take reasoning procedure. This method of problem-solving does not really vault the reasoning process. However, it does fall short of the empiric test requirement. Pure library research is incomplete in this regard.

OBSERVE THE SITUATION

It has been stated previously that very few solutions or pieces of knowledge are man-made. Instead, they exist in the real world and wait upon man for discovery. Then why not explore the world of actual events, locate and describe a solution to a problem? The procedure may satisfy the requirement for empiric testing.

Suppose this process were followed exactly as stated. It would be implied that the researcher actually circumvents the thinking phase to observe the world about him directly. In essence, he would make random observations. The pitfalls of this procedure were discussed in part in Chapter 3.

Let us pick up again the situation of the head nurse and her problem and review, by example, some of the difficulties to be encountered by the chance observation method of approach. We will assume that she will survey the world for a chance solution to her problem.

Where Does the Observer Look?

Where, by chance alone, will she look for a solution to her problem? What is the probability that she will locate a problem situation that contains an appropriate solution? It is highly improbable that she will find the situation in short order. As a matter of fact, it is inconceivable that she or any other researcher would follow the implied procedure literally. If such were the case, the progress of man would have come to a halt long ago.

What Does the Observer Look For?

If, by chance, the appropriate problem-situation is located, what, by chance, would be observed as the solution? Many solutions to problems are not obvious. As a matter of fact, they are quite obscure. This is one of the reasons why we have problems. In addition, prior knowledge and understanding often are necessary for the acquisition of new knowledge. One of our difficulties is that we tend to take for granted the large amount of knowledge that has been assimiliated to date.

We can claim, indeed, that we "see" the fixed stars, the earth eclipsing the moon, bees gathering nectar for honey, or a storm approaching. But we shall be less ready to maintain that we simply and literally *see* these things, unaided by any theory, if we remember how comparitively recent in human history are these explanations of *what* it is we see.[1]

How Does the Observer Select the Appropriate Solution?

If, by chance, a solution is observed, how, by chance alone, will the observer be assured that this is a reliable solution? The researcher could have chanced upon a situation in which circumstances were favorably disposed toward any given assignment of nurses: the patients were not severely ill and were making excellent progress toward recovery; each nurse displayed an unusual amount of skill; a number of interns were transferred to the nurses' unit. Without prior knowledge or thought, the head nurse could not assess the situation before her adequately. The hidden biases of selecting this particular problem situation will have influenced her choice of a solution.

How Does the Observer Determine Unique Solutions?

If we assume that all the world's knowledge lies before us to be unfolded and discovered, what is the role of invention and creativeness? Does man simply imitate what already exists, or is it possible for him to create other, and perhaps better, solutions to his problems? Could not this head nurse or some other head nurse develop solutions to the assignment problem that are superior to those already in existence?

In reality, the researcher does not circumvent the thinking process and go directly to the observable world. He does not observe by chance alone. Actually, he may engage in considerable thought and preparation prior to observation. As a matter of fact, the authors reason that there is a relationship between the kind of preparation and the role of chance. That is, the problems incurred by chance observations would tend to be minimized as the factors to be studied are deliberately isolated and controlled beforehand.

It would appear that each of the processes discussed thus far—asking the expert, perusing the literature, and observing the situation—involves the thinking phase. The question is whether the process is performed formally or informally. The point of view will be expressed here that deliberate and formal consideration of this matter constitutes an integral part of the research process. We will term this phase of research "formulating the hypothesis." It is an established procedure and may involve any one or all of the three processes discussed.

The Hypothesis—What Is It?

We cannot take a single step forward in any inquiry unless we begin with a *suggested* explanation or solution of the difficulty which originated it. Such tentative explanations are suggested to us by something in the subject matter and by our previous knowledge. When they are formulated as propositions, they are called *hypotheses*.[2]

Thus Cohen and Nagel expressed the need for formulating a hypothesis. They also defined the term as a "tentative explanation or solution" to the problem. There seems to be agreement among researchers regarding this tentative characteristic. The hypothesis also might be called a paper solution, because the researcher generally will arrive at his hypothesis on paper through some process of thought construction. The hypothesis is tentative, therefore, because it is only a paper solution to a problem.

All kinds of tentative solutions for problems can be devised. They may represent different levels of thought. Each level relates to the degree of certainty with which the researcher may express his solution. The degree of certainty or assuredness, furthermore, can be construed as a function of the fund of available knowledge and understanding of the problem situation that the researcher has acquired or can acquire.

Picture the strange new world of a little 2-year-old boy. It is replete with blank spaces and unanswered questions. It is a small world whose boundaries include only his immediate environment. It is a small world because he has experienced little and has acquired insufficient knowledge. Furthermore, his partially developed intellectual capacities will not permit him to absorb and integrate the abundance of new experiences that occur just outside his world boundaries.

If you asked this boy—"What is the moon?"—how would he respond? "The moon is a marshmallow!" "An orange!" "A bag of peanuts!" If you asked him the color of an obviously red house, what would he say? "Yellow!" "Green!" "Red!" If you inquired— "How much is 25 times 49?"—what would he reply? "A bunny rabbit!" "A horse!" "Two!"

This boy is guessing. In a sense, he also is hypothesizing. His guesses are hypotheses—tentative solutions to the questions that have been asked him. Perhaps they even are the best solutions that he can offer. But they are guesses nevertheless.

A pure guess is a hypothesis based essentially upon chance. The solution is not really derived. It is selected helter-skelter from nowhere. The problem-solver, like the 2-year-old, could offer almost any response. If the choice point, like a fork in the road, narrowed the field to a small number of possible alternatives, he might have a good chance of guessing correctly. Chance favors the prepared mind. On the other hand, a broadly stated problem may yield almost any response. (If you must guess, it is advantageous to state your problem appropriately.)

The child must guess because he cannot determine his hypothesis by other means. He does not have available a fund of possible solutions to the particular question that is posed. He cannot comprehend what is to be expected as a solution. Therefore, he cannot scrutinize what little he does know, or seek information from other sources.

The more mature adult also guesses. He cannot possibly know all that there is to know, nor would he be able to comprehend all that there is to know. Adults also vary in their ability to acquire and comprehend knowledge. Some people must guess more often than others.

Fortunately, most adults do not have to rely heavily upon

guesswork. Through the joint processes of acculturation and maturation, they can acquire knowledge and the ability to think about solutions to problem situations. Lacking the required knowledge, they are more aware of and able to approach the expert sources.

The more knowledgeable and mature person can advance more readily to the next level of hypothesizing—the level of speculation. A speculation can be considered as a guess based upon some prior knowledge and some understanding. However, the knowledge employed may be incomplete and inaccurate. Furthermore, the thought processes may be inconsistent.

We speculate about many things. Consider the motorist, for example. As he drives, he must speculate about other motorists. Often there are three or more other motorists to consider: the one in front of him, the one behind him and the one on the other side of the road. He does not know these people, yet he speculates what they will do. His speculations are based upon his knowledge of the rules of the road and the feeling that the other motorists also understand the rules of the road. His prior driving experiences reinforce his thoughts in this regard. More often than not, he will speculate correctly. There are occasions, however, when he will be wrong; an "accident" is said to result. It could be said also that some motorist speculated ineptly.

Observers generally agree that a hypothesis represents informed rather than sporadic thinking. The thought processes have been established quite specifically as "the formulation of the deduction."[3] A particular kind of logical process wherein one proposition (or hypothesis) is derived from other propositions has been considered.

Hypotheses also pertain to given sets of facts or some fund of previous knowledge. They may be conceived as connecting links between or one or more known sets of facts. The hypothesizer should be aware of the facts that are being studied.

. . . the valuable suggestions for solving a problem can be made only by those who are familiar with the kinds of connections which the subject matter under investigation is capable of exhibiting . . . The hypotheses which occur to an investigator are therefore a function, in part at least, of his previous knowledge.[4]

A guess or a speculation probably would not be considered to be a hypothesis. Each may fail to satisfy either or both of the two attributes discussed above. The guesser usually is so devoid of knowledge that any basis for informed thinking is lacking. The speculator may reason adeptly, but be so limited in knowledge as to be unable to draw reliable conclusions. On the other hand, the speculator may have access to a sizeable number of facts, but may fail to assimilate his materials and correctly deduce the connecting mode.

There is a question as to when we move from the realm of speculation to the sphere of hypothesis. That is, at what point does the researcher acquire sufficient knowledge to derive adequate hypotheses; at what point is a system established to yield productive thinking and provide adequate hypotheses?

As the 2-year-old boy grows up, he moves gradually from a world of the unpredictable to the predictable. He becomes aware of relationships, that certain events occur with other events. In essence, he acquires knowledge. He learns to give other than purely random responses to questions. He develops the ability to forecast solutions to problems with a certain degree of confidence.

How does the child learn? What is the character of the knowledge that he will acquire? How will it differ from the guess or the speculation?

One day this child may run to his mother and cry out, "I hurt my finger!" The mother will perceive that the tip of the little finger is red and inquire what happened. Since the child may not be able to verbalize his experience, he will lead his mother to the radiator in the next room and reply, "I touched that." The mother will realize immediately that the child touched the hot radiator and was burned.

The child had sensed two events: touching a hot radiator and being burned. The parent deduced a connection between the two events, which she had not witnessed: touching a hot radiator caused the burn. Furthermore, she could predict that her child will be burned each time that he touches the hot radiator. If he can become aware of the connection or relationship, he may learn to stay away from that hot radiator. How can the mother assist her child to deduce this relationship? How did the mother learn to make the deduction herself?

The mother simply may have had several experiences with the two events in the past. She also may have observed similar consequences. Therefore, she had some highly probable factual evidence with which to establish the relationship. In addition, it was linked rather closely to the observable events. It was an empiric relationship.

The mother may say to her child, "Stay away from hot radiators or you will be burned." The child has already experienced such an event. It was meaningful to him. One such confirmatory statement by the mother at this time might be sufficiently reinforcing to establish the relationship indefinitely.

If the mother could have made this statement to the child before the initial experience, she might have prevented the burn. However, could the child have appreciated the stated relationship without benefit of experience, without factual information? It is highly improbable that he could have done so. He may not even have been aware of the sensation of a burn. Yet there are circumstances in which it is mandatory that he learn vicariously, without benefit of experience—the avoidance of fires, speeding automobiles, poison.

The relationship may be established by other means. The mother could have accumulated an extensive array of pertinent facts or information during her lifetime. These facts could be arranged systematically by the learner to produce the relationship without benefit of experience. For example, the mother may have learned that skin tissue will burn when exposed to heat conditions above a certain point. She also knows that a radiator is sometimes heated above this point and will constitute, on these occasions, a heat condition conducive to skin burns. Skin contact with this radiator will lead to a burn.

If the mother has the facts available and assimilated, perhaps she could deduce the relationship without benefit of experience. In addition, she will have a basis for understanding how the events occurred above and beyond the mere fact that they were experienced. This mode of thought construction would be extremely valuable to her young child. Unfortunately, she cannot transmit her resource of information and the ability to think as easily as she can say to her child, "Stay away from hot radiators or you will be burned."

Two additional levels of hypothesizing can be considered now. We may hypothesize or deduce empiric relationships that are derived directly from experience. We also may hypothesize relationships without direct experience through the mental manipulation of an organized system of other related events (or empiric relationships). Each level presupposes the prior acquisition of factual information; each level requires systematic thought.

The former level might be considered to be a more primitive

process of hypothesizing. The empiric relationship requires fewer facts and less thought. The connection is tied so closely to the observed events that it almost can be experienced itself. It is close to the concrete and may be inferred from the process of experiencing the events.

The reader may be able to conceive of a vast number of empiric relationships that the child can absorb through the process of daily living. These become the foundation of his resources of common-sense knowledge. In addition, formal education may enable him to be cognizant of empiric relationships that also may be useful to him during his later life.

Many of the empiric relationships acquired formally may be more difficult to comprehend. This may be particularly true of those relationships that the child has not actually experienced. For example, he may be told that "Cows give milk." Being a city boy, he may have observed cows only in picture books. However, he will have seen milk in bottles or cardboard containers. To link the cow in the book to the milk in the container may constitute a formidable problem for an inexperienced, unknowledgeable young child.

In a sense, he is asked to hypothesize that this relationship is true. Until he actually experiences or observes "cows giving milk," it will remain only a paper solution. He may accept the proposition because other people have observed the event happening. Neverthless, some residue of doubt may remain.

The more advanced level of hypothesizing circumvents the problem of blind acceptance of a proposition without understanding.

When facts are assembled, ordered, and seen in a relationship, they constitute a theory. The theory is not speculation, but is built upon fact. Now, the various facts in a theory may be logically analyzed, and relationships other than those stated in the theory can be deduced. . . . *The formulation of the deduction* . . . constitutes a hypothesis.[5]

The child also may learn to reason that the proposition is true. He may acquire a body of knowledge dealing with the life cycle of mammals. This body of knowledge may be assembled and ordered into a system revealing how the substance "milk" is produced within the female organism to provide nourishment for her most recent offspring. The child will learn that the system is applicable to the mammalian order. He will reason or deduce that a cow is a mammal.

Therefore, under the circumstances described by the system, the cow will give milk.

The child will hypothesize again that "cows give milk," but upon a totally different basis. He need not accept the proposition simply because other people have observed the events happening. Instead, he may learn to understand how the events have occurred. He can place them in their proper perspective. He even may deduce other relationships such as "goats give milk," "dogs give milk," "cats give milk," and "humans give milk," and neither he nor anyone else need have experienced these events happening.

We may recognize a close affinity between the two levels of hypothesizing and the developmental stages of the research process: to describe and to explain. The establishment of empiric relationships is akin to the descriptive level, while the level of explanation actually entails hypothesizing from theory.

But as explanation feeds upon descriptive material, so theory is built upon previously established empiric relationships. The researcher needs facts before he can develop a theory. Therefore, he may be required initially to hypothesize and develop a core of empiric relationships from which to deduce other relationships. Both levels of hypothesizing may be necessitated throughout the development of a specific area of knowledge.

Once the basic core of empiric relationships has been established, theory development should begin. It already has been suggested that we can predict with greater assurance from the level of explanation than from the level of description. So we can hypothesize more adeptly from theory than from sheer experience. Theory, in essence, embodies many experiences, more factual information. Theory organizes the facts and, in the process, employs a more logically consistent system of thought. Theory may assist the researcher to hypothesize a solution that is less tentative.

The final attribute of a hypothesis is that it is testable. The solution remains tentative, regardless of the level at which it was formulated, until it satisfies the requirements of an empiric test. This is true even of the empiric relationship that supposedly is derived from experience. The experience that gave rise to the empiric relationship was antecedent to the establishment of the hypothesis. It was not necessarily a crucial test. The hypothesizer still must determine that his or someone else's initial experience was perceived properly.

Thus, the hypothesis also serves to direct the inquiry or study. That is, it later becomes the purpose of the project to dispel the tentative character of the hypothesis and determine whether or not it is the actual solution to the problem. The hypothesis becomes the "investigator's eyes in seeking answers to questions."[6]

THE HYPOTHESIS—HOW IS IT FORMULATED?

The formulation of a hypothesis may be described as the mental manipulation of some known entities or facts to uncover the unknown. The hypothesizer starts with facts. Something is given. He employs reason to investigate what is given, to provide some interplay among the facts, to yield what is not given. He uses other facts and reasons to test what have been offered as solutions.

Formulating a hypothesis is like building a model. It could be any kind of model: a mathematical representation, a diagram or a blueprint, a miniature version, a nursing-care plan. The purpose of the model is to simulate and test the final product without undertaking the hazards and the expense of actually erecting the real thing. The model builder first simulates the parts in scaled or model form. He then interlocks the pieces in various combinations to determine the best fit, the most workable arrangement or configuration. The value of the model, therefore, will depend upon the builder's ability to identify, simulate and fit the parts together.

The worth of a hypothesis will depend upon some analagous characteristics of the researcher. What is to be derived will be a function of what is given and how it is represented by the researcher. This characteristic will relate to his ability to acquire and assimilate the subject matter. What is to be derived is also a function of his capacity to reason or to manipulate the facts logically to produce the best fit or solution. Although the authors will offer some suggestions in this regard, what happens often is dependent upon the idiosyncracies of the individual researcher.

Start With the Problem

The formulation of the hypothesis is initiated by the statement of the problem and the definition of terms. The problem statement should indicate the kind of solution to be made known or the kind of hypothesis to be formulated. The terms of the problem should describe what is already known or given. The researcher's task in formulating the hypothesis then is to investigate what is known in order to produce what is to be made known.

The discussions of the problem and the definition of terms in Chapter 4 really are pertinent here. They were separated merely for convenience in presentation. The reader might review that chapter and, in particular, the section on model building (p. 205). He may note that each configuration suggested the kind of hypothesis to be formulated, the given or known facts, and the manner by which they could be employed to produce the unknown.

The reader should review also the section on the definition of terms (p. 208). He should be aware that the terms of the problem are analogous to the parts of the model. The ability of the researcher to isolate, identify and define the terms will have considerable influence upon the erection of the model or the formulation of the hypothesis. It will regulate the amount and the kind of knowledge to be made available for problem-solving. The reader should be cognizant that the definition of terms actually serves a dual function: to clarify the problem and to facilitate the development of a hypothesis.

Some consideration was given to the conception of the problem and its respective terms as "specific," "common" and/or "underlying." It was suggested that the fund of known facts will expand or contract accordingly. Briefly, a "specific" description may narrow the available facts to what is present in the situation to be observed. A "common" description will expand the resource to what is known within a given field of practice and some closely related applications. An "underlying" description will open the doors to a body of fundamental knowledge that is universal in application, and thus to many fields of inquiry and practice.

The definitions may be related also to the level of hypothesizing. That is, the terms may be stated as a form, amenable to the formulation of a hypothesis directly from experience or theory. The terms may be described as they can be experienced by an independent observer. They may be defined also as a concept denotable within a given body of systematized knowledge or theory.

Consider the case of a patient who has been confined to her bed for X many days. She has become irritable and demanding. The researcher may question whether or not there is a relationship between patient confinement and irritable behavior.

The terms may be defined as they can be experienced—hospitalized patients who have been confined to bed for X many days, and behavior such as crying, shouting at nurses and other patients, rejecting food, visitors, etc. (The reader should note that "irritable behavior" may require extensive description.) The researcher then may compile two lists of information pertinent to each term. On the one hand, he may attempt to depict what generally has been observed to happen when patients are described in accordance with the definition. On the other hand, he also will ascertain and list the sources of irritable behavior during hospitalization. His ultimate objective is to interrelate the two lists of information, determine common properties and derive a relationship.

The terms also may be defined to fit the concepts depicted within a given and established theory of behavior. This would enable the researcher to employ some previously established rules suggestive of a relationship between his known terms.

The examples illustrate a major difference in approach to hypothesis-development. Each approach should be scrutinized carefully and its possible consequences observed.

In dealing with strictly empiric evidence, the researcher begins problem-solving with essentially unassembled and, as yet, unrelated sources of information. He will be required to organize his data and assemble his model from scratch. He actually is engaged in theory-development of a primitive nature. He may be required to disassemble and reassemble his parts several times before striking what appears to be the best configuration.

In dealing with theoretic data, the researcher utilizes organized knowledge. He employs something more than sheer facts. He uses a system of reasoning in which the facts have been interrelated. He takes advantage of knowledge that has been arranged in a network of relationships and tested (perhaps) to produce other knowledge or relationships.

The difference in approach is analogous to building a house with and without plans. He who builds with plans knows in advance how much and what kind of material to secure. He also knows how the parts will be assembled and what the final product will look like. He who builds without plans takes chances. He is never certain of what he needs. He is never sure of what he is building.

Manipulate the Terms

What is given by the terms of the problem are the necessary, but not the sufficient, ingredients to formulate a hypothesis. Previous knowledge, including theory, may describe the terms and even suggest possible relationships; however, it does not necessarily interrelate the parts. Formal reasoning provides a basis for interrelating the parts by suggesting some rules for manipulating the terms, but the rules do not yield the relationship.

The problem is a human one. It involves thinking. When it was said that "research is a person," it was implied that research involved the act of thinking. Thought-production is a process unique to man. Furthermore, creative thinking is a process unique to certain men. It is at the point of generating hypotheses that the true researcher often is separated from his fellow man.

But the act of creative thinking has defied description. It is more descriptive of the creative man than of the creative act. It may occur differently in different men, and at different times in the same man.

One of our eminent thinkers has described the process as a random act.

A problem is posed for which we must invent a solution. We know the conditions to be met by the sought idea; but we do not know what series of ideas will lead us there. In other words, we know how the series of our thoughts must end, but not how it should begin. In this case it is evident that there is no way to begin except at random. Our mind takes up the first path that it finds open before it, perceives that it is a false route, retraces its steps and takes another direction. Perhaps it will arrive immediately at the sought idea, perhaps it will arrive very belatedly: it is entirely impossible to know in advance. In these conditions we are reduced to dependence upon chance.[7]

The authors are not inclined to feel that the process is *entirely* random, as the above quotation would imply. Instead, creative thought is more apt to be generated when the array of circumstances is ripe.

Thomas Henry Huxley is reported to have exclaimed, on reading Darwin's *Origin of Species,* "Oh, what an ass I was not to have thought of that!" Even if the story is apocryphal, it is pertinent, for Darwin had assembled many facts which had been known for at least 2 generations. In addition, he had added many observations on his famous 4-year voyage on H.M.S. *Beagle.* Nevertheless, this enormous body of data did not take on any systematic order until a fortuitous event occurred. Darwin was pondering the problem of understanding what caused species to change, when he happened to read Thomas Malthus's notion that a population tended, in the absence of certain other checks, to overwhelm the resources for the sustenance of that population. In other words, the physical environment itself was always snapping at the heels of any species. If individuals change in certain directions they will be at an advantage; if they change in other directions, at a disadvantage. This, then, combined with Darwin's other information, resulted in the notion of the struggle for survival of the species. After its public expression and in spite of the fierce theological controversy it aroused, this explanation was quickly accepted by scientists. Huxley was simply exclaiming, because "anyone could have seen it." This was indeed the "right" man at the "right" time.[8]

If we read between the lines of the illustration, we may observe that there are several factors above and beyond chance that enabled the "right" man to create some useful thoughts. Darwin was armed with information that had been gathered systematically. He fitted his knowledge to the conceptions of someone else and developed a new idea. These were not necessarily random events.

Therefore, some useful hints to assist the researcher to propel ideas and develop hypotheses may be offered. The hints will not substitute for actual thinking. Only the individual researcher can do that. However, they may aid him to organize his thoughts in the process of formulating a hypothesis.

Briefly, we will propose that the researcher generate several hypotheses, scrutinize each carefully and select what would appear to be the most satisfactory. In a sense, the process can be likened to trial-and-error learning. However, it is more stringent and formalized.

Generate Several Tentative Hypotheses

As the researcher scrutinizes his backlog of information, he may initiate not one but several tentative hypotheses. There is usually more than one way to solve a problem. Therefore, the researcher may propose several solutions. His ultimate task is to determine the best solution.

A researcher conversant in the field of patient care may generate a number of ideas relating "patient confinement for X days" to "irritability."

He may consider that patient confinement leads to irritability, that it is a source of frustration. The patient has been confined to a hospital bed and cannot perform the activities of normal daily living. He has a need to earn a living, be with his family, care for his belongings. He has not been able to satisfy these needs and does not know when he will be able to do so. He reacts by becoming irritable.*

The researcher may consider that the relationship between the two terms is a spurious one. Their point of occurrence is coincidental. The patient is irritated because he is in pain, does not like the food

* Refer to Chapter 7 for a discussion of the problem of variables in subjects selected for research.

or has been disturbed by the nurse. "Confinement to bed for X days" was just an added factor.

The researcher may determine that "confinement to bed for X days" leads to "irritability" as well as to "despondency" and "infantile behavior." There are several relationships to be considered. There also may be several exceptions to the rule.

Where do the ideas come from? They usually are developed from an analysis of previous knowledge. This source comprises all the pertinent, written materials: studies, descriptive accounts, authoritative opinions and theoretic and interpretive analyses. It also includes the common-sense knowledge of the researcher: his experiences and his depth of understanding. What has been learned from the past is often the key to the future.

Previous knowledge will not necessarily provide the answers, but offers a basis for securing the answers. Otherwise there would not be a problem, but a matter of inquiry. The researcher must think about his problem situation and the related sources of knowledge, and somehow interrelate the two. Knowledge assists but does not replace thought.

The researcher also may resolve the issue with both informal and formal thought. Informal thought is characteristic perhaps of the random processes mentioned in the descriptive passages. Formal thought refers to the processes of reasoning and includes both induction and deduction.

No doubt the beginning stages of generating ideas are informal. The researcher has to begin somewhere, and perhaps he will begin with what he already knows and can understand. He may start with a flurry of ideas—some new and some that were considered ages ago. Or he may start with a complete blank and, in the course of running back and forth mentally, pick out and assemble the pieces systematically or in a helter-skelter fashion.

What happens here usually does not appear in print. Furthermore, the sources of common-sense knowledge that may be employed seldom are referenced. What the reader sees as the final product has been formalized beyond recognition. However, it is difficult to imagine that any study, developed and publicized by man, circumvented the informal thinking phase and happened in the manner described by the printed release.

Formal thinking may be considered then to occur after the fact. That is, it will begin after the initial onset of ideas. In a sense, it will put the house in order, set the ideas in appropriate form and evaluate them accordingly.

Formal thinking, regardless of the mode, may be described as the development of an argument. A series of propositions, premises or evidence is presented, from which a conclusion is drawn. The argument or conclusion is our hypothesis.

How would an argument be developed? The manner of approach would depend partially upon the nature of the evidence or the validity of the premises. This is another way of stating that it would depend upon the state of previous knowledge—whether the previous knowledge was organized or disorganized; whether or not some theorization had taken place.

Let us assume that the state of previous knowledge was essentially unorganized. It consisted of numerous descriptive statements regarding each term but lacked a set of general rules that might be employed to suggest a relationship or to link the terms together. The task may be expressed formally as the need to establish the premises and derive the conclusion.

Now we can refer back to the definition of terms. The illustration suggested that two lists of information descriptive of each term should be drawn up. In scrutinizing the lists, the researcher may perceive several instances in which irritable behavior occurs following "confinement to bed for X days." He may infer and generalize as a result that "confinement to bed for X days" leads to "irritable behavior."

This form of reasoning is known as induction. It has been defined as a process "by which we pass from evidence concerning *some* members of a certain class of objects to an assertion concerning *all* members of that class."[9] The evidence is contained in the premises that "some patients become irritable after X days of confinement." The assertion is the conclusion or hypothesis that "all patients will become irritable after X days of confinement." This is an example of the way in which empiric relationships are formulated.

The same solution could have been determined also by deduction. Cohen and Nagel interpreted deduction as "a search for a *general rule* which asserts a *universal* connection between facts of (one) kind and other facts of (a) different kind."[10] Their premises would consist of the rule suggestive of a relationship between the facts and a series of observations descriptive of the facts. An inference (or conclusion) is drawn from the observations as a function of the general rule.

This process implies the presence of a theory in which knowledge has been systematized, and that some general rules have been formulated. Reference will be made now to the second example, in which the terms are defined within the context of a theory of behavior. The general rule—"Frustration leads to aggression"—has been established within the theory and is given. It is observed and established that "confinement to bed for X days" is a form of frustration, i.e., the needs of normal living are not satisfied. It is observed and established also that "irritable behavior" is a form of aggression toward the nurse and other patients. Therefore, the inference, conclusion or hypothesis can be deduced that "confinement to bed for X days leads to irritable behavior."

Thus, the researcher could arrive at the same conclusion by different methods of reasoning. However, the processes are not interchangeable, nor is one a poorer substitute for the other. Deduction assumes that the premises are true and that the conclusion is valid if it is consistent with the premises. Induction does not make any assumptions regarding the premises. They are treated as probable. The conclusion is valid to the extent that the premises are true.

Induction actually is concerned with the establishment of valid premises. If the state of previous knowledge is such that valid premises have not been established, the researcher must rely upon the inductive process. For instance, there may be some question regarding the validity of the premises in the example of deductive reasoning.

Deduction deals in explanations. It seems to explain how the generalization was derived and, in addition, to provide for exceptions to the generalization. Therefore, it elaborates upon the generalization and, as a consequence, may yield other generalizations. However, the deductive argument also relies upon the existence of organized knowledge or theory.

Determine the Best Hypothesis

Which of the tentative hypotheses is to be selected for the empiric test? It is inexpedient and expensive to test each idea in this way. It would be more expedient to select the best hypothesis by other means and then arrange for an empiric test.

Previous knowledge also is employed to test the thoughts that are generated and to select from them the most appropriate hypothesis. This generation of ideas is somewhat akin to trial-and-error learning. The learner confronts a problem with a variety of responses. The one that secures the reward (overcomes the obstacle) remains, while the others are discarded. The selection of a response is based upon the actual experience of success. The selection of a suitable hypothesis also is based upon a success experience—the success of being compatible with previous knowledge.

Therefore, the researcher employs previous knowledge to test his ability to think. In this regard, he must seek evidence or knowledge not only to support his contentions but, if possible, to refute them. He desires his hypothesis to stand unrefuted ultimately. Those ideas or hypotheses that fail to do so may be eliminated; the others may remain for further testing.

How is previous knowledge employed? Let us re-examine the example of inductive reasoning. The premises are considered to be probable. The conclusion—that confinement to bed for X days leads to irritable behavior—will be refuted if only one negative instance occurs. The previous literature may reveal a single negative instance and eliminate the hypothesis on this account.

As a matter of fact, the other two hypotheses that have been suggested are examples of negative instances. One suggests that the two terms are unrelated, while the other considers that "confinement to bed for X days leads to irritable as well as to other forms of behavior." If any evidence is presented in support of these hypotheses, then the initial hypothesis can be refuted. Suppose we assume this to be the case. How can the deductive argument be resolved?

The premises may be re-examined in the light of the evidence. Accordingly, it may be determined that, while "frustration may lead to aggression," "not all frustration may lead to aggression." Furthermore, it may be reasoned that "confinement to bed for X days may lead to varying degrees of frustration." Therefore, "confinement to bed for X days may not always lead to aggression."

The theory perhaps is not inclusive and should be reformulated to account for the exception. In this regard, the following premises may be proposed:

1. There are varying degrees of frustration.

2. The different degrees of frustration may lead to different responses or behavior: aggression (or irritable behavior); regression (or infantile behavior); resignation (or despondency).

3. Frustration-induced behavior varies in adaptiveness.

4. The degree of frustration will vary inversely with the level of adaptiveness.

5. Confinement to bed for X days will lead to varying degrees of frustration.

The following conclusion can be deduced or inferred from the above: "Confinement to bed for X days will lead to varied frustration-induced behavior: irritability, infantile behavior, despondency." This deduction may serve as a satisfactory explanation of the third hypothesis and suggest to the researcher that this is his best alternative.

Two comments should be made at this time. One refers to the need to make assumptions. The other considers the nature of theory development.

There is an obvious need to explain or resolve the hypotheses caught in the midst of conflicting evidence. It is evident also that the premises employed to re-establish the theory and provide a more inclusive explanation may not be entirely valid. We have made the assumption, nevertheless, that they are true and will await additional evidence to support or refute them.

Assumptions of this kind often are made to establish theories and promote explanations. However, the validity of the explanation will be a function of the number of assumptions that are made.

A theory is by no means the final word. Theories are sometimes little more than collections of hypotheses. Occasionally a hypothesis may be formulated that cannot be explained by the theory, in which case either the hypothesis or the theory has been formulated incorrectly. If the former situation prevails, then the hypothesis has not withstood the test. If the latter is the case, then the theory is incomplete or incorrect. It should be modified or supplemented to explain the exception, or discarded. There have been several occasions in the history of science when some highly regarded theories have been rejected on this basis.

THE HYPOTHESIS—HOW IS IT STATED?

This section is a summary of some of the conditions for stating a hypothesis. They are by no means inclusive, but should serve as key check points.

The hypothesis should answer the problem as stated. The problem statement should specify the kind of answer that is expected. Does the hypothesis reflect this kind of answer? If not, then the researcher has gone astray. He has not fulfilled the requirements listed by the statement of the purpose.

The hypothesis should be testable. It will have been scrutinized in the face of fact and reason. An empiric test is also warranted. Has the hypothesis been stated in testable form? Can the paper model be erected in actuality? If not, the total requirements for research have not been satisfied.

The hypothesis should be compatible with previous knowledge. It should fit the facts or be explained as an exception to the facts. Is the hypothesis in accord with other knowledge? If not, the researcher should be able to account for the differences.

THE PLACE OF THE HYPOTHESIS IN NURSING RESEARCH

Nursing, like others of the younger disciplines, comprises a body of knowledge striving for maturity. The art and the practice of nursing may span the history of mankind. But the development of a systematized resource of constructs that define practice is only partially complete. It seeks to come of age.

What symbolizes maturity? Growth? Is there a finite body in which all of nursing is known? Transition? Is there an ultimate form into which all nursing knowledge is cast? Let us summarize the previous discussions with regard to the concept of the maturity of nursing knowledge.

The growth of knowledge is measurable in terms of the size or the number of components. As such, it always has been expanding. In fact, expansion fosters expansion. As each new relationship unfolds, the groundwork for additional inquiries is bared. For all practical purposes, each body of knowledge ultimately may comprise an infinite number of components.

However, the growth of knowledge is a function not only of numbers but also of kinds of configurations. A body of knowledge may be measured by its power to predict. In this respect, there are some relationships whose predictive powers transcend many situations. Their individual strength may be greater than the combined powers of a large number of independent single relationships. Thus qualitative differences also characterize the maturation of knowledge.

Accordingly, maturation is denotable by something more than expansion of knowledge. It may imply a change in the form of knowledge. In other words, we may gather that research not only contributes additional knowledge but also reshapes existing forms. A state of knowledge can be modified in several directions. Growth can be acclaimed as knowledge in transition achieves its most adaptable state.

GROWTH AND TRANSITION OF NURSING KNOWLEDGE

Several movements have been observed in the growth of nursing knowledge. There has been a transition from reliance upon the person to reliance upon the recorded experience. There has been a movement toward the formalization of knowledge. There has been a change in the direction of understanding.

Toward Reliance Upon the Person

Societies, as they become more complex, tend to lean naturally toward the idea of an expert or an authority as knowledge personified. It is a simple process to place confidence in persons who have acquired knowledge and proficiencies in problem-solving in special areas. The procedure is not time- or method-bound. Solutions are provided with relative ease.

Authorities emerged in nursing as they did in other fields of endeavor. Initially, the voices of a few personages could be heard above the crowd. They came essentially from the field of nursing itself. However, authorities from other fields, such as physicians, also were available to direct action and issue food for thought. These people were self-motivated—reformers who took up the obligation to bring order to some of the chaotic conditions that existed at the time.

When confronted with problems in later years, nursing societies themselves took deliberate action to convert the experts. They often brought together groups or committees of authorities who had acquired specialized knowledge in particular areas of nursing practice.

What has been the role of the expert or the authority in nursing research? The historical review has suggested that expert opinion was employed almost exclusively in the early years of modern nursing research. In recent years, the utilization of experts has been confined generally to some of the more grandiose projects such as the curriculum studies[11]; the establishment of functions, standards and qualifications for nursing practice[12]; and the place of nursing in modern society.[13] However, the influence of purely authoritative judgments in problem-solving still can be observed in many of the lesser-scaled projects.

Let us examine some of these projects:

Administrative Organization of Collegiate Schools of Nursing.[14] The purpose of this study was to determine patterns of administrative organization in collegiate schools of nursing as they involve the interrelationships among the school, the college or university, and the hospital and the community agencies utilized as teaching fields. Solutions were provided by the administrative heads of the college or university and the department or school of nursing and the medical and the surgical nursing instructors of 16 collegiate schools of nursing in the northeastern part of the United States.

Science Principles Applied to Nursing.[15] The objective of this study was to identify major facts and principles from anatomy, physiology, chemistry and physics that apply to nursing care. The authors first isolated and listed the facts and principles to be identified, and then submitted the listing for evaluation by a jury of nurses and science faculty.

A Study of the Educational Programs of Hospital Schools of Nursing.[16] The specific aim of this study was to identify the strengths and the weaknesses of the present programs of education and training in the hospital schools of nursing. The researchers were furnished with the opinions of various groups, gathered in response to a mailed questionnaire. The judgments covered 14 areas of concern and were stated in terms such as "highly satisfactory" or "not satisfactory." One hospital administrator, a director of nursing, a director of nursing education, 5 physicians, 3 faculty members, 5 alumnae members and 10 nursing students in each of 26 hospitals responded to the questionnaire.

What can the reader observe in scanning these illustrations? He may note that the studies entail the determination of a large number of simple and complex relationships. They do not deal with the development of a single relationship. This practice may be typical of studies that employ expert opinions for problem-solving. The use of the expert seems to circumvent the requirements for controlled tests and measures. It also appears to save a considerable amount of time.

The reader may infer that the researcher has several roles to perform. He serves to isolate and pinpoint the particular areas for study. These compose the items of the questionnaire or the interview form. What is selected for study and how it is presented definitely will influence the outcome. The researcher also serves to compile and summarize the resulting opinions.

In this sense, he may evaluate the findings and suggest that some judgments are weighted more heavily than others.

The reader may have observed that several different categories of experts were employed. Their respective roles were 2-fold. In two instances they offered opinions concerning the many issues under study. In the other instance, they evaluated the opinions or judgments of the researcher.

How can we evaluate the utilization of expert opinion in these cases as a source or a form of knowledge? What are the opinions? They may be considered as tentative hypotheses. They have been derived in most cases on an informal basis in which the expert may have employed, as supportive evidence, experience or knowledge readily at hand. The researcher or other experts may be employed to substantiate or eliminate some of the hypotheses offered. The opinions or tentative hypotheses may be weighted by the repute or the prestige of the expert or by the number of experts in concurrence. They are not tested by formal logic or evaluated in the light of previously acknowledged evidence. They are not subjected to empiric testing.

Toward Reliance Upon Experience

A reaction against expert opinion or reasoning is followed sometimes by a movement toward reliance upon sheer experience. This is a transition toward supposed objectivity. It ushers in the fact-gathering age.

There is a tendency to treat the reasoning process, model-building and hypothesis-formulation with suspicion. The researcher's ability to formulate relationships in advance of observation often is questioned. There is some fear that such practices bias observation, i.e., the observer sees only that which will support his hypothesis.

Fact-gathering, on the other hand, may be considered to be a sign of purity in research. The researcher will rely only upon what is observed or actually is known to be the case. He will not hazard a guess, a speculation or a hypothesis. He will describe only what he sees. In this, he may feel certain.

Fact-gathering also may appear to be the means by which a young body of knowledge, such as nursing, can get started. Facts become the basis upon which a body of knowledge is built. The researcher must begin by observing and recording what is.

It may be recalled that the middle period of the era of modern nursing seemed to be the period of the fact-gathering age in nursing. Plans were implemented to gather annual statistics on the numbers of nurses, students, patients and facilities. These facts have been supplemented by information accumulated by other related health fields. This endeavor flourishes currently on a large scale.

In addition to these annual enterprises, there also have been a number of smaller though more highly concentrated studies focusing upon more restricted questions. These studies were not founded upon any formal hypotheses. The problems were stated and solved directly by observation.

Institutional Nursing in New Hampshire.[17] An observation program focused upon the activities and the functions performed by different levels of nursing personnel—registered nurses, practical nurses and nurse aides—was employed in the study. Two research teams of two persons each observed the nursing personnel during at least some portion of each shift for 1 week. In addition, interviews were held with a sample of the patients on the wards under supervision, and with the nursing personnel.

A Time Study of Nursing Activities in a Psychiatric Hospital.[18] To answer questions relating to the proportion of attendant nursing time spent with patients, and in tasks related to their care, and on non-nursing tasks, two methods of observation were employed. These were: (1) the continuous method of observation (over the shoulder) and (2) the work-sampling method. To ensure and facilitate observation, a system of classification of the activities to be observed was worked out and forms were derived for recording observations. Each classification and activity was defined so as to describe a nursing action.

The Nurse's Thursday in a Psychiatric Ward.[19] The actual nursing situation in the psychiatric wards in a selected hospital was studied preliminary to the establishment of an affiliating program for nursing students. Each nurse's every action on two psychiatric wards was observed and recorded according to a prearranged classification in consecutive intervals of 1 minute during 24-hour periods. Fifteen nurses were trained as observers. The observers were scheduled for 2-hour observation periods during the day and the evening and for 3-hour periods during the night. An open and a closed psychiatric ward were surveyed on 3 days of the same week—Monday, Thursday and Saturday.

Nursing Observations of 100 Premature Infants and Their Feeding Programs.[20] The amount of formula that premature infants of a given weight and age could tolerate while at the same time maintaining a satisfactory weight record was determined through nursing observations. The amount and the kind of food offered to each of 100 premature infants, the behavior associated with their feedings, the infants' birth weights and ages in days, their daily changed weights, all were carefully recorded on specially devised forms for the period that each infant was in the hospital.

There appears to be one outstanding characteristic among the examples—the observations were not performed casually. In each case, the researcher seemed to take deliberate pains to specify beforehand how, when and where the observations were to be made. These were to be orderly studies. Specific forms were developed, instructions were detailed, subjects and times were denoted. In many cases, follow-up efforts were made to confirm the observations.

Two general issues are of concern here. The first pertains to the development of the observational procedures. The second deals with the validity of the observations.

Upon what basis were the researchers able to pinpoint their observations? Upon what basis did they determine how, when and where to observe? The forms and the procedures apparently were developed with considerable forethought. What did the researchers think about?

Could the researchers draw valid conclusions from their findings? Despite the care taken to record precisely what happened, can the researchers state that what was observed will hold true generally? Unless the conditions for selecting observable situations were known in advance, it is possible that these situations were not truly representative of the factors under study. Upon what basis were the factors ascertained?

The authors would venture the thought that preliminary or tentative hypotheses were formulated in advance by each of the researchers. The hypotheses were unstated, contained in the unwritten thoughts of the investigators. The procedures were developed as a function of these hypotheses. This would have to be the case. Otherwise, why one format rather than another? Unfortunately, the reader has not been given formal presentations of the hypotheses. Therefore, he cannot understand fully the implications of what transpired. Would it not have been possible for the researchers actually to formulate and state their hypotheses formally? Would such statements really bias the outcome?

Toward Formalization

Perhaps the true reason for lack of formalization is that the process of formulating a hypothesis is a difficult one. We have suggested from time to time that the process really is informal. The feeling of formality is expressed only in the final copy, which often may omit many of the intervening steps.

A vast amount of preparation actually characterizes the process of formulating a hypothesis. The researcher may make a number of false starts. He may be required first to grapple with the actual situation rather than with his thoughts in the search for hypotheses. This sometimes is considered to be the pilot-study stage. It usually is omitted from the final product. But should it not be included? Are not statements such as the following of assistance to the reader?

The pilot study was conducted during the fall of 1956. The preceding months encompassed the frustration of developing an instrument which could be used with nursing students in various types of schools, and with patients who were subject to the highly unpredictable happenings of illness and hospitalization. To ignore this instrument developing phase of the study would be to present an unrealistic picture and leave unanswered many questions relating to the lack of rigorous controls over the selection of students, patients, and the clinical assignments of students. Consequently, the first half of part 1 describes the proposed methodology and the factors which changed or influenced the original planning, and the second half describes the revision of method, analysis of data and findings of the pilot study. . . .

Although the pilot study afforded a method of selecting students and patients and a technique which could be used to determine the extent of agreement between the perceptions of patients and students, there was the obvious need for further refinement of techniques and for the testing of hypotheses.[21]

Perhaps the first stage toward formalization is informality. A recognition of this requirement may be viewed as a mark of progress.

It would appear also that a certain amount of sophistication is required by the researcher before he can formulate a hypothesis adequately. That is, he must become sufficiently aware of the subject matter to prescribe alternate courses of action. A pilot study may enable the researcher to become more sophisticated. In addition, the general state of knowledge at the time may either enhance or deter the researcher's abilities in this regard.

It may appear, however, that the character of nursing knowledge gradually is becoming amenable to formalization. Instances of completed studies can be cited more frequently. Let us examine a few and observe their qualities:

The Relationship Between Authoritarian Attitudes and Attitudes Toward Mental Patients[22]

Problem. What is the relationship between an authoritarian personality tendency and a negative attitude toward mental patients?

Hypotheses. (1) Authoritarian individuals will express more negative attitudes toward mental patients than will nonauthoritarians. (2) Authoritarian individuals will see mental patients as less like themselves than will nonauthoritarians, in terms of response to certain situations. (3) Authoritarians will show less susceptibility to changing their attitudes toward mental patients following psychiatric orientation and association with them than will nonauthoritarians.

Procedure. Two groups of nursing student affiliates in psychiatric nursing were classified as authoritarian and nonauthoritarian. Their attitudes toward mental patients were determined prior to and after instruction and clinical experience in psychiatric nursing.

Conclusion. Hypotheses 1 and 3 were confirmed. Hypothesis 2 was not confirmed.

Play Interviews for 4-Year-Old Hospitalized Children[23]
Problem.
1. Are 4-year-old hospitalized children able to use clinical equipment to express their feelings about intrusive procedures?
2. How do 4-year-old hospitalized children tend to interpret intrusive procedures?
3. What attitudes do 4-year-old hospitalized children tend to show toward personnel who administer intrusive procedures?
4. What methods do 4-year-old hospitalized children use to cope with their feelings about intrusive procedures?

Hypotheses. When given opportunity for play with clinical equipment and other accessories for projective play, 4-year-old hospitalized children are able to express their feelings concerning the procedures they experienced. Individual children show characteristic patterns of coping with these feelings.

Procedure. Play interviews were held with 22 four-year-old hospitalized children at a time when they were allowed to play with clinical prototypes of equipment required for intrusive procedures. The play behavior of each child was recorded.

Conclusion. The data presented clear evidence that the majority of the children studied perceived no protective intent of the adults behind the intrusive procedure but rather considered them as hostile in intent with the exception of the procedures in the oral area.

Favoritism in Personnel-Patient Interaction[24]
Problem. What are . . . the differences in nurses' relationships with patients they like and their relationships with patients they dislike?

Hypotheses. (1) Personnel will contact preferred patients more frequently than nonpreferred patients. (2) Personnel's interactions with preferred patients will be primarily personal or social in nature, whereas their interactions with nonpreferred patients will be primarily procedural, i.e., concerned with physical needs and necessary routine of ward care.

Procedure. Sixteen nursing personnel were very closely observed on one ward for 2 hours each over a 2-week period. Their interactions with patients for whom they felt attraction and with patients for whom they felt no attraction were analyzed and compared. Preferences and nonpreferences of personnel for patients were elicited by means of a sociometric technique—the Morenian choice process.

Conclusions.
1. Personnel made more contacts and spent more time interacting with favored than with nonfavored patients.
2. Personnel gave as much attention to the physical needs of nonfavored patients as they did to those of favored patients. They grasped

the socializing opportunities afforded by such contacts more readily when dealing with patients they preferred.

3. Personnel interacted on a personal, friendly level more freely and more frequently with preferred than with nonpreferred patients. . . .

In a word, the nonpreferred patient is treated as a patient while the preferred is recognized as a person.

These examples might be classified as more complete studies than any of the illustrations previously cited. The reader may secure the feeling that the researchers have shared their total experiences. There are links with the past. The hypotheses have resulted from previous knowledge. There is an eye to the future. The conclusions may be placed within the current framework of knowledge and are suggestive of further avenues of study.

Specificity rather than diffusion is the order here. The researchers limited their studies to the determination of a small number of relationships. They have been stated clearly and specifically.

These clearly derived statements served to direct or guide the main bodies of the studies. The quality of direction seems to permeate the papers. There was a single-mindedness of purpose as expressed in the statements of the problem or problems, the hypotheses, the procedures and the conclusions. Each followed in natural sequence.

Above all, the outcome of the studies seemed more conclusive. This was apparently the case despite the fact that some of the conclusions were negative. At least the researchers were able to reject their hypotheses rather than to say nothing at all. It is a form of assurance that may feed the confidence of the consumer of nursing knowledge. It provides the essence upon which researchers can build.

Toward Understanding

The attainment of understanding is the ultimate pathway toward the realization of environmental control and manipulation. Under these circumstances, the nurse practitioner does not merely indulge in a series of isolated predictions such as:

1. Assisting the patient to accept bodily change may require highly professional nursing service.

2. Trauma can be expected following surgery.

3. People can be prepared for change.

4. People react negatively to bodily disfiguration.

5. The nursing care of patients in trauma requires highly concentrated technical nursing services.

6. People can learn to accept change.

7. The spread of cancer can be arrested by removal of the affected tissue.

Instead, the nurse practitioner can perceive the total situation: A radical mastectomy has been employed successfully in the treatment of cancer of the breast. However, this form of treatment has some deleterious effects. As in most cases of surgery, postoperative trauma can be expected. In addition, there will result some obvious body disfiguration that the patient may find difficult to accept. The nurse can assist the patient in several ways. She may enable the patient to overcome the effects of trauma by administering the type of professional nursing care that she has been prepared to give. She can provide a mode of teaching assistance to help the patient to accept and compensate for the bodily disfiguration.

Furthermore, the nurse practitioner can make changes: Preparation for change in advance of the change itself may result in less harmful attitudinal effects. Thus, the nurse may alter her plan of care and provide extensive teaching prior to surgery.

Above all, the nurse practitioner will know what she is doing. The events are not treated as a series of independent, isolated entities in which each occurs without regard to the other. They occur together and, in harmony, become meaningful. She knows why the initial preparation, the surgery, the concentrated technical care, the teaching assistance are necessary.

Understanding is fostered by the integration of knowledge. It involves bringing together the various contributions regarding a particular area of concern. It involves a realization of the total configuration. It involves the development of a network of connections that serve to link the independent contributions into a meaningful whole.

Nursing research has concentrated on several areas of concern: the nurse's contribution to patient care, the organization of nurses, the education and training of nurses, the supervision of nurses, the recruitment and selection of nursing students. Any survey of the nursing research literature will uncover a wide variety of small- and large-scale studies to satisfy particular segments of the various areas. In addition, knowledge from some basic and applied fields outside nursing also may lend support to particular segments. A step in the direction of understanding is obtained when the particular segments can be brought to bear upon the total area of concern.

The integration of this knowledge requires a realization of what is demanded by the particular area of concern. The researcher must be able to conceptualize the end-product—what the system will be required to yield. For example, some knowledge of patients and their requirements for nursing care and some knowledge of organizational patterns matching groups of nurses with groups of patients are needed to understand the organization of nurses for patient care. The ability to foresee these requirements will influence the kind of knowledge that is selected for study.

However, the mere accumulation of related knowledge about a particular area of concern is insufficient. In addition, the system must compose a network or a chain in which the component parts can be linked. It does not suffice only to gather knowledge of patients, nurses and organizational patterns. The researcher must have the wherewithal to relate the patients to the nurse and to the organizational structure. He must be able also to integrate knowledge secured from other fields and expressed in unrelated terminology. He must be able to synthesize this knowledge.

This alludes to a peculiar problem of integrating knowledge in nursing. It was suggested earlier (see Chap. 2) that nursing was a practice that embodied several disciplines and utilized resource materials from several areas of knowledge. The problem entails the integration of the various source materials into a system of nursing practice.

Nursing needs a fusion of concepts identified from nursing practice with those extracted from the sciences, and adapted or recast to the purposes of nursing, in order to describe the phenomena of nursing practice. Nursing can be expected to achieve a modification and a specification of concepts appropriate to nursing needs.

In order thus to evolve appropriate knowledge for effective nursing practice, two developments are necessary. The activities of nurses and the problems with which they deal need to be conceptualized, and the nature of nursing needs to be identified. Hand in hand with this endeavor must go the extraction of those concepts from related scientific knowledge that are pertinent to nursing practice.

Such endeavors should lead to the development of a nursing practice theory. Such a theory should lead to the development of a theory of interrelationships of psychological, social, biologic, physical and medical factors, for this is what explains nursing practice. This is the task that only nursing can do. Sciences cannot do this for nursing. This, of course, presupposes that nurse theorists will have to be developed. Only isolated attempts have been made so far to relate pieces of knowledge from a variety of knowledge domains in such a way that they become an organized body of knowledge, the pieces of which are sufficiently cohesive to form some sort of system. The nursing profession must reach the point of making conscious applications and tests of theoretic propositions from the sciences and of contributing knowledge refined from its own practices.

That the integration of nursing knowledge has not been achieved is clearly evident. However, the movement in the direction of integration and toward the ultimate understanding of nursing practice has been apparent for some time. The writings of Florence Nightingale are suggestive of this notion. The idea of a system of nursing knowledge has gained increasing prominence in more recent times.

Here are some examples of what has been accomplished to date:

Nightingale presented a simple framework to explain and develop the basis for nursing action.[25] It has been reduced by the authors to diagrammatic form and described in Figure 4. The system is centered about the general notion that disease is really a reparative process employed by nature to remedy bodily ills. The process is promoted by conditions of fresh air, warmth, cleanliness, food, etc., and hindered or interrupted by the absence of one or more of these qualities. Symptoms such as pain and elevated temperatures, which often are regarded as parts of the reparative process, are considered, in reality, as

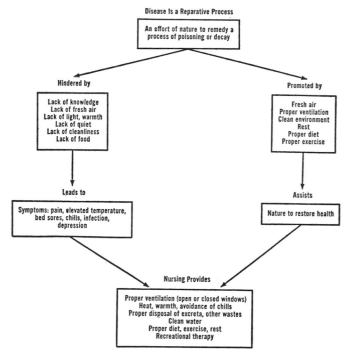

Fig. 4. A model for research. (Based on Nightingale, Florence: Notes on Nursing: What It Is and What It Is Not, Harrison, 1859; Philadelphia, Lippincott, 1946)

incidental to the disease. They tend to arise in the absence of the conditions promoting repair. Nursing can assist nature by arranging conditions to ensure the continuing presence of these factors.

Nightingale did not conceive of this miniature system as a basis for research. However, it could have been utilized to assist the researcher to formulate appropriate hypotheses. An entire series of nursing functions related to the reparative process can be derived and tested. The researcher can hypothesize the nursing care required to circumvent barriers or obstacles to the reparative process. The researcher also can reason and stipulate the services that may promote repair.

Johnson developed a model to synthesize the contributions of many disciplines, including nursing, toward the maintenance and/or the re-establishment of health.[26] A variety of sources were employed: the sociologic analysis of the nurse role by Johnson and Martin,[27] sociologic studies of related professions, concepts from the basic sciences, and a knowledge of nursing. Within the context of this framework, she attempted to explain the nature of nursing and to identify the knowledge essential to nursing practice.

The model focuses upon the central idea that illness is a form of stress that casts the patient into a state of disequilibrium. The component parts of the system include the patient, the doctor, the nurse and their respective roles in maintaining equilibrium through the management of tensions resulting from stress.

An interpretation of the system has been described briefly and pictorially in Figure 5. Stress emanating from illness, treatment activities and the doctor-patient-nurse social system cast the patient into a state of disequilibrium and produce tensions and discomfort. The nurse's primary function in giving care is to relieve tension and discomfort and restore a state of equilibrium. The activities listed under nursing services are directed toward this end.

This conceptual framework has never been tested. Furthermore, it may not have been the intent of the author to employ

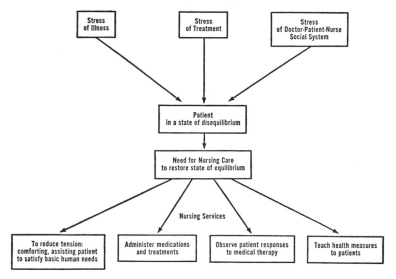

Fig. 5. A model for research. (Based on Johnson, Dorothy: Nurs. Outlook 7:291-294, 1959)

the model in a research setting. However, the researcher may use such a system as this to formulate some fruitful hypotheses regarding the functions of the nurses. The authors have inferred and derived the following to serve as illustrations:

Problem. What are the effects of the physical acts of nursing care (bathing, feeding, toileting) on the maintenance of the motivational equilibrium of the patient?

Explanation. The physical acts of nursing care have expressive significance to patients in addition to primary-need satisfaction. The nurse conveys an attitude of caring for the patient through these acts. The nursing acts symbolize and give direct gratification to the patient, which, in turn, serves to maintain his motivational equilibrium.

Hypothesis. The physical acts of nursing care (bathing, feeding, toileting) in a health-illness stress situation will tend to reduce the tension level and maintain the motivational equilibrium of the patient.

Problem. Does the approach employed by the nurse in the administration of medications or treatments (hypodermic injection, colostomy irrigation, etc.) affect the tension level of the patient?

Explanation. The motivational equilibrium of the patient may be disturbed by the presence of tension generated through treatment activities. The tensions will be affected by the nurse's approach in administering the treatment. The use of explanation, reassurance and empathy will assist in the reduction of tensions. Failure to explain a procedure, or the performance of a treatment in a cold, detached manner will generate further tensions.

Hypothesis. The nurse who approaches the patient expressively when administering treatments will reduce the tension level of the patient.

It should be noted that the models represent two different approaches to the development of nursing functions. They differ mainly because of their underlying structures. In many respects, however, they are at greater variance with the empiric approach than they are with one another.

The empiric approach describes nursing practice by observing the nurse at work. It states, in essence, that the nurse does what she does because she does what she does. There is always the question of what comes first—the patient, the nurse or the practice—and why.

The approaches through understanding begin not with the nurse but with a set of principles denoting the nature of the illness and of the curative process. These principles have been derived from other sources of knowledge and exist independently of nursing. They will be judged for their own sakes and not by whether or not they justify the existence of current nursing practices. The questions do not concern what the nurse does but what needs to be done by someone to satisfy the requirements of the stated principles.

The approaches are similar because each provides a rational basis for nursing. They may start with different premises but can eventuate into the same set of nursing practices. Each could also suggest a different array of practices. This could happen because the systems may be incomplete; each may deal with a different segment of the total health structure. The basic premises and/or the logical system also could be incomplete. In this case, the model rather than the practices will be judged. The system will stand because the premises are valid, and it is logically consistent. It will not rest upon the contention that the derived practices have been performed by so many persons in so many nursing situations.

These are approaches to the study of nursing through understanding. They represent a composite of many studies inside and outside nursing. They have endeavored to integrate diverse sources of knowledge into a meaningful whole. They are suggestive of fruitful hypotheses.

REFERENCES

1. Cohen, M. R., and Nagel, E.: An Introduction to Logic and Scientific Method, p. 215, New York, Harcourt, 1934.
2. *Ibid.*, pp. 200-201.
3. Goode, W. J., and Hatt, P. K.: Methods in Social Research, p. 56, New York, McGraw-Hill, 1952.
4. Cohen, M. R., and Nagel, E.: *Op. cit.* (see Ref. 1), p. 202.
5. Goode, W. J., and Hatt, P. K.: *Op. cit.* (see Ref. 3), p. 56.
6. Good, C. V.: Introduction to Educational Research, p. 77, New York, Appleton-Century-Crofts, 1959.
7. Souriou, P.: Théorie de l'invention, p. 17, Paris, Hachette, 1881. Translation by D. T. Campbell *in* Blind variation and selective retention in creative thought as in other knowledge processes, Psychol. Rev. *67* (No. 6):385, 1960.
8. Goode, W. J., and Hatt, P. K.: *Op. cit.* (see Ref. 3), pp. 66-67.
9. Black, Max: Critical Thinking: An Introduction to Logic and Scientific Method, p. 276, New York, Prentice-Hall, Inc., 1946.
10. Cohen, M. R., and Nagel, E.: *Op. cit.* (see Ref. 1), p. 202.
11. Shields, M. R.: A project for curriculum improvement, Nurs. Res. *1*:4-31, 1952.
12. Past, Present, and Future of FS&Q: A Guide for the Interpretation and Implementation of the Statements of Functions, Standards, and Qualifications for Practice, New York, American Nurses Assn., 1957.
13. Brown, L. E.: Nursing for the Future, New York, Russell Sage Foundation, 1948.
14. Thielbar, Frances C.: Administrative organization of collegiate schools of nursing, Nurs. Res. *2*:53, 1953.
15. Nordmark, M. T., and Rohweder, A. W.: Science Principles Applied to Nursing, pp. 3-9, Philadelphia, Typescript, 1959.
16. Williams, K. R., Covey, F., and Greene, J. E.: A Study of the Educational Programs of Hospital Schools of Nursing, pp. 1; 24-34, sponsored by The National Organization of Hospital Schools of Nursing, 1954.

17. Theriault, G. F.: Institutional Nursing in New Hampshire, p. 7, Final Report to the New Hampshire State Nurses' Assn., July, 1958.

18. Burke, C., Chall, C. L., and Abdellah, F. G.: A time study of nursing activities in a psychiatric hospital, Nurs. Res. 5:27-30, 1956.

19. Stevens, P. B., and Halpert, P. W.: The nurse's Thursday in a psychiatric ward, Nurs. Res. 6:29-30, 1957.

20. Iffrig, Sister Mary Charitas: Nursing observations of 100 premature infants and their feeding programs, Nurs. Res. 5:71-73, 1956.

21. Boyle, Rena: A Study of Student Nurse Perception of Patient Attitudes, pp. 1; 23, Washington, D. C., U. S. Department of Health, Education, and Welfare, Public Health Service, 1960.

22. Carter, F. M., and Shoemaker, R.: The relationship between authoritarian attitudes and attitudes toward mental patients, Nurs. Res. 9:39-41, 1960.

23. Erickson, F. H.: Play Interviews for 4-Year-Old Hospitalized Children, pp. 8; 66, Monograph, Society for Research in Child Development, Inc., 23, Serial No. 69, No. 3, 1958.

24. Morimoto, F. R.: Favoritism in personnel-patient interaction, Nurs. Res. 3:109-112, 1955.

25. Nightingale, Florence: Notes on Nursing: What It Is and What It Is Not, London, Harrison, 1859; Philadelphia, Lippincott, 1946.

26. Johnson, Dorothy: The nature of a science of nursing, Nurs. Outlook 7:291-294, 1959.

27. Johnson, M. W., and Martin, H. W.: The sociological analysis of the nurse role, Amer. J. Nurs. 58:373-377, 1958.

CHAPTER 6

The Design of the Test

THE GENERAL CASE

It has been reiterated from time to time that the hypothesis is only a paper or tentative solution to a problem. Although the hypothesis will have been exposed to the rigors of logical thought and scrutinized carefully in the face of facts, the tests are not considered crucial. The researcher also will desire to evaluate his hypothesis in a realistic situation.

How is a crucial test of a hypothesis developed? This is the procedural problem. It includes several steps:

1. The development of an appropriate study design

2. The identification of a pertinent problem situation, including subjects and materials

3. The construction of methodology to collect and analyze data.

The steps are interrelated and tied directly to the hypothesis, the problem and the terms.

If the researcher was requested to select the one step upon which each of the others is most dependent, it would have to be the development of the study design. The design is the medium intervening between the statement of the hypothesis and the procedure. It serves to identify the relevant elements to be tested, which, in turn, are suggestive of subjects and materials.

280

It depicts what should constitute a crucial test and, accordingly, specifies the methodology for data collection and analysis.

Therefore, the authors chose to initiate the procedural problem by considering the matter of design. This chapter will deal with the need to design an adequate test situation. It will examine the elements of a crucial test and discuss some general methods of controlling them.

The Need To Design a Crucial Test

Why is it necessary to design a special test of a hypothesis? In common-sense problem-solving or trial-and-error learning, the problem-solver usually does not effect special testing conditions. He simply may try his deduced response within the context of the specific problem situation. If it works, he may be satisfied. If it fails to work, he may try some other response.

Why can the researcher not return to or locate a specific situation illustrative of the problem statement and try his hypothesis? If it has been deduced that "confinement to bed for X days led to irritable behavior," is it not sufficient merely to investigate a situation in which patients are confined to bed for X days? Why devise special conditions?

Let us assume that the researcher did not devise special conditions. He simply observed a patient confined to bed for X days and found, to his dismay, that the patient did not become irritable. Does he then reject the hypothesis?

Suppose the researcher refused to yield to these circumstances and observed a second patient under similar conditions. On this occasion, the patient was irritable. Does the researcher now accept or reject his hypothesis?

Is the researcher in a position to draw any conclusion? If so, what can he state? If not, must he go on observing patients? How many? Under any circumstances, how can he account for the differences in observations?

The questions may be rephrased in more technical language. The first pertains to the nature of the valid conclusion. In essence, it inquires: What is truth for the researcher? The remaining questions concern the conditions under which valid conclusions may be drawn. The researcher asks: What constitutes a crucial test of a hypothesis?

What Is Truth for the Researcher?

All hypotheses are forecasts or predictions. The researcher forecasts in advance a description, another prediction or an explanation concerning the relationships of two or more events. His purpose in doing so is to identify the exact nature of the relationship and then to establish appropriate testing conditions to verify his forecast.

The researcher actually desires to establish his hypothesis as a truth. Webster suggests that truth implies "agreement with reality."[1] And this is the purpose of the test: to determine that the hypothesis is in "agreement with reality."

However, truth for the researcher may be relative. We seldom obtain full agreement with reality. "Confinement to bed for X days" may not always lead to irritable behavior. Perhaps it will occur most of the time, or in varying degrees just some of the time. Truth for the researcher may be purely a statement of probability.

Two problems confront the researcher and limit his ability to establish his hypothesis as an absolute truth. One concerns the nature of reality; the other deals with the hypothesis itself.

A primary task of the researcher is to establish or find a test situation or a criterion measure as an index of reality. And herein lies a paradox. On what basis is the criterion measure to be considered valid or real? The researcher may determine that it was attested to be the case in some other study. How? The criterion measure was compared with some other criterion measure, which, in turn, had been validated by other criterion measures and so on, ad infinitum. The gist of the problem is that the criterion measure or what is real itself may be little more than hypothetic. With what assurance, then, can it be stated that the hypothesis or the criterion measure is real?

The hypothesis is also a limiting factor. It may be measured in terms of its ability to account for all the events in a total configuration. When an observer sees a patient who has been confined to bed for X days, what does he really see? Does he just see a patient in bed? Does he see an intelligent or a dull person in bed? Does he see a person with outside interests? Does he see a person who has seen a member of his family recently? Does he see a person who is in pain? Does he see a person who is confined in a room with other persons? Does he see a person who has been cared for by other people? There are many events to be accounted for in the total situation. What is established as truth will be a function of the ability to account for these events.

Let us re-examine the nature of the hypothesis as a function of accountability. Accordingly, we might suppose that the researcher has devised a list of a hundred different descriptions of the patient confined to bed for X days. It may be assumed that the list provides every possible combination of events that can be expected to transpire at this time. Furthermore, the researcher has determined and listed the probability that a given combination of events will occur.

However, the researcher will derive his hypothesis predicting the flow of events in one of several ways to be described. Consider the probability that the various hypotheses will be verified.

A Guess

The researcher could place each combination on a slip of paper, which is folded and inserted in an open box. Then he could request any casual observer to select one of the papers at random. What is selected will be the researcher's hypothesis. It accounts for one of a hundred different possibilities. And, by chance, it may have a high or a low probability of occurrence.

A Speculation

The researcher might arrange the listing in random sequence on a sheet of paper and omit the probability statements. This time he might stop some independent observer in the hospital corridor and say: "Patient M has spent X days in bed. Which one of this list of behaviors describes what the patient is doing currently?" What is speculated will vary with the observer's previous knowledge of hospital patients. However, he will have an opportunity to make a cursory comparison among the events listed. Therefore, it is not unlikely that the speculation would be closer to reality than a pure guess.

An Empiric Relationship

The researcher might arrange his list in order of the probability of occurrence. He notes that the pair of events at the top of the list has a considerably higher rate of occurrence than the remaining combinations. These events would tend to account for the patient's behavior much of the time. If he hypothesizes that these events can be expected to occur on the next observation, he will do so in accordance with the statement of probability. However, he has accounted for only one pair of events in the total configuration. He cannot state the remaining circumstances under which the events will or will not be expected to occur.

A Theory-Derived Deduction

Consider that the researcher determined and stated the conditions under which each of the events on the listing would occur. Then he could account for any possible combination of events. That is, if he knew all the conditions surrounding Patient M on P occasion, he could deduce the events to follow with absolute certainty. A statement of probability would not be required.

To the extent that a theory is complete, it will account for all the events of the total configuration. A deduction derived from a theory should not only specify a relationship, but should also list the conditions under which it is or is not expected to occur. Unfortunately, theories are seldom complete. Therefore, the theory-derived deduction also will be a statement of probability. However, in terms of accountability or understanding, perhaps the researcher may express greater confidence in the deduction than in the empiric relationship derived as a statement of sheer probability.

What is truth for the researcher is actually a point on a probability continuum. This continuum is an expression of the researcher's confidence in his findings. It will vary with his ability to formulate complete hypotheses and identify appropriate test situations. Although the researcher may strive for certainty, there will be times when he may have to be satisfied with much less than absolute truth.

What Is a Crucial Test?

A truly crucial test of a hypothesis should permit the researcher to ascertain the validity of his hypothesis with an unqualified "yes" or "no" answer. He would desire simply to state: "Yes, we have reasoned correctly" or "No, our solution is erroneous." In view of our statements about the nature of truth and reality for the researcher, it might appear that very few truly crucial tests actually can be effected. However, man strives in the direction of the truly crucial test and has developed technics to minimize or, at least, to account for the errors in prediction.

What can the researcher do to effect a more crucial test of his hypothesis? He can develop more valid criteria. He can formulate more comprehensive hypotheses. He can establish procedures to effect more adequate controls over his test situation.

The task of identifying and developing adequate criterion measures is concerned more directly with the identification of a pertinent problem situation. It deals in subjects and materials and will be considered in the next chapter.

The task of formulating more comprehensive hypotheses already has been discussed. The reader might reconsider the matter as it affects the problem of the test. Since the subject was by no means exhausted, he might augment these thoughts with the selective writings of others.

The crux of the influence of subject matter on design is concerned directly with the problem of control. A crucial test may be considered more realistically as a controlled test. It is a test in which the researcher attempts to exercise some measure of restraint over the events to be observed.

In a controlled test, the researcher may try deliberately to organize the events to be observed so that he can effect an adequate test of his hypothesis. A controlled test implies that he may not permit all the events to be observed to begin normally. Instead, he will identify the requirements for testing his hypothesis and make the situation conform to these requirements.

It was noted previously that several different kinds of events can be observed in the situation of the patient confined to bed for X days. These are the conditions of which the behavior that follows is a logical consequence. Unless controlled, the events could combine to effect different types of behavior. Unless controlled, "confinement to bed for X days" really will describe the particular combination of events that were operative upon the occasion of the observation. And this could be a chance circumstance.

In a controlled test, the researcher may tamper with and prearrange the events deliberately so that only a particular combination occurs or is recognized. "Confinement to bed for X days" will be considered to have the same meaning in each of the observations. What is controlled is a function of the hypothesis. In essence, the researcher attempts to re-establish his paper model in a real situation. He acts to make the situation to be observed follow the specifications of the model.

It can be observed that control focuses about the events or the factors present in the problem situation. These events have been described previously as the terms of a problem or the elements of a model. They are designated also as "variables." What is controlled is the variable.

A variable, a term, a factor, or an element is a person, a thing, an event, a trait or a way of behaving. It possesses the characteristics of change and measurement. Perhaps the variable has been manipulated or acted upon and observed to vary. Furthermore, the variable should possess different values as a function of the change. In other words, the effects of change are measurable.

There are different kinds or categories of variables. Two classifications will be discussed in particular: dependency and relevancy. They reflect directly upon the problem of control.

Variables can be classified, with regard to their positions relative to one another, as independent and dependent. An independent variable is said to stand alone; it will affect but not be affected by other variables. On the other hand, a dependent variable is dependent upon or affected by independent variables.

Levine characterized this relationship as a stimulus-response connection.[2] The stimulus may exist independently of the response but is considered to influence the nature of the response. The response is dependent upon or will occur as a result of the stimulus. The authors have suggested a cause-and-effect relationship or a condition of antecedence and consequence.

The stimulus, the cause or the antecedent condition have the characteristics of the independent variable. "Confinement to bed for X days" is such a condition. It is an antecedent event, and behavior such as "irritability" may be said to follow as a consequence. The latter is, therefore, a dependent, variable, response or effect, or a consequent event.

Direct control can be exercised by the researcher over the independent variable. It can be manipulated and made to change in varying degrees. The dependent variable is not controlled directly. Instead, the hypothesis will state that, if it is truly a dependent variable, it can be influenced by a change in the independent variable. A crucial test will determine if variation in the independent variable produces a corresponding change in the dependent variable.

Our hypothesis states that the independent variable, "confinement to bed for X days," may result in the dependent variable, "irritable behavior." The researcher may effect a test of his hypothesis by influencing the presence, the absence or the degree of confinement and determining the type of behavior that results as a consequence.

However, these tests usually are confounded by the presence

of more than one independent variable. In addition to "confinement to bed for X days," the patient may expect variations in "nursing care," "pain," "problems at home," etc. Each of these variables may be independent of the others, but affect the dependent variable, "irritable behavior." The question is: Which affected the dependent variable and to what degree?

Enter the component of relevancy. Some of the variables are relevant to the hypothesis under test and others are not. The researcher is interested only in the relevant variables that are expected to be present in the problem situation. These will affect the outcome of the test.

Relevant variables may be categorized further as a function of their relationship to the hypothesis. Levine has classified the terms of the hypothesis as the "explanatory variables."[3] It includes both the independent and the dependent variable. He states in addition that "every research study contains variables that are not of interest to the researcher, but must be taken into account since they can vitally affect the relationship between the explanatory variables."[4] These are called "extraneous variables."

The researcher also desires to maintain control over the "extraneous variables." He wishes to eliminate them from the test, or at least to hold them constant while he manipulates the independent "explanatory variable" that is under study.

The conditions for a crucial test of a hypothesis can now be summarized. It is a controlled test. Control is exercised in two ways over those variables that are relevant to the hypothesis. Independent variables extraneous to the hypothesis are maintained or stabilized as constants. At the same time, the independent variable that is pertinent to the hypothesis is manipulated to study and test its effects upon the dependent variable.

Some General Methods of Design

The problem of hypothesis development is to formulate a relationship between two sets of events. It has been termed a cause-and-effect relationship. Cohen and Nagel would consider such a relationship to be invariable.[5] If the relationship has been formulated aptly and the conditions are appropriate, the presence of one event, the effect or the dependent variable, always will infer the presence of the other event, the cause or the independent variable (or the cause always will be attended by the effect). The problem of the test is to establish the hypothesis as an invariable relationship.

The problem of design is to effect such a test when conditions or events (extraneous variables) in addition to those provided in the hypothesis (explanatory variables) may be present. The test situation must be designed to evaluate the relationship between the explanatory variables independently of the extraneous variables. The task may become complex when some of the extraneous variables are also directly related to the explanatory variables.

Each project actually will contain its own problem of design. The specific requirements for testing may necessitate the invention and/or the development of specific conditions for the particular study. The creative abilities of the researcher will be taxed again.

However, most studies can be reduced to some variation of one of a few basic design patterns. These were elaborated many years ago by John Stuart Mill.[6] This section will consider three of the classic models:*

1. The Method of Agreement
2. The Method of Difference
3. The Method of Concomitant Variation.

These methods were proposed by Mill as canons or rules for the discovery of hypotheses as well as canons for proof. Our discussions will pertain only to the latter.

The Method of Agreement

The method of agreement, as a canon for proof, stipulates that the dependent explanatory variable always will be attended by the independent explanatory variable despite the presence or the absence of extraneous variables. If the rela-

* The reader is referred to two other methods developed by Mill: The Joint Method of Agreement and Difference and The Method of Residues.

tionship of "confinement to bed for X days" to "irritable behavior" is formulated as being invariable, the latter always will be accompanied by the former, no matter what else is present in the situation. A test may be designed in which instances of "irritable behavior" are isolated and the presence of other variables is observed. While the number and the kind of extraneous variables (nurse, home condition, pain, other patients, etc.) may be observed to vary, "confinement to bed for X days" should always be present. The researcher also may provide or locate instances in which "confinement to bed for X days" is present with different combinations of extraneous variables. If an invariable relationship holds, "irritable behavior" should occur in each instance of "confinement to bed."

The researcher who employs the "method of agreement" design will encounter many problems. Some of these concern practical considerations. Others deal with the method as a truly valid test.

The invariable relationship stipulates that the explanatory variables always should occur together. However, the researcher can examine only a limited number of instances. How can he conclude that what was found to be the case in a limited number of instances will occur indefinitely? This is a practical problem.

It is also possible to draw erroneous conclusions from this test. The chance of observing "irritable behavior" to occur with each instance of "confinement to bed for X days" really is remote. And the authors would question the validity of this relationship even if it were confirmed in a limited number of instances. Does "confinement to bed for X days" lead to "irritable behavior" in all instances? What of the patient in a state of coma for the X days? Does "confinement to bed for X days" lead to "irritable behavior" in all instances, or is the former simply associated with an array of other circumstances, such as discomfort, pain, inability to satisfy certain needs, that actually provoke the irritable behavior?

Black cautioned the researcher who employs the method of agreement to be aware of the following dangers:

1. The inaccurate classification of relevant variables

2. The presence of other unnoticed but relevant variables in the situation.[7]

"Confinement to bed for X days" actually may occur in association with "irritable behavior" in a limited number of observations. As a result, it may be classified as a relevant explanatory variable. However, it is possible also that some of the other variables, such as those mentioned above, were present in each instance but were unnoticed by the observer.

These issues pertain to the discussion of accountability. Several conditions seem to relate to the same effect. The problem is to separate conditions that are necessary and sufficient from those that just happened to be present in the situation. Some of the conditions, such as discomfort, may be sufficient to produce the given effect (irritable behavior). However, it also may contain conditions (confinement to bed for X days) that are present with the effect. And the latter (confinement to bed for X days) is observed more easily than the former (discomfort). Thus, the more obvious and spurious relationship is apt to be formulated.

Two suggestions are offered to the user of the method of agreement. One is "to vary the conditions as much as possible."[8] This maxim may allow the truly sufficient conditions to be present or to fail to be present. When "failure to be present" occurs, a negative instance of agreement or a condition of no relationship may become apparent also. And this becomes the second suggestion: to employ the method of agreement as a negative test and eliminate false hypotheses.

The Method of Difference

The method of difference is based upon the proposition that the dependent explanatory variable will not be present in the absence of the independent explanatory variable. Therefore, it suggests that all extraneous variables be held constant or controlled while the independent explanatory variable is manipulated, i.e., placed into and withheld from the situation. Under these circumstances, an invariable relationship is said to occur in the presence or the absence of the dependent explanatory variable.

This design would permit us to test hypotheses such as "confinement to bed for X days leads to irritable behavior" with a limited number of observations. The researcher needs only to find or to develop instances in which each of the relevant, though extraneous, factors is present. "Confinement to bed for X days" could then be varied and its effect (presence or absence) upon "irritable behavior" observed. The indefinite number of observations required by the method of agreement is not important to the method of difference design.

However, this method also has severe limitations. They are such that Cohen and Nagel cast doubt upon the method as a canon of proof.[9]

The major issue concerns the plurality of cause or the partial cause factor. If there are several conditions that relate to "irritable behavior," it may continue to be present despite the absence of any one of the other factors. In other words, "irritable behavior" may continue in the absence of "confinement to bed for X days" if "discomfort" or "pain" or "inability to satisfy need" also is present.

Cohen and Nagel suggest, however, that the negative use of the method of difference may be of value.[10] That is, it also can serve to eliminate hypotheses. If it can be determined that the presence or the absence of "irritable behavior" does not relate to the presence or the absence of "confinement to bed for X days," the researcher may cast doubt upon the tenability of the hypothesis.

The Method of Concomitant Variation

The two technics discussed thus far suggest that the explanatory variables appear or fail to appear as an all-or-none affair. That is, they will be either completely present or absent but not partially present. The technics treat the variables qualitatively.

However, the idea of a multiple or a partial cause indicates variation in degree. The presence of an independent variable may cause a partial variation in the dependent variable rather than merely effect its complete presence or absence. The quantitative aspects of the variable are to be treated also.

The method of concomitant variation deals with the measurable characteristics of the variable. It considers that the dependent explanatory variable varies or changes in degree as a function of the independent explanatory variable. Increases or decreases in the latter will be accompanied by corresponding increases or decreases in the former. As "the number of days of confinement to bed" increases, "the amount of irritable behavior" will increase also if an invariable relationship holds.

The technic does not negate the presence of other variables. Extraneous variables also may influence the degree of relationship. There even are times, Black suggests, when variation in the independent explanatory variable will produce a corresponding variation in an extraneous variable and compound the effect upon the dependent explanatory variable.[11] As "the number of days of confinement to bed" increases, "the amount of discomfort" also may increase to increase further the degree of "irritable behavior." Thus, the researcher must continue to account for or control the influence of extraneous variables.

THE IMPLICATIONS OF DESIGN

The implications of the foregoing discussion of the development of a true test of a hypothesis are that the researcher always must deal in the realm of probability and that a true empiric test of a hypothesis can never be exacted. These are some of the limitations imposed upon the acquisition of knowledge even with the utilization of research technics. These are some of the negative aspects of the discussion.

Some positive implications also may be derived: that the researcher can effect a test of only two variables at a time in an empiric relationship; that there is a need to exercise some measure of control over all other variables; that some measure of control may be effected by systematically varying the relevant independent variables.

Each of the models has been designed to determine the existence of an invariable relationship between only two variables in the presence of other relevant variables. Each design attempts to effect some measure of control over the other relevant variables. Control is exercised by systematically varying the conditions of the test. In the case of the method of agreement, the number and the kinds of extraneous variables are altered, while the researcher ascertains whether or not the explanatory variables remain in a state of constancy.

In the case of the method of difference, the researcher strives to maintain constancy in the extraneous variables. A similar kind of control is exercised in the case of the method of concomitant variation, where the specific concern is the determination of relative rather than absolute effects of change.

Systematic variation implies that the researcher will develop artificial rather than actual conditions for the test. That is, the researcher will not investigate just any situation or circumstance but only those that satisfy the requirements of his design. As a matter of fact, he may deliberately create conditions in accordance with his design that never may occupy or have occupied a true place in reality.

The special conditions of the test may be augmented in one of two ways: by the method in which data is collected or by the method of analysis. In the former, the researcher may develop, observe and record only those instances that satisfy each of the particular conditions of his design and must eliminate all others from consideration. With the latter method, he may obtain some measure of the effects of each relevant variable upon the dependent variable and extract the effects of the extraneous variables. These problems will be considered in the chapters to follow.

IMPLICATIONS OF DESIGN FOR RESEARCH IN NURSING

The problem of design pertains to questions relating to the establishment of truth. Through design, the researcher seeks to bring understanding to knowledge. He endeavors to identify and establish exact relationships dealing with the pertinent events and with nothing else.

The problem of design is also a problem of organization. Through design, events can be reoriented so that they can be studied in their proper context. The pertinent events under study are separated from those extraneous events that otherwise would impinge upon the outcome.

With design, the events studied are organized, and statements of truth can be ascertained. Without design in research, there always will remain the question of truth.

ESTABLISHING TRUTH IN NURSING

The acquisition of absolute truth under ideal circumstances is a formidable, almost a prohibitive, task. Consider then the possibility of attaining truth in nursing. The problem is confounded by the complex nature of the variables and the situation. There is also a question regarding the stability of truth in an area of practice.

The nature of the typical nursing situation (if there is any such thing) makes the search for truth a herculean task. Examine, for example, the following description of a patient situation in a hospital that was used for an experiment in nursing education.

A variety of social and economic backgrounds were represented among the patients. Approximately 60 per cent of the patients were Negroes, the remainder being whites. A few adolescents were present; but in keeping with national trends in tuberculosis, the older age group predominated. There were a few patients with drug resistant organisms, for whom there was little hope of eventual release from the institution. For patients who responded well to drug therapy, the length of stay varied from 2 to 8 months. Patients receiving chest or orthopedic surgery were transferred to the adjoining medical center on the day of operation and returned to the chest hospital within 48 hours. A few pregnant tuberculous women were transferred from other state hospitals to await delivery. Severity of illness ranged from the moribund to a completely ambulatory state.[12]

It contains not one but many variables, each impinging upon the other: variations in social and economic conditions, status, age, race, response to treatment, length of hospital stay, severity of illness, prognosis, and in types of patients—medical, surgical and maternity. And each variable may be a complex maze of many components. They are difficult to isolate; they defy description; and many are impervious to measurement. How can a researcher reorganize the events contained within situations such as the above to single out and study a pair of events independently of all others? This is a major obstacle in the search for truth in nursing.

It must be considered also that the essence or place of nursing is in the area of practice. All efforts—recruitment, education, supervision, administration, consultation and research—are peripheral to practice. Nursing is practice, the provision of patient care. Practice is the paramount reason for the existence of nursing and its peripheral activities, which feed upon nursing practice and exist only because of their intent to improve it.

However, the art of nursing practice is an ever-changing one. The typical nurse of 50 years ago might not survive in many aspects of the modern milieu of nursing practice. And practice lives for today. It feeds upon quick and useful answers that serve current needs. It cares not for the past nor even for the future. It pays little heed to the profound solutions that may gain prominence only in the future.

Research, on the contrary, is a slow, plodding effort to build from the past to serve the future. It disregards the quick and useful answers and concentrates upon the everlasting solution, the so-called truth. How can two such mutually opposing forces serve one another? How can the researcher ascertain the truth in an ever-changing situation, one that will not stand still, one that defies control?

An Analysis of Two Approaches to Truth

Two avenues to truth in nursing research will be traced. On the one hand, the design problem was only partially satisfied. In the other instances, the researchers took more deliberate pains to control some of the pertinent elements of their studies. Consider the effects of each approach.

The Partial Design Approach

One of the authors was once engaged in what might be called "a partially designed study."[13] The study was not completely devoid of design. However, it did fail to consider and control some highly revelant variables.

The intent of the study was to determine or identify nurse staffing patterns in the "progressive patient care" elements of various hospitals. A survey was conducted by questionnaire of hospitals that had indicated previously that they had established one or more of the elements.

The study was patterned after the method of agreement design. The rationale implied the following: given a particular element of progressive patient care, e.g., an intensive care unit, a particular nurse staff pattern should follow. The relationship can be characterized in variable form as:

	Independent	*Dependent*
Explanatory	A particular	A particular
Variable	PPC element	nurse staffing
		pattern

Furthermore, the relationship was expected to be maintained regardless of the conditions (extraneous variables) surrounding the hospitals surveyed.

Thus, the explanatory variables were treated while the extraneous variables were essentially uncontrolled. Accordingly, an attempt was made to devise definitions of the progressive patient care elements and the necessary nursing personnel. The hospitals were instructed also to submit their answers in a prescribed form, listing the numbers of nurses, patients and beds in the various elements during a given 24-hour day (exclusive of week ends).

A tremendous amount of variation in nurse staffing was uncovered among the hospitals surveyed. For example, the professional nurse hours for intensive care units varied from approximately 1 to more than 10 hours per bed per day. This type of result may not have been highly useful or encouraging to the nurse administrator who planned to staff such units.

However, were the units actually staffed so diversely? A follow-up visit by members of the study team suggested that several extraneous factors may have influenced the results. The hospitals appeared to have different concepts of progressive patient care. The patients in some of the intensive care units were acutely ill; in others, they were up and about. The patients also had different types of illnesses. Some of the units were open wards; others were composed of private rooms. The hospitals were of different sizes and their units varied accordingly. The hospitals utilized nursing personnel differently. Some made greater use of practical nurses; others of nurse's aides. Some hospitals employed the same staffing pattern throughout the 24 hours; others decreased their staffs during the evening and night tours of duty.

Each of the extraneous variables and perhaps many more may have influenced the outcome of this study. It appeared improbable that the relationship between progressive patient care and nurse staffing was as highly varied as the results indicated. However, how far the results departed from a true or actual state of affairs will not be ascertained until such studies can be repeated with adequate controls.

A More Complete Design Approach

The three studies that follow appeared to develop more deliberate and complete approaches to the problems of design and control. While it cannot be said that any was a model of perfection, each yielded results that perhaps were closer to a true state of affairs.

1. *Observer Factors in the Measurement of Blood Pressure*[14]

Variation in the measurements of human blood pressure has long been recognized. In part, fluctuations are due to normal differences among subjects—wide fluctuations in blood pressure readings can be expected among different subjects and within the same subject at different times. It is known also that variation sometimes is due to errors of measurement. In this regard, the researcher expressed concern that most studies had concentrated upon instruments and procedures as error-producing factors. She hypothesized that the observer also may contribute to errors of measurement.

The hypothesis can be expressed diagrammatically as follows:

	Independent	*Dependent*
Explanatory Variables	Observer or reader	Errors of measurement of human blood pressure
Extraneous Variables	Subjects Instruments Procedures	

A problem of design was the issue here. How could the researcher determine the influence of the observer (the independent explanatory variable) upon the measurement of human blood pressure independently of subjects, instruments and procedures (the independent extraneous variables)?

Actually, two designs were employed, but only one will be discussed here. This was termed the "double stethoscope experiment." The author employed a situation in which two observers could measure blood pressure simultaneously. Inter-observer comparisons could be made while the instrument and the procedure variables remained relatively constant.

How was the subject factor controlled? A variation of the method of agreement was employed to separate the observer and the subject contributions. Five blocks of experiments were planned, each of which involved five subjects and six observers (nurses). The blocks were arranged so that "each nurse measured each subject just once and measured in combination with every other nurse just once."[15] The order of readings and pairings were arranged randomly. Thus, independent measures were obtained of the effects of the observer and the subject variables as well as of the chance or random effect of being paired with a particular observer and observing a particular subject at one time.

In summary, many observations were made to determine that error of measurement (as expressed by inter-observer variability) is a function of the observer. The instrument and the procedure variables were held constant, while the observer and the subject pairings were allowed to vary randomly.

The subjects were matched in sex, age and other characteristics. However, half the groups were normotensive, while the other half were hypertensive. It was expected that better quality readings could be obtained from the former group.

This design permitted the researcher to extract statistically the effects of the subject variable and the random selections from inter-observer variability. She concluded, as a result, "that the inter-observer variability was random rather than systematic."[16] However, any systematic variability that did occur was apt to be a function of the subject. "Observer differences seem to be generally small if one is measuring the blood pressure of subjects with distinct, sharply defined sounds; with subjects where the sounds are muffled, indistinct or fade into background noise, the differences are larger and a very aberrant reading may occur."[17]

2. *An Investigation of the Relation Between Nursing Activity and Patient Welfare*[18]

In 1956, the University of Iowa undertook a series of studies designed to investigate the relationship between nursing care and patient welfare. This investigation took place in an actual practice situation where many problems of control existed. The more exacting type of design developed to satisfy the requirements of the preceding study could not be instituted here. Nevertheless, some controls were effected. How they managed and what happened as a result will be illustrated.*

The group was concerned with the question of how nurses would spend their time if the size of their staff was increased. Accordingly they formulated the following hypothesis:

	Independent	*Dependent*
Explanatory Variables	Increasing the size of the ward nursing staff ⇨	1. More time spent with patients 2. Improved patient welfare
Extraneous Variables	1. Number and kind of patients 2. Number and kind of nurses 3. Physical setting 4. Time	

It was reasoned that an increase in the size of the ward nursing staff should result in a reallocation of duties so that more time would be spent with patients. An improvement in patient welfare was expected as a consequence.

The group recognized that many extraneous variables also would influence the dependent variables. Only a partial listing of some of

---

* The author took the liberty of making a slight modification in the actual design for ease in presentation.

the more pertinent factors has been made. Of particular concern was the influence of hourly, daily and weekly fluctuations that were apt to occur in a practice area. The element of "time" has been used to symbolize these fluctuations.

A variation of the method of difference was employed to test the relationship between explanatory variables independently of extraneous variables. The design may be pictured as follows:

Change Group	Base Staff	Increased Staff
No Change Group	Base I Staff	Base II Staff

The underlying rationale suggested that observations should be made of a female medical ward under two conditions: one in which a base nursing staff was maintained and the other in which the size of the nursing staff was increased. However, in recognition of the expected fluctuations in the practice area (the "time" factor), a second female medical ward—the "no change" group—was selected to serve as a control or a base population for each time period. Adjustments were made in the "no change" group to compensate for fluctuations in numbers and kinds of patients. In essence, this group composed a shifting base population in which each of the extraneous variables, including "time," was controlled.

In the analyses that followed, comparisons were made of observations of the "increased staff" situation and each of the corresponding "base" situations. The hypothesis was not confirmed by the results. With additional time available, nurses did not allocate a greater proportion of their time to patients. Furthermore, an improvement in patient welfare did not occur.

3. *Effect of Nurse Staffing on Satisfactions With Nursing Care*[19]

This study was made because of the general belief that feelings of inadequacy of nursing services remained despite sizeable increases in nursing staffs. It was an attempt to isolate the relationship between feelings of inadequacy and the number of nursing personnel employed in hospitals. In comparison with the other two illustrations, this project involved a much wider sampling of practice situations. Since rigid controls could not be adopted, statistical manipulations were relied upon more heavily.

Several hypotheses actually were explored. However, this illustration will consider only one: that feelings of satisfaction will be a function of the daily hours of professional nursing care. The explanatory and the extraneous variables are displayed as follows:

	Independent		*Dependent*
Explanatory Variables	Variation in the daily average hours of pro- fessional nursing care	⟹	Variation in the feelings of satisfac- tion with nursing services
Extraneous Variables	1. Variation in the daily average pa- tient census 2. Variation in the ownership of the hospital 3. Variation in the daily average hours of total nursing care	⇧	

It was expected that size, ownership and total staffing of the hospital (extraneous variables) also would affect the dependent variable.

A modification of the method of concomitant variation was employed here to effect adequate controls and test the hypothesis. (This accounts for the inclusion of the time variation in the descriptive statement of the hypothesis.) An instrument was developed that yielded a score of patient satisfaction. It was expected that any one of the independent variables would cause a rise or a fall in the satisfaction score. However, the score differences obtained were expressed as a function of the composite effect of all the identifiable independent variables and those that were not identified. If the effects of all the extraneous variables (including those not identified) could be determined and extracted from the satisfaction scores, the remaining residual score could be attributed to the effects of the explanatory variable. The data were treated substantially in accordance with this rationale.

The results of the analysis showed a high positive relationship between satisfaction and the number of professional hours available. The patients who were provided with a higher number of professional nurse hours tended to be more satisfied with the nursing services.*

From the point of view of design, the following cursory analysis of 4 independent studies is limited severely. The sampling is small and highly selective. The studies were chosen deliberately to satisfy the peculiar biases of the authors. Never-

* This was not the case with obstetric patients.

theless, a summary suggests the following implications for nursing research:

1. Design Is Seldom Perfect. Each study offered only tentative statements of truth. The researchers did not state emphatically that the hypothesis was absolutely correct or incorrect. Instead, they dealt in terms of probability.

However, the researchers appeared to be aware of the limitations of the particular design. It might even be supposed that those researchers who effected better designs were more cognizant of the shortcomings of the study. A recognition of discrepancies is also a step closer to the truth.

In addition, these researchers were able to suggest further avenues of study and more appropriate designs. The reader might obtain this feeling from an examination of the actual source documents. In this respect, research may be viewed as a series of successive approximations of the truth. With each step, it is desirable to move closer to reality.

2. Designs Can Be Effected in Practice Situations. Each illustration was concerned with an area of nursing practice. They comprised many variables, some of which were expected to change in point of time independently of the researcher's actions. The researchers solved the problems of design in different ways. Some were more successful than others.

Control or design was essentially disregarded in the first illustration. Some of the more pertinent factors could have been isolated and controlled in anticipation of their effect. They were not, and the results were inconclusive as a consequence.

The researcher of the second example simulated the actual practice situation in a laboratorylike setting. The most effective controls may have been obtained in this manner. She actually was able to manipulate and control many of the pertinent variables. Perhaps her results were most meaningful in this regard.

The group of investigators of the third illustration attempted to work within the confines of an actual practice situation. They fostered controls by adjusting a portion of the practice area (the patient census and the staffing of the control ward) to conform with the changing requirements of the experimental unit. They were not wholly successful, and their study was limited to this extent.

The final study also took place in practice areas. However, the researchers elected to accept the array of circumstances as they found them and to institute statistical controls. The practice areas were selected deliberately to satisfy the requirements of a statistical or mathematical model. Data were fed into the model and manipulated to effect an appropriate test. The authors were aware of the limitations of this approach and suggested that the results were not to be treated as final, but as hypothesis-building.

3. Design Pertains to a Complex of Activities. The reader will have observed that design does not comprise a single problem. It pertains to a variety of activities: the selection of subjects and appropriate situations, the development of materials and procedures for collecting and analyzing data. Each activity was interrelated by the design mechanism.

If a single element can be isolated, it is that of organization or systematization. Design really comprises the organization of subjects, materials, situations and data for the purpose of answering the question: Is the hypothesis true? Each component should have a place in the design configuration and contribute toward this end. Components are not to be construed as independent entities.

4. Design Is an Individual Affair. Each study had problems of control peculiar to itself. They were treated in various ways, or not treated at all. Other researchers might even have effected different designs for these studies.

Design is an individual problem. It is to be custom-fitted to the requirements of the particular study. A researcher cannot expect to exchange designs or borrow them from other studies, however effective they may have been. The development of the most satisfactory design is another test of the creative capacities of the researcher.

REFERENCES

1. Webster's New International Dictionary.
2. Levine, Eugene: Experimental design in nursing research, Nurs. Res. *9*:204, 1960.
3. *Ibid.*, pp. 204-205.
4. *Ibid.*, p. 204.
5. Cohen, M. R., and Nagel, E.: An Introduction to Logic and Scientific Method, pp. 245-249. New York, Harcourt, 1934.
6. Mill, J. S.: A System of Logic, Ratiocinative & Inductive, Book I, London, Longmans, 1889.
7. Black, Max: Critical Thinking, An Introduction to Logic and Scientific Method, pp. 265-271. Englewood, Prentice-Hall, Inc., 1946.
8. *Ibid.*, p. 271.
9. Cohen, M. R., and Nagel, E.: *Op. cit.* (see Ref. 5), pp. 257-261.
10. *Ibid.*
11. Black, Max: *Op. cit.* (see Ref. 7), pp. 286-303.
12. Gifford, A. J. (ed.): Unity of Nursing Care: A Report of a Project to Study the Integration of Social Science and Psychiatric Concepts in Nursing, p. 110, Chapel Hill, N. C., Univ. North Carolina, 1960.
13. Abdellah, F. G., Meyer B., and Roberts, H.: Nursing patterns vary in progressive care, Mod. Hosp. *95*(No. 2):85-91, 1960.
14. Wilcox, Jane: Observer factors in the measurement of blood pressure, Nurs. Res. *10*:4-17, 1961.
15. *Ibid.*, p. 7.
16. *Ibid.*, p. 16.
17. *Ibid.*, p. 10.
18. An Investigation of the Relation Between Nursing Activity and Patient Welfare, pp. 2; 141; 181, Nurse Utilization Project Staff, Ames, Iowa, State Univ. Iowa, 1960.
19. Abdellah, F. G., and Levine, E.: Effect of Nurse Staffing on Satisfaction With Nursing Care, pp. 4-6, Chicago, American Hospital Assn., 1958.

CHAPTER 7

The Selection of Subjects

THE GENERAL PROBLEM

For the researcher, truth is relative. It depends on his ability to formulate hypotheses and design conditions for testing them. It is also a function of his ability to depict reality and to provide appropriate measurements of his observations.

Thus far, the discussions have related to abstract matters. The problem may have represented the symbolic counterpart of a multitude of actual problems; but problems stated in abstraction do not have a place in reality. The hypothesis may have been formulated as a tentative solution to this problem, derived only on paper. The design may be only a plan to establish a setting in which the pertinent components of the problem can be identified and separated for testing purposes.

However, the purpose of the test is to determine that the hypothesis is real. The test must be made in an actual situation. It must deal in specifics, with what can be observed to happen. Yet the specific testing situation also should conform to the requirements of the problem stated in abstraction—that is, the elements or the components of the problem must be interpreted and reconstructed as they were conceived by the researcher to appear in reality. Otherwise, the hypothesis cannot possibly be tested.

How does the researcher represent the variables under consideration in a specific and observable setting? How can such terms as "confinement to bed for X days" be expressed in reality? Upon what basis does he determine that such a variable as "irritability" has or has not occurred?

In many respects, the development of the test is similar to the production of a play. The playwright develops a series of ideas in the form of a running narrative or plot. His contribution is a script that may be conceived as a set of directives, issuing words and actions to a cast of characters. Reality is achieved when actors are selected to play the roles in the setting prescribed by the author.

The test may be construed as a series of productions featuring the re-enactment of an incomplete play. As a series, it is to be performed repetitively but with different sets of actors. It is incomplete in the sense that the climax or what happens when the plot unfolds remains to be revealed. The hypothesis is a prediction of what will happen. The question posed by the test is: How often will the prediction come true?

What is needed to produce the test are actors or subjects. The subjects are the medium through which the variables may be introduced and expressed. They serve as the vehicle in which changes can be denoted.

Reality or the specific test situation can be described in part as a function of the subjects selected for study. The selection process will influence what happens and, therefore, should occur in accordance with the strict requirements of the design. Among the major concerns of the researcher are who or what the subjects are, how many are to be selected, and how they are to be selected.

WHO OR WHAT ARE THE SUBJECTS?

When the researcher inquires who or what will be the subjects of his study, he is not looking for just anyone or anything. He wishes to be highly specific in this respect. As the playwright may be very concerned about casting the proper actor in the appropriate role, so the researcher desires to select sub-

jects who will satisfy the requirements of his study. Just anyone or anything will not do.

How does the researcher know whom or what to select? The
selection criteria should be inherent in those portions of his
paper developed to this point. Whom or what to select should
be revealed in the statement of the problem, the definition of
terms, the hypothesis formulation and the design.

He will examine his problem statement to determine the
point at which the results of his inquiry are applicable. As will
be recalled, the problem may be at a specific, a common or an
underlying level. The subjects for the test may be conceived
accordingly, and the results will be applicable to those in the
particular study group and others like them.

If the problem was stated specifically, e.g., if it is concerned
with the confinement of a group of patients in Ward A of Hospital B, then the population of subjects is almost self-defining.
The study will deal directly with the group implied by or
stated within the context of the problem. Any conclusions will
pertain only to this body of subjects. The typical, everyday
problem-solving situation is of this order.

If the problem was stated at the common level of inquiry,
e.g., if it is concerned with the confinement of a group of
medical patients in open wards of general hospitals, then the
population definition becomes more complex. While this population is real in one sense, it is also hypothetic or abstract. It
is real because subjects of this order have been observed to
exist in several specific situations. This is the manner by which
the problem came to light in the first place. It is hypothetic
because the population is represented in the problem statement
as a composite of the common characteristics of each specific
grouping, i.e., confinement, medical patients, open wards, general hospitals. The need is to define the limits of this population, specify its characteristics, and then relocate it in specific
situations.

The point of application at the common level of inquiry is
highly elastic. It may be described as a narrower body of subjects, e.g., the confinement of hepatitis patients in open wards

of 50-bed general hospitals; or a wider body of subjects, e.g., the confinement of people in hospitals, prisons, etc. As the level of inquiry fluctuates, the characteristics of the populations of subjects will be altered.

If the problem was stated at the underlying level of inquiry, e.g., if it is concerned with frustration due to confinement, then the point of application is even more elastic. Confinement could occur anywhere to anyone, and the population definition will be less complex. The implication here is that the same results can be expected if the explanatory variable is introduced to any group of subjects under controlled conditions. The subjects of the illustration may be humans, animals or any creatures to whom the variable, frustration due to confinement, can be introduced and on whom it can take effect.

The statement of the problem at any level of inquiry will indicate to the researcher the population from which his subjects may be selected. This population becomes his *universe*. It may be small or large in number; it may even be of infinite size.

The universe will be defined by a number of traits or characteristics that may pertain to both the explanatory and the extraneous variables under study. It may be a universe of almost anything or anyone: people, animals, insects, plants, other living or inert matter, behavior, events, etc.

The major determinant of the universe of subjects will be the explanatory variables. Subjects may be conceived as an expression of the variables. They represent the mode through which the independent variable or variables are or have been introduced and the changes in the dependent variable or variables have been uncovered. "Confinement to bed for X days" is an event in the process of happening. By itself it means nothing, for it happens to people. Thus, people will be required as subjects who will be or have been confined to bed for X days. Their resultant behavior is to be studied to denote the presence or the absence of "irritability."

Who are these subjects? They could be any order of people: young, middle-aged or elderly; male or female; very ill or not so ill; with or without families. There are many different categories of persons that could be selected.

The principal characteristics of the universe will be implied within the definition of terms. For example, if the term is defined as "confinement to bed due to illness," then the state of being a patient (being ill) will be construed as a major characteristic, and a "patient" universe will be indicated. If it is defined merely as "confinement," then the universe need not contain only patients. It may consist of anyone who is confined, including animals. The question is: Do they serve as an outlet for the expression of the variables, as a means through which new variables can be introduced and by which changes can be observed and recorded?

The secondary characteristics of the universe will be determined as a function of the extraneous variables. They will indicate whether or not the population should vary in such traits as age, sex, degree of illness and family relationships. These will pertain only to those factors that impinge upon and cause changes in the dependent variable.

The extraneous variables suggestive of secondary characteristics should be uncovered in the process of formulating the hypothesis. In carefully scrutinizing the ensuing hypothesis, the researcher may figure out or learn of exceptional instances when the hypothesis would not satisfy the requirements of the problem, when the dependent variable would change as a function of other relevant variables. It may be reasoned that "irritable behavior" resulting from "confinement to bed for X days" will occur more readily in older than in younger patients, in men rather than in women. Any factors of this order, which are determined by the researcher to influence the nature of the hypothesis, should be considered when defining the universe of subjects. They represent some of the other characteristics that will compose the selection criteria.

It may be surmised from the illustration that subjects can and usually do represent the presence of more than one variable. When mention was made of different orders of people, the presence of additional variables in the same subjects was implied. Age, sex, degree of illness and family relationships were just a few of the other variables suggested. When animals are employed for study purposes in place of men, the researcher is aware also that other variables have been introduced into the study.

Thus, who or what are selected as subjects is often an integral part of the design complex. The focus is not merely upon an expression of the explanatory variables, but also upon any relevant extraneous variables. As a matter of fact, design is achieved partially or wholly through the selection of subjects.

Ideally, the researcher may desire to design a study in which a "pure" group of subjects is selected. In its rarest and truest form, a "pure" group represents solely the explanatory variables. If a group of subjects devoid of all factors but the explanatory variables could be isolated or created, a "pure" group would be constituted. Here, the researcher might conceive of the basic chemical elements in isolation and in a vacuum. The introduction of a change or of an additional variable would be reflected immediately as a function of that variable only. But imagine attempting to study the effects of "confinement to bed for X days" in isolation! Such conditions can be achieved only in test tubes, if at all.

In a more practical sense, it is recognized that subjects are composed of many variables. An attempt to obtain purity is made by matching on all variables, by determining that the variables are distributed proportionately among the subjects. The problem is to separate and extract the effects of the extraneous variables from any changes that may have occurred in the dependent variable.

By the method of agreement, the researcher attempts to assure the presence of the explanatory variables in equivalent amounts. He attempts to vary all other conditions as much as possible. Therefore, he may select subjects only as a function of the explanatory variable. It is argued that the presence of the independent explanatory variable is a sufficient condition to ensure the presence of the dependent variable, no matter what else is in attendance.

The method of difference does not necessitate a variety of extraneous conditions. A more effective design may even suggest that the subjects be matched or equated only in terms of the extraneous variables, and initially in terms of the dependent explanatory variable. Therefore, any changes in the latter may be said to occur when and if the independent explanatory variable is introduced.

The idea of a *control* group (illustrated in Chap. 6) is to have an arrangement or a design to effect control through the selection of subjects. Here, more than one group of subjects is selected for study. The groups are chosen so that each represents the equivalent attributes of the extraneous and dependent variables, i.e., they may be of the same age, sex and degree of illness, and may behave initially at the same level of irritability. The treatment or the circumstance prescribed by the independent explanatory variable (confinement to bed for X days) will be introduced among the subjects of one group and not among the subjects of the other. The latter is considered as a *control* group. Any changes in the dependent explanatory variable (level of irritability) among this population may be attributed solely to the presence of the extraneous variables. Any difference between the two groups in this regard may be a reflection of the presence of the independent explanatory variable (confinement to bed for X days) in one group rather than the other.

Who or what are the subjects? They represent a universe or a general population to whom the results of a study may be applicable. The subjects are selected to embody an expression of the relevant variables under consideration and, therefore, may be anyone or anything that can serve in this capacity. A universe of subjects usually is described by more than one variable, sometimes by many variables. In this regard, subjects also may be selected to institute the necessary controls suggested by the study's design.

How Are the Subjects Selected?

The researcher is ready to select subjects. He has determined who or what will be selected. Does he then choose the first person, thing or event that satisfies his selection criteria? Or are there specific rules that may govern the manner by which subjects are chosen?

As the specifications of the universe of subjects are determined in advance, so the rules for selection also must be ascertained and described. How the subjects are selected will influence the outcome of the test. For example, suppose we are interested in pursuing a study of the effects of confinement to bed and decide to observe the behavior of a group of middle-aged males who have been confined to bed for X days. Accordingly, we proceed to the nearest community hospital, relate our plans to the director, and request permission to study a group of his patients. He is more than willing to be of assistance. He obliges us to the extent that the most co-operative middle-aged male patients are suggested. Immediately, a source of variation—"co-operation"—is introduced, which may not have been considered in the formulation of the hypothesis. Not only who or what, but how subjects are to be selected should be specified in advance as part of the procedure.

Several conditions will affect selection standards. These pertain to the universe and to other requirements of the study. Once the parent population has been determined, it should be described numerically and qualitatively. How large is the universe? How many variables does it encompass? How are these characteristics distributed among the population?

The Size of the Universe

The number of subjects in the total or parent population will influence the requirements for selection. If the universe is sufficiently small and accessible, then the entire population may be selected for study. Under these circumstances, the researcher does not have a problem of how to select. He merely chooses everyone.

However, it is more probable that the universe will be excessively large and inaccessible. It may even be infinite in size and spread throughout the four corners of the earth. Under these circumstances, the researcher must consider sampling the universe—taking a portion of the population for study.

The process of sampling creates the problem of how to select. It becomes a question of how many subjects will be chosen, and in what way. "How many" is discussed in the next section. "In what way" is a function of the qualitative characteristics.

The Number of Variables

In a truly practical situation, it will be difficult to obtain an equitable or proportionate distribution of all relevant variables among the groups of subjects. This is particularly the case when selection is based on a large number of variables. The researcher may be able to identify, select and match subjects on one or perhaps two variables, such as age and/or sex. He is usually hampered, however, when he attempts to build up his list of criteria to include additional variables, such as degree and type of illness, family relationships, income, level of intelligence, etc. The problem is pertinent to the study of humans, when a fairly extensive number of variables often is relevant.

The idea of a *random* population is offered as a solution to this problem. Here the researcher may select, match or equate his subjects on a few principal secondary characteristics and assume that the remaining characteristics are distributed randomly or by chance among the universe. That is, he makes the assumption that individual members of the universe, as defined by the few principal secondary characteristics, would exhibit an entire range of other relevant traits, and, furthermore, that the other relevant traits would be spread among the universe in accordance with the features of a chance distribution. If subjects were selected at random from the universe, they would be expected to differ in regard to other relevant traits by chance alone.

In reality, a "chance" or "random" variable is added to the extraneous group of variables relevant to the hypothesis. Errors or differences due to random selections can be estimated. Thus, the effect of the independent "chance" variable upon the dependent variable can be determined and extracted from the results.

Random sampling implies that every subject in the universe

has an equal chance of being selected for the study. We might conceive that the entire universe was cast into a large receptacle that was jostled and turned over many times. A blindfold researcher then stepped forward, reached into the receptable and chose one individual. The selection was recorded and placed back in the receptacle. It was jostled again and another subject was chosen, placed back in the receptacle, and so on, until the entire sample was selected.

Of course this procedure is not practical. The total universe generally is not known and, furthermore, cannot be accumulated in one place at one time. Second, even if the universe were identified and could be listed on individual slips of paper, the technic is a cumbersome one.

In more practical circumstances, a known portion of the universe is isolated—e.g., patients in general hospitals in five communities—and the researcher selects randomly from this segment. He may do this by listing everyone in the total segment and selecting every n^{th} name for the sample. He could also number the individuals in the universe segment serially and then select individuals in an order corresponding to a table of random numbers designed for this purpose.[1] The researcher might consider or devise other methods to serve this end.

The Nature of the Distribution

Before the researcher can begin or even specify how to select his sample, he must determine the distribution of the variables among his universe. Is each variable distributed equally? If the researcher wishes to sample a patient population by sex, should he choose an equal number of male and female patients? He should not do so if 60 per cent of the universe is male. The proportionate breakdown of the variable in the universe should be determined before the selection process is begun.

One of the shortcomings of the proposal to select a random sample is that the variables concerned may not be distributed by chance among the universe. For example, if we assume that age is distributed randomly or normally among the professional nurse universe, we would expect to obtain a distri-

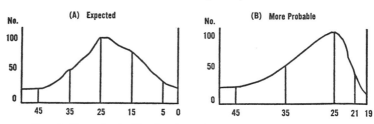

FIG. 6. Hypothetic distribution of professional nurses by age.

bution similar to that displayed in Figure 6 (A). However, the distribution more probably approximates that of Figure 6 (B). The assumption of randomness will have been violated. The researcher would be grossly in error if he treated the subjects as if they were selected from a random population.

The stratification of the universe into proportionate components is a procedure that has been advanced to deal with this problem. That is, the general population is divided into what has been described as "a series of homogeneous subuniverses," based upon the requirements of the study.[2] First, each of the subuniverses is sampled independently, and then they are combined for the analysis.

Let us propose the need to select a sample of adult patients and control such extraneous variables as sex, age, degree and type of illness. The universe has been stratified into sex and age groups as follows:

	Sex		
Age	Per Cent Male	Per Cent Female	Total Per Cent
20-40 Years	.20	.20	.40
40-60 Years	.30	.10	.40
60 Years and over	.10	.10	.20
Total	.60	.40	1.00

The proportionate distribution of patients into six subuniverses (2 sex × 3 age groups) has been identified in the above table. A stratified sex and age sample will evolve if patients are selected from the total universe in accordance with the proportionate values stipulated. In a sense, they will constitute "pure" sex-age patient groups.

We could go on and designate additional subcategories for degree and type of illness. However, the number of subuniverses would multiply many times. It would become impractical to select subjects in this manner. Instead, the researcher could limit the study to a single degree-and-type-of-illness group or make the assumption that all additional variables are distributed randomly. In the latter instance, patients would be sampled by chance from within each subuniverse. In essence, the procedure comprises stratified random sampling.

The Design of the Study

Let us suppose that the study's design dictates that more than one group be employed for testing purposes. Specifically, it suggests that a control group be used that initially will be similar in every respect to the experimental or study sample. The problem then becomes one of selecting two or more equivalent groups.

A simple extension of any one of the previously described methods for selecting a single group of subjects can be utilized to select more than one group. After the researcher has made his initial selection, he will reach back into the pool or universe to choose subjects for each of the equated groups. The subjects will be selected in exactly the same way. If the samples are sufficiently large, it is highly probable that they also will be equivalent. Nevertheless, the researcher may compare his samples beforehand to determine that equivalency exists.

A more rigid method is to match subjects on a one-to-one basis. That is, the researcher will define his universe and select one group of subjects. Then he will examine each subject in this sample and locate and draw another subject from the universe who has equivalent characteristics. Thus additional samples, so selected, will be equivalent to the first sample.

The matching procedure is useful when a small number of subjects is required for study and the number of variables to be equated is low. However, the difficulty of finding and matching subjects will increase as the number of variables upon which selection is based is increased.

The problem of how to select subjects is an important one and also should be considered in advance by the researcher. It relates specifically to the numbers and the kinds of subjects to be selected for study. It considers the size of the universe, the number and the distribution of the relevant variables descriptive of the universe, and the number of groups required by the study's design.

How Many Subjects Will Be Studied?

It usually is not possible to determine the exact number of subjects to be employed for a study. This will be known only when the researcher decides to use the total universe. Therefore, estimates of numbers are important when sampling is in order.

Perhaps the most general statement that can be made about estimating sample size is "the more the better." This notion is based upon the contention that truth or the results of the test will be a statement of probability—that the events will occur as predicted. Coinciding with this thought is the earlier inference that there is not one test to be conducted but a series of tests, the total number of which usually will be dependent upon the sample size.

The researcher attempts to build up the probability value that the hypothesis will or will not occur as anticipated. He does so by accumulating a number of confirmatory or "failure-to-confirm" responses. This value will be altered as the results of each test are added to one pile or the other. Sampling should continue until a pattern has been established and the researcher can state with confidence (the probability value) that the hypothesis has or has not been confirmed. In general, each new response should increase his confidence in one direction or the other.

However, there are limiting conditions to this proposal. In many instances, it is both inexpedient and unnecessary to sample extensively. Additional sampling beyond certain minimal requirements may not contribute substantially to the over-all results. We will consider first the establishment of minimal requirements and then some of the limiting conditions. The latter will include sampling technics and practical considerations.

Establishing Minimal Requirements

Two results are to be expected from the test: a measure of the change or the effect upon the dependent variable under study; and a determination of how the change was effected, i.e., what produced it. The validity of the prediction or the probability that the hypothesis is true will be a function of the researcher's ability to detect the change and to denote relationships producing change. A hypothesis such as "confinement to bed for X days leads to irritability" contains precise specifications for change—from a nonirritable to an irritable state, resulting from confinement to bed for X days and from nothing else. The test should serve to ascertain that these specifications have been observed.

The minimal requirements for sampling will be a function of the need to satisfy these specifications. They will be partially dependent upon the definitions of the universe in terms of over-all size and numbers of variables. They also will be influenced by the testing conditions.

Consider first the effect of the total universe size upon the expected dimensions of the sample. Suppose the researcher is given an underlying population of 100 patients. A sample of 30 patients selected randomly might be highly representative of this group. On the other hand, how closely would the same 30 patients typify a universe of 100,000 patients?

Numbers will have an effect upon the selection of a random sample and upon the interpretation placed upon any observations recorded among the subjects. In general, the observations are evaluated by comparing the results with some predetermined standard of expected values.* A purely random popula-

* This topic is discussed in Chapter 9 under Method of Analysis.

tion that actually is hypothetic and infinite in size has a reference standard with a characteristic shape and a derived set of values. This is expressed in Figure 7. A variety of standards for randomly selected samples differing in number also is included in the illustration. It can be observed how each distribution deviates in shape from the population based upon infinite sampling. In general, results from smaller samples (less than 30 subjects) tend to be less stable. They may begin to stabilize as they increase in number, suggesting some minimal requirements for selection.

However, the most salient point of this illustration may not be the numbers themselves but what they represent. A random population may be descriptive of a complex variety of traits. Thus, large numbers may be required to ensure that each member of a combination of traits is represented. On the other hand, a "pure" or genuinely homogeneous population, one made up of identical members, may be represented by a single case. The number of variables rather than the actual or the estimated size of the universe may be the determining factor in estimating sample size.

The concept may have a dual but opposing effect upon sample size. The best test of the hypothesis will attempt to account for all the relevant variables. This may imply that the population should be stratified into several subuniverses. As the number of variables or subuniverses increases, so the expected sampling requirements also may be increased. But the researcher may elect to minimize the number of subuniverses by lumping the distinct groupings into a so-called general random population. However, when he does so, he also sacrifices his ability to denote the clear lines of relationship between variables as formulated in the hypothesis. A larger number of observations may be required to clear the muddle.

Minimal sampling requirements are dependent on the discriminating power of the test. This is a function of the observer and the materials employed as the medium to detect change. The problem of developing adequate materials will be discussed at greater length in Chapter 8.

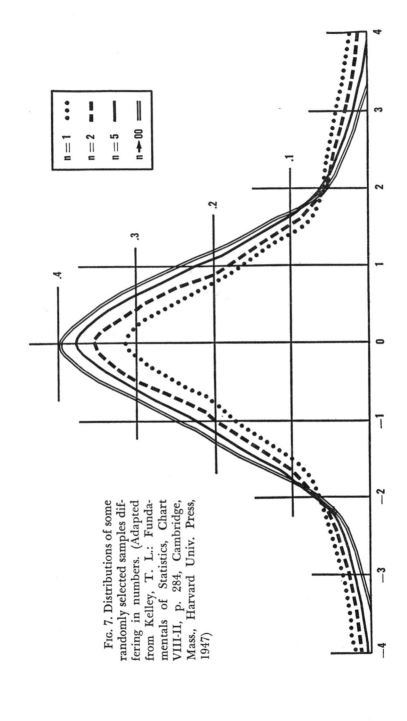

Fig. 7. Distributions of some randomly selected samples differing in numbers. (Adapted from Kelley, T. L.: Fundamentals of Statistics, Chart VIII-II, p. 284, Cambridge, Mass., Harvard Univ. Press, 1947)

As more subjects are required when variables are fused, so more subjects will be required also to detect change when the discriminating power of the test is low. The number of observations can be minimized where clear-cut, discrete, "yes" or "no" answers regarding the appearance of change can be obtained. But, if the pattern of change is one of degrees, the effects of small differences are denotable when accumulated in large amounts. For example, a small variation in "irritable behavior" may be regarded as a real change only when it has been observed consistently in a large number of patients.

Statistical designs and controls have been developed to assist the researcher with a multivariate problem to work with smaller samples. This form of analysis has been employed most successfully in the field of agriculture.[3, 4] It has been applied extensively also in the social and/or behavior sciences, where it is difficult to obtain "pure" groups and effect precise measures of change.[5, 6]

Practical Considerations

Practical considerations often are paramount in the determination of the numbers of subjects. Researchers operating on limited budgets may not be able to afford many observations. Furthermore, such subjects as rare species of insects or birds may be inaccessible or difficult to locate. The nature of the study may be such—flying into space for instance—that specially equipped, trained and willing volunteers are few. Humans often are unwilling or unable to serve as guinea pigs.

Sampling Procedures

The selection procedure will be a more influential criterion of the test than sheer numbers of subjects. Good sampling practices may clarify the issue earlier and with fewer observations. Poor sampling procedures only tend to confuse matters, regardless of the number of observations.

The adherence of the researcher to good sampling practices may lower his requirements for subjects and, in many instances, make possible the use of small or restricted samples. If subjects can be selected who are clearly illustrative or representative of what is suggested by the hypothesis, and of nothing else, the researcher may be able to base his conclusions upon fewer observations. This suggests the selection of "pure" or relatively "pure" groups, free of other factors that may contaminate the lines of change.

Selection practices that pay little or no attention to the expected lines of change tend to result in inconclusive findings. These are the studies into which other factors may enter and contaminate the lines of change. However, since control by selection will not be in evidence, the expected changes may not be detectable, or at least cannot be attributed to any single factor. What may result is a population, selected at random (but unintentionally so), in which the predictive probability values oscillate back and forth with each new observation, as chance would allow. The researcher never is certain of what he has found. Additional observations only perpetuate the cycle of oscillation.

THE SELECTION OF SUBJECTS FOR NURSING RESEARCH
(A Discussion of Two General Problems)

The preceding discussions were stated to be guidelines for the researcher. But they deal in abstract matters. They are illustrated by hypothetic cases devoid of and uncomplicated by the realities of the actual research setting.

Yet the problems of the nurse researcher are real. Sometimes guidelines must be reinterpreted when applied to specific situations. Sometimes the researcher even may dispense with the guidelines in bowing to the practicalities of the situation.

There are two general problems to be discussed here. They arise in consideration of nursing as a specific application for research. One problem relates to the identification of subjects and the other to the selection of subjects.

IDENTIFYING THE SUBJECT

Nursing is a many-sided practice. It is a maze of interactions of persons, events and things. People may interact with other people, with events and with things. And, in this maze, it may be difficult to determine who plays what role. Are there several universes participating in a single study? Are there several groups to whom the derived relationship will be applicable? Or do the various participants serve different functions, of which the role of the subject is one? If so, how does the nurse researcher identify the subject role?

We have taken the position that the subjects are the media through which a test of the hypothesis is effected. The hypothesis may state that something happens, has happened, or is to happen to produce a change in something else. What happens or happened is related by the independent variable. It happens to a dependent variable in which a change is expected. The question of the test is: Does the dependent variable change as directed by the hypothesis? In order to know this, a vehicle—subjects—must be interposed to signify realistically the events that are transpiring. Subjects serve as an expression of the change that may take place in the dependent variable after exposure to the independent variable.

Something Happening

Independent Variable

Happens to

Dependent Variable

As Expressed by

(Subjects)

Subjects are not employed as the independent variable (something happening). This is to be a standard condition performed repetitively throughout the test series. Instead, subjects relate more directly to the dependent variable. They are or have been treated or affected by the independent variable, and their condition is or has been altered as a result. It is implied that the results of the test will apply to other subjects from the same universe—i.e., they will be affected similarly when exposed to the same independent variable.

A Simple Case

The initial example deals with a fairly simple situation. It has a single purpose. The study's design is not cluttered with an array of interactions.

Nursing Observations of 100 Premature Infants and Their Feeding Programs[7]

The intent of this study was "to determine the amount of formula that premature infants of a given weight and age will tolerate and at the same time maintain a satisfactory weight record." The independent variable or variables may be denoted as the feeding program or programs or, specifically, the varying amounts of formula. The tolerance reaction (dependent variable) of premature infants was studied as it was affected by the independent variable. Thus, the setting could be diagrammed as:

Independent
Variable(s)

Amount(s) of formula

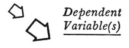 *Dependent*
Variable(s)

| Tolerance reaction while maintaining weight | *Subjects* (Premature Infants) |

It was expected that the extraneous independent variables, age and weight, would also influence the tolerance reactions. The universe of subjects was limited to a population of infants classified into two weight groups—(1) from 840 to 1,340 grams, and (2) from 1,400 to 2,500 grams—and premature births.

Complex Cases

The examples that follow relate to studies in which the identification of subjects is less evident. The studies are complicated by the interaction process. They may be characterized also by a multitude of purposes.

Here is a study with a single purpose that involves more than one group of persons. The question is: Who plays the subject role?

Nursing Service Staffing and Quality of Nursing Care[8]

Staffing studies such as this consider the interaction of various combinations of nursing personnel with different numbers of patients. One of the primary objectives of this study was to test the hypothesis "that quality of nursing care provided selected groups of patients decreases when numbers of patients assigned to nurses increase." In other words, it was expected that the dependent variable, "quality of nursing care," would be influenced by the independent variable, "numbers of patients assigned to nurses."

"Quality of nursing care" is an entity or a characteristic that is exhibited by nurses who give care or by patients who receive care. Who would play the subject role? Nurses? Patients? If direct observations or measures are taken, either group probably could be sampled as an expression of the dependent variable.

Independent Variable

> Numbers of patients
> assigned to nurses

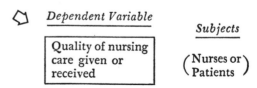

Dependent Variable

> Quality of nursing
> care given or
> received

Subjects

$\left(\begin{array}{l}\text{Nurses or}\\\text{Patients}\end{array}\right)$

It was determined, however, that the "quality of nursing care" would be rated indirectly by patients, nurses and physicians. In reality, it may be conceived that the dependent variable was observer ratings of the "quality of nursing care" as expressed by subjects representing patient, nurse and physician universes.

Independent Variable

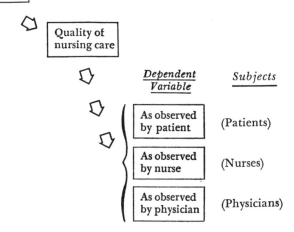

The next example contains three purposes and really should be considered as three studies. It also involves more than one group of participants. It should be observed how certain characteristics of the subjects become independent variables intervening to affect another characteristic.

The Evaluation of Nurses by Male Physicians[9]

How do physicians regard nurses? The daily interaction of the nurse and the physician has molded the role of the former in the eyes of the latter. This study has inquired into: What is "the image of the professional nurse held by the male physician?" In addition, it sought to determine the influence of age and medical specialty (of physicians) upon the dependent variable.

Who are the subjects of the study—nurses or physicians? The intervening elements or characteristics are the nurse, the aging process, and medical specialization experiences. Each was considered to have effected a change in the physician, specifically in his picture of the nurse. The results will represent the viewpoints of several subuniverses of physicians from whom the subjects of this study were drawn.

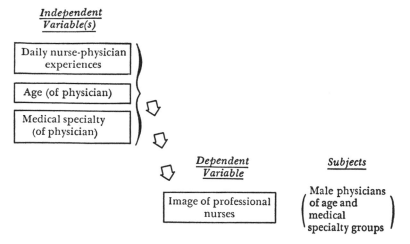

Independent
Variable(s)

| Daily nurse-physician experiences |
| Age (of physician) |
| Medical specialty (of physician) |

Dependent Variable   *Subjects*

| Image of professional nurses |

Male physicians of age and medical specialty groups

Here is another example of a multipurpose study. In this situation, the independent variable has effected changes in more than one dependent variable.

Play Interviews for 4-Year-Old Hospitalized Children[10]

This study attempted to determine the reactions of children to intrusive procedures. Several forms of behavior or reactions were investigated.

Three characteristics of the same subjects were studied in the reaction to the administration of intrusive procedures. Four-year-olds were

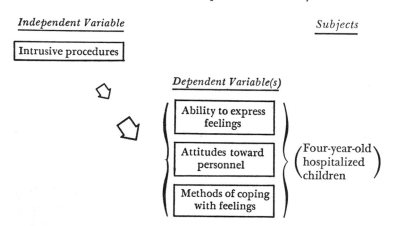

Independent Variable   *Subjects*

| Intrusive procedures |

Dependent Variable(s)

| Ability to express feelings |
| Attitudes toward personnel |
| Methods of coping with feelings |

Four-year-old hospitalized children

selected because this was considered as the "intrusive age." The results would be applicable to other hospitalized children in the same age group.

The complexities of the study may be magnified in proportion to the objectives of the research project. The former study was an illustration of a multitude of changes expressed by the same universe of subjects. The following illustration is offered as an example of a study series in which a single issue has been evaluated in terms of three criteria. Each appeared to utilize different subjects. It should be noted that there was a role reversal in which the items implement both the independent and the dependent variables.

Disposable and Reusable Surgeons' Gloves[11]

The question of substituting disposable for reusable gloves in the operating room was the concern of this study. It was explored from several points of view: costs, durability and acceptability. The authors hypothesized that: the substitution of disposable gloves will result in greater economy to the hospital; the elimination of glove processing (substituting disposable gloves) will save nursing time in the hospital; operating conditions will have a comparable effect upon the durability of the gloves; and the use of either type of glove will be equally acceptable to the wearer.

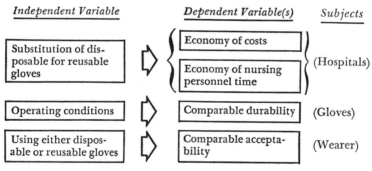

Independent Variable	Dependent Variable(s)	Subjects
Substitution of disposable for reusable gloves	Economy of costs Economy of nursing personnel time	(Hospitals)
Operating conditions	Comparable durability	(Gloves)
Using either disposable or reusable gloves	Comparable acceptability	(Wearer)

Who assumed the subject role? Different groups of subjects were required to satisfy the varying needs of the hypotheses. Thus, the economy to hospitals, the durability of gloves and the acceptability to the wearers composed the points of application.

A reversal of roles should be observed. Samples of gloves represented the subjects as an expression of the durability test. In addition, they may be interpreted as the materials intervening to influence the test of acceptability to a population of wearers.

This brief review is indicative of the problems that may be encountered in merely identifying subjects for nursing research. These problems may be typical of the applied research field where the concern perhaps is oriented more toward problem-solving than knowledge attainment. There is a tendency to perform many functions in a single study. There is a feeling that everything possible must be utilized and the utmost exacted from the study situation and the participants.

A fusion of roles can result. It may become difficult for the researcher and any independent observer to determine the true functions of the participants. The preceding analysis may provide a formula that will assist the reader to isolate the study parts. However, even this proposal is subject to interpretation. The authors are not certain that they truly have isolated the subject roles in each of the illustrations.

OBTAINING SUBJECTS

The realities of the applied situation also reflect upon the problem of obtaining subjects. The researcher may design a study and establish the requirements for selection in neatly defined capsules. But the task of fulfilling the requirements is another matter.

The best laid plans of many researchers in nursing have fallen prey to the exigencies of the practice situation. At times, too many elements are beyond the control of the individual researcher. They force accommodations to practice and the acceptance of less stringent requirements for study.

Such interferences often occur intermittently throughout the course of a study. They may occur initially and necessitate a change of plans. They may recur during the later stages and make it necessary to alter the conditions of the test.

Available Population

Typically, the applied problem may consider the effects of an ongoing practice upon a client population. The study usually will take place after the practice has been implemented for a period of time. For example, the researcher may evaluate the nursing services of hospitals that employ professional nurses predominantly. In these cases, the researcher must locate his subjects among those who already have been exposed to the treatment under concern.

Unfortunately, clients do not often distribute themselves in conformity with the design of the study. Their presence results because they require treatment. And the treatment itself may be inviting only to particular kinds of people.

The Personal Adjustment of Chronically Ill Old People Under Home Care[12]

It was the original intent of the author to relate such factors as social class, amount of care and family attitudes to the adjustment of the chronically ill aged, living at home. Her initial attempts to locate a study population in hospitals and clinics were frustrated. She ultimately resorted to a group who received care from a Visiting Nurse Association. But the V.N.A. provided services to those who could not manage without assistance, and these were generally lower-class, foreign-born women. They were not necessarily incapacitated but required essentially minor technical services such as injections for anemia.

The author apparently revised her plan and restricted the actual study population to a selection of native-born whites. It was biased in several respects. The group was neither randomly chosen nor representative of a general universe of chronically ill aged. It was simply an available population and forced changes in the study's design to include an investigation of factors other than those initially considered.

The Hidden Agendas

The applied researcher has several constituencies. The selection procedure and the implementation of the study plans often must be cleared through many channels. Indirectly, each step in the process may force an alteration of plans.

Peter New listed four groups intervening in his study of nurse staffing.[13] There was, of course, the investigator, who was conscious of the design stipulations. He had to capitulate, however, to the hospital administrator, whose sanction was necessary but who had little understanding of the investigator's needs. The investigator also had to accommodate to the nursing service administrator, who was fearful that the daily routine of patient care might be disrupted. Lastly, he had to encourage the nursing staff, who were the study's participants. Each person had his or her hidden agenda. Each influenced the selection process and the study itself.

The Intervening Events

In addition to the foregoing, other events may interpose during the course of the study to influence the outcome. These are normally beyond the control of the researcher. However, it is possible to anticipate some extenuating circumstances and to provide compensations.

A rather normal expectancy is the loss or the diminution of the sample size. This is particularly characteristic of human subjects, who may withdraw for many reasons. If the attrition is sizeable and occurs in some systematic fashion, then the entire course of the study may be altered.

The researcher seldom expects complete returns from mailed questionnaire surveys. Nevertheless, he can compensate for withdrawals by oversampling. The authors of a study of career patterns among professional nurses followed this procedure.[14] They determined the analytic requirements in advance and anticipated the need for a working sample of 2,500 cases. Questionnaires were sent to 3,866 professional nurses, and 2,643 were returned. Some of the returns were not used because they were atypical, incomplete, or late in arriving.

Attrition should be expected also among subjects of studies lasting over a long period of time. Courtney experienced this while investigating the effects of the classroom laboratory upon student learning.[15] She initiated her study with a group of 96 students from a beginning class in a nursing program. The students were assigned randomly to one of several experimental or control groups. In the course of the project, 46 subjects were lost, due to illness and normal withdrawal from school.

Thus, there are many factors that may influence the selection of subjects. Some of these are self-evident. Some are not so apparent. In any case, they will have a bearing upon what is regarded as truth.

Some researchers recognize the inherent weaknesses in their selection procedures and caution their readers to be aware of the shortcomings.

It was recognized that a more random, or less selective method of sampling would permit more meaningful interpretation of the results. However, . . . it was felt that the proposed relaxation in the sampling procedure was warranted in the interest of trying to maintain a high degree of motivation in the personnel who were to be in direct contact with the patients. If the results proved encouraging, a more rigorous sampling procedure could be employed in a subsequent study.[16]

Some researchers tend to disregard rather obvious discrepancies in sampling or hope that they may dissipate during the course of the study.

A control group and an experimental group of children aged 2 to 6, and their parents, were selected for the study. There were 23 cases in the control group and 27 in the experimental. . . .

No attempt was made to match the groups according to age, sex, diagnosis, previous hospital experience, previous emotional adjustments, length of present hospital stay, or the number of children in the hospital room. It was hoped that the sampling of patients in both groups would be large enough to minimize these variables.[17]

Unfortunately, there is no magic solution in numbers. Sampling, and in particular random selection, is a deliberate and carefully planned procedure. It is based upon a prior determination of the nature of the variables and the related universes. It is governed by a set of conditions stipulated in accordance with what has been learned. No amount of excessive numbers really can compensate for gross violations of the conditions. This is as true of applied research as it is of basic research.

It is also true that the applied researcher cannot possibly attain the ideal circumstances of the basic researcher. Perhaps she is not sufficiently practical. She may attempt too much at one time and, in effect, complicate rather than solve the problem.

REFERENCES

1. Pearson, Karl, (ed.): Tracts for Computers, No. XV, New York, Cambridge, 1947.

2. Goode, W. J., and Hatt, P. K.: Methods in Social Research, pp. 221-222, New York, McGraw-Hill, 1952.

3. Fisher, Sir Ronald A.: The Design of Experiments, Edinburgh, Oliver & Boyd, 1937.

4. Snedecor, G. W.: Statistical Methods, Ames, Iowa, State College Press, 1946.

5. Edwards, A. L.: Experimental Design in Psychological Research, New York, Rinehart, 1950.

6. McNemor, Quinn: Psychological Statistics, New York, Wiley, 1949.

7. Iffrig, Sister Mary Charitas: Nursing observations of 100 premature infants and their feeding programs, Nurs. Res. 5:71-81, 1956.

8. Safford, B. J., and Schlotfeldt, R. M.: Nursing service staffing and quality of nursing care, Nurs. Res. 9:149-154, 1960.

9. The Evaluation of Nurses by Male Physicians: Part I of a Study of The Registered Nurse in a Metropolitan Community, Pub. 93, Kansas City, Mo., Community Studies, Inc., 1955.

10. Erickson, Florence: Play Interviews for 4-Year-Old Hospitalized Children, Monograph of the Society for Research in Child Development, Inc., Vol. XXIII, Serial No. 69, No. 3, 1958.

11. Struve, M., and Levine, E.: Disposable and reusable surgeons' gloves, Nurs. Res. 10:79-86, 1961.

12. Mack, M. J.: The personal adjustment of chronically ill old people under home care, Nurs. Res. 1:9-30, 1952.

13. New, Peter Kong-Ming: The hospital researcher walks a tight rope, Mod. Hosp. 93:93-95, 1959.

14. Bressler, Marvin, and Kephart, William: Career Dynamics, p. 10, Harrisburg, Pa., Pennsylvania Nurses Assn., 1955.

15. Courtney, M. E.: The effectiveness of the classroom laboratory in the teaching of nursing arts, Nurs. Res. 8:149, 1959.

16. Carpenter, H. A., and Simon, Ralph: The effect of several methods of training on long-term, incontinent, behaviorally regressed hospitalized psychiatric patients, Nurs. Res. 9:18, 1960.

17. Godfrey, A. E.: A study of nursing care designed to assist hospitalized children and their parents in their separation, Nurs. Res. 4:57, 1955.

CHAPTER 8

The Selection of Materials

THE GENERAL PROBLEM

The testing procedure is an exercise in concrete reporting. The researcher should take nothing for granted. He must leave little to the imagination of his readers. He must report the events exactly as they transpire.

The testing procedure is also an exercise in objective reporting. The researcher will minimize his own or the observer's role in interpreting what happens. The reader desires assurance that what was reported to have occurred actually took place in the manner described. He wants proof that any trained observer or reporter would have recorded the events in the same way.

Materials are employed to foster the observer-reporter role of the researcher. They are used to ease the observation and recording process. They also may provide for greater objectivity by permitting the researcher to remain relatively aloof from the judgmental or interpretive aspects of the test.

The Need for Materials in Research

A universe consists of a set of traits or qualities descriptive of an aggregate of persons, events or things. For instance, a sample of patients represents certain age, sex, illness, family and behavioral qualities that are characteristic of a universe of patients. The outcome of the test and the interpretation of the results will be affected by the extent to which these traits do or do not appear as indicated.

The researcher states that the extraneous variables or qualities—age, sex, illness and family condition—will have an effect upon the patient's behavior. However, he wishes to isolate this effect from what may result if only "confinement to bed for X days" is introduced into a patient situation. Therefore, he conceives of two groups of subjects who are selected from the same universe and have in common the former set of qualities. These traits are to remain relatively constant. The groups are to be equated also with regard to the behavioral characteristic "irritability." If the groups truly are similar with respect to these qualities and only one group is confined to bed for X days, then any differences in behavior may be attributed to the additional condition.

However, the researcher and his readers may raise many issues. They may question the selection of subjects: Do they represent the universe? Are different groups of subjects matched or equated? They may voice concern about the problem situation: Has the independent explanatory variable been introduced in the manner prescribed by the hypothesis? Have other extraneous variables been controlled? They may inquire about the effects of the test: Has change taken place in the dependent variable? Can any change be attributed to the action of the independent explanatory variable?

All the relevant variables should be thoroughly described, measured and recorded:

The researcher requires adequate initial descriptive measures of the extraneous variables. He desires to know that his group of subjects is representative of the universe and is equated with other groups of subjects representative of the same universe. He also may appreciate a running account of changes that occur in these conditions. Theoretically, they may be expected to remain constant or to change in the same manner for all groups.

The researcher is required to record what happens in the problem situation. In particular, he is concerned about the actual implementation of the independent explanatory variable. It must be remembered that the term was defined initially in conceptual or model form. It may undergo reinterpretation or modification in the transition to a realistic state.* Whatever actually transpires becomes the concept that is tested. This should be imparted to the reader exactly as it occurs and related back to the original definition.

The ultimate question of the test is whether or not, how much and in what direction the dependent variable has changed. Does the patient who has been confined to bed for X days become irritable? Is he more irritable than patients who have not been confined to bed for X days? The researcher must have some index of the subjects' states prior to the introduction of the independent explanatory variable. He must determine that they have been or can be equated with respect to the dependent variable, i.e., the patients are equally irritable. He must later re-examine his subjects to determine the extent of change. These measures or observations are most critical to the outcome of the study.

Some of the qualities just discussed can be described or measured with relative ease. Independent observers probably would have little difficulty in determining the appropriate age and sex characteristics of the patients. Other qualities are not described or measured as easily. Thus, the same observers may not be able to make uniform, extemporaneous descriptions of illness, family and behavioral qualities. The observers may not agree on what is to be observed. They may not be able to perceive some of the proposed observations.

Special devices, instruments or materials may be needed to ensure accurate and objective measures or descriptions. They can be employed to establish the sequence of observations, specify what is to be observed and permit observations that ordinarily evade human perception. They are required more often to secure the appropriate descriptive measures of the extraneous and the explanatory variables.

ATTRIBUTES OF MATERIALS

The discussions above concern the need to obtain and record information and to measure change. If the researcher desires to construct or locate devices for performing such services,

---

* An operational definition serves as a transition from conceptual to actual form.

what essentials should be satisfied? Five attributes of materials will be considered: communicability, recordability, measurability, validity and reliability.

Communicability

Some materials may be viewed as a set of written directives to subjects or observers. As such, they provide a uniform and standardized set of testing conditions. This is an important feature of the procedure. The idea of a test series implies repetitive observations of similar situations. If the conditions of the test are not stated uniformly, then unique and discontinuous observations rather than a series may be obtained. Under these circumstances each observation must be judged as a distinct study and cannot be accumulated with the others to develop a probability value.

A classic example of what happens when concrete directions are not provided is displayed by John Godfrey Saxe's "The Blind Men and the Elephant":

> It was six men of Indostan,
>   To learning much inclined,
> Who went to see the Elephant
>   (Though all of them were blind),
> That each by observation
>   Might satisfy his mind.
>
> The *First* approached the Elephant,
>   And happening to fall,
> Against his broad and sturdy side,
>   At once begun to bawl:
> "God bless me! but the Elephant
>   Is very like a wall."
>
> The *Second,* feeling of the tusks,
>   Cried, "Ho! what have we here
> So very round and smooth and sharp?
>   To me 'tis mighty clear
> This wonder of an Elephant
>   Is very like a spear."

The *Third* approached the animal,
  And happening to take
The squirming trunk within his hands,
  Thus boldly up and spake:
"I see," quoth he, "the Elephant
  Is very like a snake."

The *Fourth* reached out his eager hand,
  And felt about the knee.
"What most this wondrous beast is like,
  Is mighty plain," quoth he;
" 'tis clear enough the Elephant
  Is very like a tree."

The *Fifth,* who chanced to touch the ear,
  Said: "E'en the blindest man
Can tell what this resembles most;
  Deny the fact who can,
This marvel of an Elephant
  Is very like a fan."

The *Sixth* no sooner had begun
  About the beast to grope,
Than, seizing on the swinging tail
  That fell within his scope,
"I see," quoth he, "the Elephant
  Is very like a rope."

And so these men of Indostan
  Disputed loud and long,
Each in his own opinion
  Exceeding stiff and strong,
Though each was partly in the right,
  And all were in the wrong!

What has happened is that the observer has become a variable. The outcome of this hypothetic study was affected by the vantage point of the different observers. Truth was influenced directly by the observers and what they were able to perceive.

Of course the reader may say, "The observers were blind. What else could be expected?" But, the seeing also may fail to see; or they may see too many things; or they may see only what they want to see. Each incident may result in inaccurate reporting. The researcher cannot establish a truth under these circumstances.

Materials may enable the researcher to remove or, at least, to control the observer as a variable. That is, they will provide a uniform set of conditions under which the observations are to take place. Therefore, the conditions of the test are not solely the property of the observer. They are to be displayed so that any trained individual can make the same observations under the same circumstances.

Materials are the means by which the researcher communicates with the subjects, the observers and, ultimately, the readers. Each is in agreement if they comprehend the instructions fully. However, any defect in the attribute "communicability" will confuse the outcome. The materials, as well as the observer, will become uncontrolled extraneous variables.

Recordability

Materials are also records. They serve as source documents in which the descriptive information about the subjects and the situation can be recorded. They yield the data to be employed in the analysis.

The process of gathering data for the test is a form of record-keeping and should be performed systematically. It will ease the task of the observer and minimize his role in the outcome. It will simplify the analysis.

Record-keeping is not necessarily a simple process. Picture a busy hospital ward of 30 patients during meal hours. Tray carts are lined up in the corridors. Nurse assistants are transporting the trays to the patients, who are both in and out of bed and may require special diets. Nurses are feeding some of the patients, while other patients are feeding themselves. An observer could have been asked to describe the behavior of four patients in this ward.

The observer may have received blank sheets of paper and have been instructed to record all instances of "irritable" behavior. This could be a formidable assignment. He is in the midst of a flurry of activities—the feeding process. He must skip back and forth from patient to patient. Each time a patient reacts, a judgment is to be made—Is this a form of irritable behavior?—and a notation of some type written on one of the sheets of paper. The observer may decide ultimately to record everything that he sees and to make judgments later—an arduous task for one series of observations and impossible for four.

Instead, the observer could have received prepared sheets listing distinct instances of irritable behavior:

1. Demands attention
2. Abuses others
3. Refuses assistance
4. Reacts excitedly.

These categories will have been described fully and will contain numerous examples. The observer is to record each instance of the various forms of behavior occurring within a given time period, and nothing else. Under these circumstances, perhaps observations of four patients may be secured with considerably more ease.

This type of records form naturally into a process for analysis. As a matter of fact, they could have been devised with the method of analysis in mind. They may fall into natural groupings and provide values to be manipulated and compared for decision-making.

On the other hand, the first type of record may yield a complex of confusion. A large variety of observations may be obtained. Each observation must be scrutinized individually and, if possible, categorized into some meaningful classification. Only then can a plan for analysis be formulated.

"Recordability" or the power of the instrument to ease the record-keeping process is another important attribute of materials. Like "communicability," its presence will limit the effect of the observer and the material upon what really happens to the dependent variable under study.

Measurability

The term "variable" is synonymous with change. When the term is employed in the context of a relationship, it is implied that variation or change in the independent explanatory variable will result in variation in the dependent variable. We might conceive also that any change in the dependent variable can be attributed to the relative presence or absence of the independent variable.

It was indicated previously that variations in degree may exist. The factors may be completely present or absent or partially present or absent. In either case, a large or a small difference is to be denoted between two observations.

Differences can be ascertained as a judgment of the observer that things have changed. A man meets an acquaintance whom he has not seen for 2 years and states, "You have gotten heavier." This is a rough estimate of the difference between two observations. It is inexact and may be wholly erroneous.

Differences also can be measured with the aid of instruments. Shoes are fitted more precisely with a foot-size indicator. Instruments can detect the less obvious differences in degree. They secure more exact measurements.

The concept of measurement is inherent in these discussions and constitutes another important attribute of materials. It is a medium or an expression for change. It is employed to foster the decision-making process.

Like other terms, "measure" has several meanings. A measure may be synonymous with the instrument that is employed, such as a foot-size indicator, a ruler, or a thermometer. It may refer to the process of measuring—taking a patient's temperature or determining the pulse rate. A measure may be the end-result of the process, e.g., the patient has a high fever, or the unit of expression, e.g., a degree, an inch, a beat per minute.

Lorge *et al.,* who presented an excellent discussion on the nature of measurement, recognized these many-sided definitions.[1] Furthermore, they felt that the term could not and should not be limited. "Measurability," as we use the term, will refer to all of these things also. It will be considered as the capability of the material or the instrument to yield a unit descriptive of the subject in point of time, and can be employed to denote change.

Change may occur in several ways. It may be suggested by differences between two groups of subjects at one time. It also may occur within the same group of subjects at different times. Measurability will connote the power of the instrument to detect these changes.

What is measured as a reflection of change is the property of the object, the event or the person. This, Lorge states, is crucial to measurement. It is defined as "some feature that is considered to be common to all objects of a given kind or class, but that need not be considered to be present in all objects whatsoever."[2] Some properties of persons that can connote physical well-being or its opposite are blood pressure, pulse rate, basal metabolism, body temperature and weight. It was suggested, by way of example, that irritable behavior can be observed by its properties: demandingness, abusiveness, negativism, excitability.

The property of the subject is what is observed and measured. It is to be defined rigorously by the researcher and understood clearly by the observer. One or more properties of the subject may be observed. However, the more careful studies attempt to restrict their observations to a single property at one time.

Two measures of the property may be derived: an all-or-none and a scaled measure. The former is descriptive of "discrete" variables. The latter refers to "continuous" variables.

A "discrete" measure comprises one of the simplest forms of observation. The event either happens or fails to happen and is categorized into a class. A patient's behavior is judged to be irritable or nonirritable. The measure of difference indicative of change is based upon an enumeration or a count of each class. Thus, there may evolve a greater incidence of behaviors classified as "irritable" among patients confined to bed for X days.

Unfortunately, observations do not fall readily into discrete categories. Observers may not determine easily that a behavior is "irritable" or "nonirritable." Instead, they may view it as "somewhat," "more," or "less" irritable. The line of discrimination between the classes may be thin.

A "scaled" or continuous measure recognizes differences in degree. It is also considerably more complex. A set of scaled values or numerical equivalents is to be derived for each differentiation in behavior. What is employed as the unit of measurement, and the interval between units, must be established with defined limits. As there is a degree of temperature, is there also a degree of irritability? Does the level of irritability increase in equal amounts? Is there a beginning point on the scale of "complete nonirritability" and a maximum point of "complete irritability"?

There are many hazards to the scaling process. Each step is imbued with unknown factors so that the investigator never is really certain of the true value of his measures. Thus, the measurement aspect imposes another restraint upon the nature of truth. The ability of the instrument to measure or its failure to do so properly is another extraneous variable with which the researcher must contend.

Validity

The test was considered previously to be an expression of whether or not the hypothesis is in agreement with reality. The validity of the test, in turn, will be a function of the ability to identify reality. That is, it will depend substantially upon what the researcher determines to be the actual counterpart of the paper situation displayed in the formulation of the hypothesis.

Reality may be considered as the interaction of the relevant variables under study. This is, what is to be observed and measured. Materials are employed to perform this requirement. They are selected to denote the presence and the interaction of the relevant variables in the subjects and the situation.

The selection of materials will strongly influence the validity of the test. What often results is a function of the descriptive and the measurement powers of the instruments. For example, patients actually may change as a result of being confined, yet the test that is employed may not provide a measurement of the type of change that is expected.

The materials for research should be relevant to the specific purpose for which they were selected. They were chosen or designed to measure particular traits or properties. They are to be used to satisfy these purposes. Validity is an index of the degree to which the material "serves the purpose for which it is used."[3]

It is said also that a material is valid when it measures what it is supposed to measure. However, some materials may satisfy this requirement but fail to meet the needs of the study. It is possible, for example, to select an instrument that purports to measure a form of irritable behavior. Nevertheless, it may fail to depict the type of irritable behavior exhibited by patients as a function of confinement. Materials for research, therefore, may be considered to be valid when they measure what they are supposed to measure and serve the purpose for which they are selected.

Cureton and others suggest that validity has two aspects: relevance and reliability.[4] The latter refers to the ability of the instrument to yield accurate and consistent measures or true scores that are free of errors of measurement. The term will be discussed subsequently as an independent attribute of materials. Relevance is an index of the "closeness of agreement between what the (material) measures and the function that it is used to measure."[5]

Relevance is determined by establishing a standard or a criterion with which the usefulness of the material's measures or scores is compared. A criterion is selected that is known to measure the function of the material. Independent observations, employing the actual material and criterion scores, are obtained from the same subjects. The direction and the degree of relationship can be reported as an index of relevance. Validity is an index of the relationship between the raw material scores and the true or perfectly reliable criterion scores (or scores corrected for errors of measurement).*

The researcher may seek to establish the validity of an instrument designed to detect changes in "irritable behavior." Two groups of patients are selected, one of which has been rated by some external measure as "irritable," the other as "nonirritable." The instrument will be judged to be valid if the patients can be separated with relative accuracy into the same two groups.

The major problem in estimating an index of validity is the determination of the criterion measure.

The question arises often, "Is the criterion valid?" and it can be resolved only by obtaining a measure of validity on the criterion, itself. A self-perpetuating process, lasting indefinitely, can be generated in this way.[6]

Upon what basis, in this example, does the researcher determine that the external measure of "irritable behavior" is valid? He may state that experts made judgments regarding the behaviors in question. Upon what basis are the expert judgments considered valid, or upon what basis are the experts considered expert? Some other materials may have been designed to measure the degree of expertness. And so the process can continue until some ultimate criterion is reached.

Unfortunately, we seldom locate the ultimate criterion. Reality or ultimate truth in these matters is sought constantly but rarely attained. Thus, different kinds of validity are estimated. For example, we may seek *empiric validity,* which is an expression of the procedure discussed above: a comparison of the score yielded by the material with observable criteria. We also can obtain *logical validity,* in which the content of the material is judged to parallel some external requirements, e.g., the content of a test to measure achievement in training parallels the training course content; and *face validity,* in which the materials simply look valid to independent observers.

* Further discussions of validity actually deal with relevance. However, to avoid confusion, it will be assumed that we are treating perfectly reliable measures and make reference to validity rather than to relevance.

It is evident that truly valid materials will be obtained infrequently. Furthermore, it may even be difficult to secure good estimates of validity. Nevertheless, some estimate of validity is helpful to the researcher: "A test score becomes meaningful when the test user knows to what degree the test measures what it is supposed to measure."[7] This is particularly true in research matters, where the investigator desires to account for all discrepancies. It is better to know that we are in error in depicting and recording reality than not to know and draw misleading conclusions.

Reliability

Errors are an inherent part of measurement. We cannot expect to obtain two identical measures of the same property of the same subjects. The validity of an instrument is limited by this characteristic of measurement. The outcome of the test will be affected accordingly.

It is true also that a certain degree of consistency in measurement can be expected. Otherwise, the measurement process would have little or no value. We may anticipate that a group of subjects will maintain the same relative standing in repeated measurements of the same property. For example, measurements of irritability by two observers employing the same instrument at the same time should yield relatively equivalent results. Patients judged as less irritable by one observer should be rated as less irritable by another observer. Patients judged as more irritable by one observer should be rated as more irritable by another observer. The degree of consistency is an index of the reliability of the instrument.

Estimates of reliability can be secured in two ways: Absolute measures of consistency can be determined and relative indices of this attribute also can be ascertained. The estimates represent two approaches to the concept of reliability.

Absolute determinants of consistency are developed from an analysis of repeated observations or measures of the same sub-

ject. Each observation is an estimate of the true measure*
and is in error to the extent that it departs from the true measure. The observations would form into a distribution of errors
whose standard size can be determined statistically. The standard error of measurement is an absolute expression of the
reliability of an instrument.

A measure of relative consistency is an expression of the
variation in scores or measures produced by a particular instrument. An instrument administered to any group of subjects normally can be expected to result in a wide distribution
of score values. Part of the variation in scores arises because
subjects are truly different with respect to the property that is
measured. Variation also occurs because of inaccuracies in
measurement. Reliability reflects that proportion of the differences in the score obtained that is "due to true differences
between individuals in the quality being evaluated."[8] (In a
negative sense, reliability suggests that a proportion of the differences in standing also is erroneous.) Thus it is manifested as
a ratio between the obtained and the true score.

Thorndike classified the two sources of variation into systematic and chance factors.[9] Systematic sources are definable
and predictable. Chance factors are vague and unpredictable.

Systematic factors do not relate to reliability. In a sense, they
exist independently of the instrument. Thus, the true or actual
differences in the property being measured can be listed as a
systematic factor. In addition, certain errors of measurement
will occur in a predictable and systematic fashion and will not
influence the reliability or the relative standing of subjects
within a group. For example, observers are known to rate
performances differently. Some observers will persistently rate
highly, others will give only low or intermediate ratings.
Therefore, the errors of measurement that occur will be distributed systematically among a group of subjects rated by the
same observer. The relative standing of the subjects will not
be altered.

* The true measure is an unknown but can be estimated as the mean
or the average score obtained.

The chance factors relate to reliability. There are many unpredictable sources that may produce errors of measurement. For example, an instrument designed to measure achievement in a particular subject area may consist of 50 items drawn from a pool of 1,000 items. By chance, some individuals at the time of administration may be more familiar with these items than some other individuals are. They may not be so favored on another occasion. Their relative standings among the remaining individuals would be altered accordingly.

The reliability of an instrument may be viewed as an index of the precision of measurement. At least it will indicate to the researcher the errors or the variations that arise as a function of chance. A certain amount of individual variation in repeated measurements not only is anticipated but, under certain circumstances, desired. Differences in behavior in point of time, for example, are expected as a consequence of being confined to bed. However, behavioral changes or differences also may occur because the instrument used to measure change was unreliable. This type of change will only confuse the issue. "The accuracy of prediction which it is possible to achieve or the amount of improvement in performance which can be shown is limited by the reliability of the measure through which the performance is manifested."[10]

KIND OF MATERIALS

The previous discussions have indicated that materials are employed for different purposes. Although they can be tailored to the requirements of specific situations, the different kinds of materials have their limitations. They should not be employed out of context. We should not expect them to perform functions for which they were not designed.

The discussions that follow have grouped the materials in accordance with their general purpose. Some are designed essentially to gather descriptive information of past events. Some are to be developed to describe ongoing events. Others are used to measure change.

For Describing Past Events

Researchers may gather evidence of past events to test their hypotheses. This information is used frequently as criteria for the selection of subjects. It also is employed commonly to survey problem situations similar to the one that is under investigation. Here, the researcher does not recreate the situation. Instead, he studies instances in which the relevant events already have been known to occur.

General descriptive information rather than exact measures can be secured under these circumstances. The data are generally secondhand and subject to problems of recall. The obtained evidence sometimes is distorted or influenced by the observer.

Interview Forms. The researcher or any of his designates may meet with the informant in a face-to-face situation. Population census information is gathered in this way. Interviewers go directly into the household and secure information relative to a prescribed set of questions. The interview form provides a modicum of control by standardizing the data collection procedure. It may serve also as a convenient form for recording the results of the interview.

Communication problems can be minimized in an interview situation. The interviewer has an opportunity to explain or convey the intent of the questions. At the same time, the form forces him to communicate with and follow the instructions of the researcher.

Questionnaires. The researcher may gather his information from remote sources by requesting his informants to respond in writing to a prescribed set of written questions. In one respect, this procedure is similar to the interview process. A form or a series of written questions is used. However, the interviewer is not present. Thus, problems of communication may abound. Misunderstandings contribute to many of the difficulties that are encountered when questionnaires are employed. The respondents may fail to understand or may misinterpret the questions. Since the researcher cannot be present, he is unable to clarify the statements. Furthermore, he may not always know or be able to detect when misinterpretations have occurred.

Questionnaires should be briefly and simply worded. In general, the researcher should not expect to secure detailed and exact information of complex situations by this means. A simplified form for recording answers also is beneficial, especially if large masses of data are to be obtained for analysis.

Anecdotal Records. Sometimes an informant is requested to speak freely about a problem situation. He is not limited by the questions posed by the researcher and may offer information that was not anticipated. A case study of a patient is an example of an anecdotal record. The respondent describes what happens to the subject as he himself experiences the situation.

Anecdotal reference materials often form poor records. Since the informants may not be restricted to precise formats, a variety of descriptive data may be offered. Some of the data may be highly relevant; other pieces of information may not be pertinent at all. Some of the data may be distorted or even omitted. The researcher ultimately must sift through the materials and separate the appropriate information for study. It is relatively difficult to organize anecdotal records for analysis.

It is not unlikely that much of the material gathered by this unstructured medium will be distorted. The anecdotal record-keeper must reach into the past and often recalls only the unusual or spectacular event. The normal incidents sometimes are blotted from his memory. He may not present an accurate description of the true state of affairs.

For Describing Ongoing Events

Researchers may decide to construct or locate actual situations descriptive of the hypothetic sequence. Materials designed to depict what happens are required. Ease and completeness of recording are major requirements.

In this respect, motion-picture and sound-recording devices can be employed fruitfully. They are manipulated easily and, together, will provide a fairly comprehensive and objective report of what happens. Unfortunately, they also are expensive and often are used sparingly. Furthermore, like the unstructured anecdotal records, they may provide a massive amount of information. The materials still must be sorted and sifted to uncover the purely relevant data.

The discussion that follows will be limited to a description of manual-recording media—the check list and the diary. They represent two opposite modes of data collection.

Check Lists. The idea of collecting only relevant and primarily objective information is represented by this type of record. The investigator becomes aware of the limitations of the observer in trying to perceive and record everything that happens. He recognizes further that it may be necessary only to restrict the observer to whatever is pertinent to the hypothesis.

The check list is a record of only the relevant information to be observed. Of course, what is relevant or pertinent is determined by the researcher and not by the observer. The form is also a convenient recording device. The observer may be required to check the incidents of occurrence only within given time periods.

The advantageous qualities of this type of instrument also are restrictive factors. A very limited segment of the total situation is observed at one time. The final record, which merely contains incidents of occurrence, may not be wholly descriptive. While it may lend itself easily to statistical treatment, the record may not be entirely meaningful.

Diaries. A diary is a running anecdotal record of ongoing events. It usually is kept by the subjects themselves. This record may circumvent some of the difficulties of the check list by providing more complete descriptions of what happens. However, it also contains the disadvantageous features of anecdotal records.

For Measuring Change

In addition to the descriptive materials mentioned, the researcher may require instruments to measure and record change. This can be achieved in two ways. Change may be measured directly by observing and recording what happens when the subject is placed in the test situation. In the event that direct indices cannot be obtained, change may be ascertained indirectly. Measures may be secured that presumably are related to what normally would be expected to occur.

Direct Measures. The most valid index of change is a measure of the criterion itself. If a person on a prescribed diet is expected to lose so much weight in so many days, then the measure of change is the weight loss. Scales have been devised to measure it. Such mechanical gadgets as scales, thermometers and sphygmomanometers provide fairly objective measures of change. They are useful to the extent that they are valid, i.e., serve the purpose of the test, and yield relatively consistent scores.

However, many behavioral changes cannot be measured directly by mechanical means. For example, what can be employed to determine that patients become more irritable after being confined to bed? Or how can it be ascertained that nurses spend more time with patients?

Performance evaluation records can be devised to measure or denote some behavioral changes directly. Check lists are employed for this purpose. They are particularly useful if they can be quantified to yield a score. To do this, sometimes rating scales are developed and attached to the items. The observer determines not only that the event has occurred but that it was performed well, fairly well, or poorly.

Problems of scaling, reliability and, perhaps, validity arise when performance evaluation records are used. The task of developing appropriate rating scales with meaningful units of measurement is fairly complex. The prominent role of the observer also must be recognized. Indices of observer as well as instrument reliability are helpful. Finally, as the investigator moves gradually into the realm of judgment and away from the true criterion, some question may be raised as to how valid the record is.

Indirect Measures. Instances may arise when it is not possible or feasible to measure the effects of change directly. For example, the effects of teaching proper foot care to hospitalized diabetics may not be uncovered for several months or even years after the patients have been discharged. Furthermore, since patients are discharged into a variety of conditions, there will be a lack of truly comparable testing conditions. "The delayed appearance of desired change," "the lack of comparable testing conditions," "infrequency and inaccessibility of incidents," and "the cost in time and effort of attaining proper measures" were among the reasons suggested by Lindquist when adequate direct measures of change could not be obtained.[11]

Indirect measures exact indices of change to situations that are samples of or which simulate the real thing. For instance, the investigator may simulate a series of anticipated home conditions that the typical diabetic may face over the course of time. Patient responses to these situations before and after treatment may be quantified as a more immediate measure of the effects of patient teaching.

Lindquist described three general types of indirect measures.[12] One, termed the "identical elements" type, presented the subject with exact duplicates of the true criterion situation. The researcher also may obtain samples that are related but not necessarily identical to the criterion. Finally, the criterion behavior may be simulated and described verbally to the subject who, in turn, will respond verbally.*

The first two involve measures of performance and may employ performance evaluation records fruitfully. They are not distinguished sharply from each other and may be used jointly in the same series. The illustration cited is an example of this: In addition to the direct application of proper foot care procedures, the researcher may infer change also by observing pa-

---

* This is useful only when human subjects are employed.

tients' reactions to more general though related hygienic practices.

The "verbalized behavior" type of test is a fairly inexpensive medium. It is a paper-and-pencil device. It does not require the construction of actual situations. The instrument may include many samples of behavior and can be administered to large numbers of subjects at one time. This procedure has been useful in measuring human achievement and some nonintellectual pursuits, such as interest and attitude change, which often are covert experiences that are difficult to measure outwardly under any circumstances.

The primary problem of materials used as indirect measures is that of validity. The researcher and any interested observer may always question whether or not the instrument provides the same measure as the criterion, since the latter cannot be observed directly. Any departure from the true measure would cast doubt upon the outcome of the test.

THE UTILIZATION OF MATERIALS IN NURSING RESEARCH

The research developments in a field such as nursing in reality are patterned upon the accomplishments of the individual practitioners. They reflect the orientations, the interests and the technical abilities of the researchers. The field will evolve as the practitioners change and gain in competence or as other researchers are permitted to lend their skills.

We propose that research in nursing has evolved accordingly. The original contributions are characteristic of what nurse-trained researchers would produce. Later advances mirror the competencies of research-trained nurses and their co-researchers.

The movement toward instrumentation or the utilization of materials is a case in point. Instrumentation is a symbol of refinement and exactitude in determining and describing what happens during the test. It represents a shift away from human judgment and a step closer to objectivity, uniformity and agreement. Nursing research is moving from a person-centered to an instrument-centered approach. It is reflective of a change in the orientation and the skills of the researchers.

The movement will be traced with regard to one of the most pressing problems in nursing: the development of adequate determinants to measure or assess the requirements for action. In particular, it will be focused upon the development of determinants of patients' needs for nursing care.

Ascertaining a patient's requirements for nursing care may be the paramount issue in nursing research. It is an objective to provide the fundamental basis for all other actions. It also may yield the final measure of success.

Determinants of the need for nursing care are both causes for action and measures of effectiveness. This is a cyclical affair. A need has been defined as an incomplete state in which a patient requires nursing assistance to satisfy some condition for living. Thus, it initiates nursing activities. Consequently, the results of the activities may be evaluated in terms of whether or not the need for nursing care persists. That is, does the nursing action diminish the need for care?

All nursing activities stem either directly or indirectly from the patient's need for care. These include educational and administrative functions as well as the ministration of actual nursing services. How students are selected, trained and evaluated, and how the nursing unit is supervised and staffed must be measured eventually in accordance with their effect upon patient need. The determinants of patient need constitute the ultimate criteria for nursing.

This problem permeates all of nursing. It is of concern to the practitioners—the bedside nurse, the supervisor and the educator—who periodically take actions influencing the care of patients. It is pertinent also to the researcher in nursing. She wishes to assist practitioners in these matters. She also desires to help herself. The researcher cannot advance much further than her ability to evaluate what has been learned already.

Solutions to this problem have been tendered from both practice and research. Each will be discussed. One, the service contribution, will be designated the patient-centered approach.

It is oriented toward the patient and the care requirements. In point of time and development, it is a precursor of the other, the research-centered approach. The latter has the primary initial function of satisfying the requirements of the researcher.

THE PATIENT-CENTERED APPROACH

Research, like teaching, administration and supervision, is ancillary to nursing. While the ultimate objective of these peripheral activities is to improve nursing service, each has some distinct and different intermediate goals. And each has developed functions that are in accord with the more immediate aims.

However, the nurse probably was a nurse long before she became a researcher, a teacher or a supervisor. Her initial interests converged in this direction. She was educated primarily to perform nursing functions. Her value system was oriented toward the fulfillment of those activities more directly associated with nursing care.

But some seeds for conflict may have been sown during the initial orientation period. As a nurse, her approach had become patient- or care-centered. What she did was done for or because of the patient. Yet, as a researcher, she must become knowledge-centered; and as a teacher, student-centered; and as a supervisor, staff-centered. The various roles have several conflicting aspects.

On the other hand, nursing is not entirely antagonistic to the other practices. For example, it has many features in common with research. Much of nursing consists of comprehensive investigations. It is a continuous study of the patient and his needs, interspersed by nursing actions. And for this purpose the nurse is trained to observe, record and evaluate—three basic skills of research.

Nursing practice may be interpreted partially as an attempt to co-ordinate the efforts of medical and paramedical personnel in behalf of the patient. The physician will make preliminary observations and prescribe the treatment or the kind of medical care that the patient needs. He predicts that the treatment will effect changes in the patient's condition and lessen his requirement for care. He will implement a portion of the plan and direct the nurse and other paramedical personnel to conduct the remainder of the plan. The nurse is generally the only member of the group to maintain constant liaison with the patient. It is she who observes what changes actually transpire and communicates these changes to the physician. The nurse acts as a medium of exchange between the physician (and other paramedical personnel) and the patient.

Once the patient care plan is implemented, the nurse becomes a primary source for the determination of patient care needs. Through observation she will gather much of the information that is necessary to assess the patient's reactions and formulate modifications in the over-all care plan. However, she performs this assignment as a nurse rather than as a researcher. Neither the patient, the physician nor she herself can wait upon the more refined procedures of research. She relies principally upon her own educational and service experiences to formulate clinical hunches as to what is required by the patient.

It may be surmised that much of the original and even current information on patient needs emanated from the clinical observations of the nurse. Some of the more perceptive and inquisitive nurse observers made detailed and complete studies of patients, which have been published and disseminated widely. These materials have served as prototypes suggestive of the nursing care requirements for particular classifications of patients.

Descriptive Analysis of the Nursing Care of Two Selected Cardiac Surgical Patients[13]

Patient A was admitted 5 days before surgery. The writer was introduced to the patient while she was visiting in the room of an 11-year-old boy who had undergone a surgical repair of an atrial septal defect and pulmonary valvular stenosis. . . .

At the scheduled time the patient, accompanied by the writer, was taken to the operating room. She was removed from the cart on a special scale; the weight was reported as 30.250 Kg. This measure is also repeated postoperatively in order to determine the fluid gain. . . .

Patient A returned via bed in a semiconscious state and was placed in the tent with an oxygen flow of 10 liters a minute and the humidifier at 4 liters/minute. A soft flannel material was used to cover the head of the patient, and another placed over her shoulders. . . .

Immediately upon return from surgery, Patient A responded with crying and restless movements; she opened her eyelids when her name was called. Six-inch blocks were placed under the head of the bed. . . .

The vital signs were taken by the nurse every 15 minutes for 1 hour, then every half hour until the end of the evening period. The patient was then prepared for the parents' first visit; . . . The parents were called into the room. At this time the patient appeared very pale, was tossing about in bed, crying as though in pain. The mother, apparently frightened, looked at her daughter and said to the writer, "She was always so active and healthy looking, I can't believe this is the same girl. . . ."

Patient A co-operated well in all nursing activities. She coughed upon request but was unsuccessful in her attempts to raise mucous secretions. She turned on either side with the assistance of the nurse. Two pillows were used to support the back and one was placed under the flexed lower extremity while the patient was on her side.

The patient continued her restlessness during the night, moaning and crying with pain when awake. She complained of being warm although her body was cool to touch and her temperature within normal limits. The vital signs were taken every 2 hours and the blood pressure remained stable at 118/65; the pulse was of strong quality. . . .

Even though the patient cried and was restless, the first medication for pain, Demerol, 20 mg., was given by injection 12 hours after surgery. Since narcotics not only relieve pain but also depress the respiratory center and coughing reflex, the surgeon ordered the analgesia in the early postoperative period to be given sparingly and with discretion. . . .

Patient B was admitted to a semi-private room; Patient A occupied the other bed. The time of admission was the regular visiting hour, so that the parents became acquainted with each other and this opened new avenues of psychological support to each of them. . . .

On the Sunday before the operation Patient B visited outdoors in a wheel chair, accompanied by her parents. She spent the afternoon with her sisters and brothers. . . .

Physical care for Patient B began on the evening before surgery. This included the preparation of the operative site, enema, tub bath, weighing the patient and giving the prescribed medications. . . .

On the morning of the operation, the writer gave the preoperative medications and antibiotics and dressed the patient for surgery. . . .

Patient B, under the care of the anesthetist, received oxygen by mask inhalation during the period of transfer from surgery. . . .

Patient B returned in an unconscious state, and was placed in the oxygen tent. Her face was extremely pale and edematous, lips cyanotic, respirations shallow and irregular. Her extremities appeared mottled and limp, and nail beds cyanotic. . . .

Because of continued cyanosis of the patient and insufficient concentration in the tent, oxygen by mask inhalation was restarted. . . .

Continuous and constant watch for any sudden change in the condition of the patient was maintained during this immediate postoperative period. One hour after return from surgery there was some response noted as the patient began to move her head and eyelids. . . .

Early on the 1st postoperative night Patient B was very restless and complained of pain in the operative area. She was given Demerol, 20 mg./H., and rested fairly well between positioning, breathing and coughing exercises every 45 minutes. . . .

On the morning of the 9th postoperative day, Patient B complained of discomfort after breakfast; she "just didn't feel good." When the writer visited she noticed that the patient appeared extremely pale. . . . The resident and the surgeon were notified of the change in the condition. . . . One hour later the apical rate decreased to 148 and respirations increased to 44. She appeared anxious and troubled by the bounding heart beats—"feeling the heart beat in my throat". . . .

This is the case-study approach. It may have been nursing's mode of entry into research. The case study is a means of probing without excessive reliance upon instruments. The expert nurse practitioner, a keen observer, presents a running interpretative account of the crucial elements. It is a continuous rather than a static study. It is an attempt to depict the patient's reactions to several factors operating simultaneously in the nursing environment. The single patient is examined over an extensive period of time so that a wide sampling of events can be observed. The person is held constant while the internal and external events about him are permitted to vary.

Nursing Environment

From Patient Care to Research

While this clinical approach is tailored to patient care, it leaves much to be desired for the researcher. Her primary concern is not the patient, but the acquisition of knowledge. These nurse observations are to be employed in research for testing purposes. They are to be gathered in strict compliance with the conditions of the test, which may conflict with those required for the administration of patient care.

The usefulness of the case-study approach is also a deterrent feature for research. In order to secure a more complete picture of the events happening, the observer is permitted wide latitudes. She generally is not confined by the specifications of recording materials. The ability to develop precise and reliable measures of any single event is sacrificed as a consequence.

The approach is observer-bound. It is a reflection of the experiences, the training and the perceptiveness of the expert practitioner. However, what one expert sees may be very different from what another expert experiences. Even her interpretations of the same person's reactions at different points of time may vary.

The case study is an uncontrolled approach. The researcher cannot truly isolate the effects of the individual environmental factors upon the person. Even the role of the observer cannot be controlled.

This poses a peculiar problem for the nurse-researcher-observer. The research-observer role is quite distinct from the nurse-observer role. While the nurse is required to act when the situation becomes unfavorable for the patient, the researcher is expected merely to describe and not effect changes herself. But the initial orientation of the nurse as a nurse may not allow her to complete the transition to the research role.

The desire or the need to participate may arise and result in a conflict. Two nurse researchers described their feelings in this regard:

> . . . resolution of the conflict was not easily implemented, particularly since full commitment to the research role seemed to necessitate relinquishment of the nurse role; neither observer was willing to make this "sacrifice." In reality they did not relinquish their nurse role. When faced with conflict, they tended to act as nurses, not research observers.[14]

The Research-Centered Approach

The newest generation of researchers in nursing has been knowledge- rather than task-oriented. While the task-oriented person is concerned with the care of patient present, the knowledge-oriented researcher primarily desires to assist patient future. The nurse on the job will use all her resources to enable the patient to progress. On the other hand, the researcher may employ this patient to develop additional resources for the care of other patients. She wishes to effect progress only under certain conditions and is willing to tolerate the lack of progress under other circumstances. Her primary assignment is to acknowledge the combination of events—that certain conditions lead to patient progress and other conditions lead to a lack of patient progress.

The shift in orientation was not merely a change in objectives. It also signified the need for a change in technic. In particular, the observational skills of the nurse clinicians were found to be deficient for research purposes. The researcher wanted to pinpoint relationships. She desired more objective and lasting assurances. She needed precise measures. Thus, the advent of research-oriented persons into this aspect of the nursing program was accompanied by a movement toward instrumentation. Many of their studies involved an instrument-development phase. Many projects were initiated for the sole purpose of constructing instruments.

The movement has progressed slowly. The acquisition of reliable and valid measures has been an arduous development. Some of the problems to be encountered will be illustrated in a review of two related studies that were discussed in Chapter 6.* The specific illustrations represent the instrument-development phases of these investigations.

Each study attempted to determine the relationship between the size of the nursing staff and the effectiveness of the care. They asked essentially the same questions: What is nursing effectiveness? and How can it be measured? The first is a question of validity. It deals with a search for criteria. The second question is a problem of quantification or scaling. It considers how effective the nursing care actually had been.

The determination of "what is nursing effectiveness?" apparently was influenced by the study design. Each project approached the subject matter differently. It would seem that the instruments were developed primarily as a function of the data-collection process.

The researchers of one study decided that nursing effectiveness could and should be measured in terms of what happened to patients.[15] They hypothesized specifically that an increase in the size of the ward nursing staff will improve patient welfare. In order to test this hypothesis, they concentrated upon a single nursing situation in which the size of the ward staff was varied. Thus, the study was designed to secure detailed information of a limited number of subjects as conditions in the nursing situation were altered. Instruments were to be developed to obtain daily observations of patient welfare made by nurses and physicians.

The question remained of what specifically was to be observed as indicative of patient welfare. A large number of meanings could be attached to patient welfare. The researchers limited the scope to include only objective measures. They stipulated that the materials should consist of identifiable and obtainable items for objectivity and quantifiable items for scaling.

The major criterion was conditioned by the hypothesis—

* An Investigation of the Relation Between Nursing Activity and Patient Welfare, Nurse Utilization Project Staff, Ames, Iowa, State Univ. Iowa, 1960; Abdellah, F. G., and Levine, E.: Effect of Nurse Staffing on Satisfactions With Nursing Care, Chicago, American Hospital Assn., 1958.

patient welfare should be expressed in terms of what could happen to a hospitalized person when the ward nursing staff had been increased.[16] The researchers reasoned that patients would be affected in one of four ways.* The action should lead to a change in "mental attitude," "physical independence," "mobility," and "skin condition." Each category was refined to include a set of adjectives or descriptive statements characteristic of the different conditions. The statements were selected and later screened by juries of experts including nurses and a psychologist.

The other study was designed as a large-scale survey.[17] It was developed to secure information from several nursing situations that varied in staff size. Although a much larger sample of subjects participated, more limited information was obtained. The researchers could not elicit the kind of detail about patients that was acquired by the first group of researchers.

A major research problem was to construct an instrument to facilitate data collection.[18] How could measures of something as complex as nursing effectiveness be obtained without making specific and detailed observations? The investigators decided that this information could be inferred from the feelings or the reactions of people who had been involved directly or indirectly in the care process. It was to consist of expressions from patients who received care, from nurses who administered care, and from other personnel, such as doctors and administrators, who observed care being administered. Nursing effectiveness was described, therefore, in terms of patient and personnel satisfaction with nursing care.

The respondents actually reacted to a series of prepared statements that supposedly described the nursing situation. This procedure furthered data collection. The statements composed a check list of items to which the participants were either to agree or to fail to agree.

Nursing effectiveness was more realistically synonymous with

*Seven scaled measures in all were used. The three measures not discussed in this chapter are special aspects of physical independence, patient's opinion of nursing care given him, and physician's evaluation of patient's condition and progress.

the check list of items and in part with the procedure for constructing the check list. A series of efforts culminated in the final forms. A sample of patients and one of nursing and medical personnel initially were requested to record and submit a list of observations that typified either satisfactory or unsatisfactory nursing care. The responses were categorized later into classifications of similar observations and reduced to two 100-item check lists (one each for patients and personnel). The forms were tried out in two groups of hospitals, and additional screening of items took place. The final check lists evolved contained the 50 items that were reported most frequently and/or ranked highest in importance.

At the conclusion of this initial effort of instrument development, the researchers of each study developed a series of definitions to conform with the requirements of their respective studies. The definitions, in turn, were qualified by and composed of a set of items or descriptive statements. The next step in the instrument-development process was to transcribe the descriptive accounts into a table or a scale of values. A set of scores was required for "mental attitude," "physical independence," "mobility," "skin condition" and "patient and/or personnel satisfaction." A change in nursing effectiveness would then imply a change in one or more of these scores.

The components of patient welfare were organized into rating scales. The observers or raters were requested to respond to each item of the scale by checking one of a group of alternatives most descriptive or characteristic of the patient. The alternatives were arranged in a graduated series and were assigned values or weight by panels of nurse experts.

Bathing, for example, was considered as one index of physical independence.[19] It was divided into a 6-point scale, ranging from complete independence to dependence:

(6) Bathes without help in the bathroom.
(5) Bathes without help in bed or at bedside.
(4) Bathes with help in bathroom.
(3) Partial bath in bed or at bedside by self.
(2) Bathes only face and/or hands.
(1) Needs complete bed bath.

The bathing behavior of the patient was depicted by its position on the scale.

The rating scales were of different sizes. The "mental attitude" scale consisted of 17 dichotomous items that were or were not characteristic of the patient.[20] Weights—from (5) "best mental attitude" to (1) "worst mental attitude"—were assigned to each item. The following is an example of the variations of behavorial traits and values:

DESCRIPTION OF PATIENT	CHARACTERISTIC	NOT CHARACTERISTIC
Co-operative	(5)	(3)
Agreeable	(4)	(3)
Irritable	(2)	(3)
Quarrelsome	(1)	(3)

"Mobility" was described by a simple 16-point rating scale, ranging from "absolute bed rest" to "up *ad lib.* most of the day." "A skin condition" weight was determined from a combination of observations in which skin lesions were rated for seriousness, size and number.

Scores were developed for the various components by totaling the item weights. For example, three items—bathing, nutrition and elimination—made up the "physical independence" scale. A "physical independence" score was secured by simply adding the values obtained for each trait.

The check lists of the second study had a format similar to the "mental attitude" scale.[21] The 50 items of each check list were arranged as dichotomies, e.g., they either happened or failed to happen. The items were also weighted on a 5-point scale of importance. The following is a representative sampling of the *patient* check list items:

ITEMS	WEIGHTS
No answer to call for a nurse for a long time	(5)
Bed was not changed when needed	(4)
Room in general was not made neat and orderly	(3)
Bed was not made right	(2)
Food trays left in front of me too long	(1)

A system of weights was developed also by expert judgment. A group of 40 patients and 57 personnel in two general hospitals participated. The procedure was somewhat more sophisticated. The researchers reasoned beforehand that, if each of 50 items was sorted repetitively into one of five piles of importance, the following distribution would tend to recur:[22]

RANKING	NUMBER OF ITEMS
Most important (5)	3
Very important (4)	12
Important (3)	20
Less important (2)	12
Least important (1)	3

The participants sorted the items in accordance with this distribution. The sortings were averaged and a weight was assigned to each item.

Satisfaction scores were derived by summing the weighted responses to each item. The total score on the check list could vary from zero to 150. A low score indicated that nursing care was adequate or effective, while a high score inferred feelings of inadequacy.

The preceding examples are good illustrations of the current stage of instrumentation in nursing research. By future standards, they probably will be classified as little more than crude efforts. As objective measures, the devices are not too far in advance of the case study materials. The criteria still comprise the judgments of experts; however, they represent the pooled judgments of many observers rather than the single observation of the case study. They do not reflect the ultimate criterion: the effect upon the patient need itself.

But these are also pioneering efforts and should be judged by present standards in this respect. They are indicative of several different approaches to the advancement of research in this area: the idea of concentrating upon a limited number of observations; the idea of standardizing and simplifying the observational procedures; the idea of obtaining quantifiable measures or more exacting descriptions. They are among the first steps taken. Advances may accompany them. The main body of nursing research probably will lag behind.

REFERENCES

1. Lorge, Irving: The fundamental nature of measurement *in* Lindquist, E. F. (ed.): Educational Measurement, pp. 533-559, Washington, D. C., American Council on Education, 1951.
2. *Ibid.*, p. 537.
3. Cureton, E. E.: Validity *in* Lindquist, E. F. (ed.): Educational Measurement, p. 621, Washington, D. C., American Council on Education, 1951.
4. *Ibid.*, p. 622.
5. *Ibid.*
6. Meyer, Burton: An analysis of the results of pre-nursing and guidance, achievement, and state board test pool examinations, Nurs. Outlook 7:538, 1959.
7. *Ibid.*
8. Thorndike, R. L.: Reliability *in* Lindquist, E. F. (ed.): Educational Measurement, p. 567, Washington, D. C., American Council on Education, 1951.
9. *Ibid.*, pp. 567-570.
10. *Ibid.*, p. 563.
11. Lindquist, E. F.: Preliminary considerations in objective test construction *in* Lindquist, E. F. (ed.): Educational Measurement, pp. 141-145, Washington, D. C., American Council on Education, 1951.
12. *Ibid.*, pp. 145-151.
13. Wierzbicki, Sister Mary Michael: Descriptive Analysis of the Nursing Care of Two Selected Cardiac Surgical Patients, Master's Dissertation, Washington, D. C., The Catholic Univ. America, 1957. (Unpublished)
14. Poulas, E. S., and McCabe, G. S.: The nurse in the role of the research observer, Nurs. Res. 9:137-140, 1960.
15. An Investigation of the Relation Between Nursing Activity and Patient Welfare, Nurse Utilization Project Staff, Ames, Iowa, State Univ. Iowa, 1960.
16. *Ibid.*, p. 2.
17. Abdellah, F. G., and Levine, E.: Effect of Nurse Staffing on Satisfactions With Nursing Care, Chicago, American Hosp. Assn., 1958.
18. ———: Developing a measure of patient and personnel satisfaction with nursing care, Nurs. Res. 5:100-108, 1957.
19. *Op. cit.* (see Ref. 15), p. 72.
20. *Ibid.*, p. 66.
21. Abdellah, F. G., and Levine, E.: *Op. cit.* (see Ref. 17), pp. 57-58.
22. ———: *Op. cit.* (see Ref. 18), p. 105.

CHAPTER 9

The Method

INTRODUCTION

Planning is the key to success in research. An investigation is not merely a fishing expedition, a blind search for the unexpected, or an excursion into a grab bag of surprises. It is a thoughtful and well-prepared endeavor to establish certain truths.

The implication is that the researcher must know what he is doing. When he derived his purpose, he recognized the need for additional knowledge. When he stated his problem, he pinpointed the difficulty. When he formulated his hypothesis, he thought he knew the answer. When he designed the procedure, he stipulated the conditions under which his hypothesis was to be verified. Each aspect of the research process contributed to the preparatory activities.

But what of the subjects and the materials—how are they to be used? This, too, must be planned. The subjects are to be cast into a situation that employs the materials in the context of the design. This portion of the procedure should be stated carefully and explicitly. It is part of the method of the procedure.

The method is a detailed accounting of what is to be done. It will be discussed in two parts. First, the question of where and how the pertinent information is to be secured will be considered. This matter refers to the method for collecting information. Second, consideration will be given to the problem of analysis. That is, we will explore what can be done with the materials that are gathered. The method of analysis will examine how the information is to be used to foster the decision that the hypothesis has or has not been formulated properly.

In point of sequence, it is probable that the development of methodology precedes the selection of subjects and materials. The researcher may decide first upon an approach to data collection and analysis and then determine the requirements for subjects and materials within this framework. In terms of reporting, it is also the culmination of the other activities. In this respect, the method laces together and summarizes the various entities in order to make a composite procedure possible.

THE METHOD FOR COLLECTING INFORMATION

There are usually many ways to collect information to test specific hypotheses. Studies on learning and motivation, for example, have been conducted by observing rats running a maze, pigeons playing Ping-pong, children in a classroom and workers in an industrial plant. Information may be gathered from each of the different situations to test the same hypothesis.

Upon what basis does the researcher select a method? In effect, each study will require its own methodology. Therefore, he does not really select but, instead, constructs a method to conform with the needs of the project. For discussion purposes, the individual plans can be grouped under more general approaches. Furthermore, certain conditions will influence the researcher to follow one mode of approach rather than another. These conditions will be discussed and related to three general approaches to data collection: the survey, the experiment and the demonstration.

CONDITIONS INFLUENCING METHODOLOGY

Several factors may persuade a researcher to adopt a particular approach. In many respects, these conditions are similar to those discussed in previous chapters, particularly in the selection of subjects and materials. However, the selection of subjects and materials is an inextricable part of the method. It is difficult to discuss one without the other. While the discussions to follow will be treated in a somewhat different context, they should serve to complement our previous thoughts on the matter.

The Problem Situation

The problem has been presented as an abstraction. It was depicted as a verbal picture descriptive of a composite series of common difficulties. The hypothesis was presented as the logical solution to this abstract situation. But it was argued also that solutions stated in abstraction may not exist in concrete reality. So it was proposed further that the problem should be perceived realistically to determine the actual workability of the hypothesis.

Consider what has been done. There has been a verbal series of transitions from the concrete to the abstract and back to the concrete again.

It began when the researcher observed a change in the behavior of a patient who had not been able to get out of bed for several days. And he noted that another patient, in somewhat similar circumstances, reacted as the first one did. "Is this a typical pattern?" the researcher inquired, as he conceived the more general difficulty. And the specific problems were reformulated in terms of what happens to people who are confined for given intervals of time. (It may be questioned whether or not being unable to get out of bed and being confined connote the same sequence of events.) The researcher concluded that people will become irritable under these circumstances. And how can he ascertain that this is true? He must reinterpret the problem in the specific sense and either return to the original patient situation or observe other patient situations or other situations of confinement. (It may be questioned whether or not being confined connotes any one of the specific situations selected for the test.)

The transition from the problem statement to the specific test situation is the problem of method. The researcher must proceed from the abstract to the specific and from the logical to the real or the empiric. Reality implies that the specific situation matches the true meaning of the abstract problem statement. Thus, a rule or a condition for selecting a general methodological approach may be formulated: *The more closely the specific situation approximates the conditions stated in the problem, the more valid is the test.*

This condition suggests that specific situations may vary in their relevance to the problem statement. Some will be related directly and others will not be. The reader will observe later that the various approaches to methodology will yield specific test situations that vary in relevancy. Each will be evaluated in accordance with this rule.

Control

The problem of control has been mentioned repeatedly in the various discussions on procedure. Briefly, it concerns the ability to observe a relationship between the explanatory variables under study, independently of any extraneous variables. The medium for maintaining control is an inherent quality of any planned methodology.

Control hinges on the capability of the researcher to minimize the number of variables in the test situation. This task pertains to both explanatory and extraneous variables. In this regard, we will suggest that a researcher can attempt too much in a single study.

Specific problem situations invariably consist of many events transpiring concurrently. So it may seem expedient to the researcher, particularly to the practical researcher, to investigate the total situation. This is a quality of general problem-solving activities: to perform a thorough and comprehensive examination.

Is this approach truly expedient for research purposes? Suppose a researcher is confronted with a multivariate patient situation. He has a variety of patients who are given a variety of nursing services and who have been confined to bed for a varying number of days. Can he actually determine the effects of each condition upon the patient's behavior simultaneously?

He cannot. The patient's behavior may result from any one or all or none of the explanatory conditions. The researcher will not be able to ascertain the relationship between any pair of variables until each pair can be separated and treated independently.

We can study the relationship between only two events at a time. All other events are to be treated as extraneous variables. We have learned from the previous discussions of design and sampling procedures that control difficulties will increase as the number of variables increases. Thus, another general condition influencing the approach to methodology may be stated: *The more completely the specific situation is devoid of extraneous elements, the more valid is the test.*

Applicability

The applied researcher often is impelled by the needs of practical situations. His problems may emanate from on-the-job occurrences. These are the recurrent difficulties that are experienced by a number of practitioners. He may visualize and study their problems at the common problem level. But he must return eventually to his clientele, the practitioners, with the answers to their specific problems.

The point of application rather than the problem statement may be the important determinant for this researcher. Therefore, he may seek to test his hypothesis in the practical situations that originally instigated the investigation. His feeling may be that if it works there that is all that he needs to know.

This form of procedure is once again a reflection of the investigator's point of view regarding research, its purpose and its practices. It becomes a function of whether the researcher is knowledge-centered or problem-centered. If applicability is paramount, then control may be sacrificed. However, the specification of a definitive relationship may not be critical to some researchers as long as the solution works.

Availability

It is entirely possible that the researcher may develop exact specifications for the test in the absence of suitable situations.

That is, he may not be able to fit what is specified to what is available. In the practical sense, he must either wait or use whatever else is available. This is an unfortunate compromise with reality that the researcher often has to make. It may be another limitation of the test.

THE THREE GENERAL APPROACHES

We will attempt to discuss methodology under the three general approaches already mentioned (survey, experiment and demonstration). Each approach symbolizes the means by which the researcher gathers evidence to support his thoughts. They are reflections of the varying influences of the conditions just considered. They differ in effectiveness.

The three approaches may be said also to represent stages in the advancement of knowledge. One is more primitive and typifies the incomplete transition from general to research problem-solving. Another exemplifies the researcher's control over the test environment. The third approach links practice to research.

The Survey Approach

It has been intimated that man does not necessarily provide unique answers to all questions. Many of his problems already have been solved. The solutions exist in the world before us. They remain to be discovered.

The survey approach represents a means to discovery. It is an exploration of the world at large. The researcher observes things happening as they ordinarily do. He does not interpose his own devices to produce extraordinary change.

However, we have asked where in the vast world he centers his attention. And it was suggested that he plans his discoveries in advance. The field of inquiry is narrowed considerably to a workable problem, and he hypothesizes beforehand what he will find. Then he surveys situations in that part of the world that is most similar to the locale of his problem and compares solutions. He will determine the number of times the solutions at large are in agreement with the hypothesis.

The researcher seeks to discover what happens to people when they are confined. And he hypothesizes that a period of confinement may lead to irritable behavior. Any number of situations of confinement could be surveyed to verify his hypothesis. He may observe confinement in the home or in an institution, such as a hospital or a prison. He will be highly selective, however, and survey only those situations reflecting upon his hypothesis and, if possible, nothing else.

The survey is, therefore, a planned sequence of discoveries. It does not imply random observation in the sense that the observer chances upon situations. Instead, he attempts to control his discoveries by deliberately selecting only those situations that relate to the conditions of his test. The survey is planned so that it will conform as nearly as possible to the study's design.

The survey is an examination of what is or has been. The researcher may obtain his information from ongoing situations. For example, he can determine what happens to people who are about to be confined for a given period of time. On the other hand, it may be more feasible to inquire about what has already happened. In this respect he surveys past events.

The subjects selected for the survey are normally those who come with the situation. The researcher accepts the total package: subjects and situation. They are not selected independently. He may choose subjects because they are within a situation, e.g., patients who are confined to bed for X days. He also may elect to observe only those situations that include certain types of subjects, e.g., hospital wards containing male medical patients.

The materials that are employed will depend upon the nature of the survey. Observational forms or records are required for ongoing surveys. The researcher must describe the events just as they occur. Surveys of past events, however, feed upon the memories of the participants. For example, the researcher may ask patients who have already been confined for X days to recall how they felt or behaved as a consequence. Interview or questionnaire materials may be employed for this purpose.

The reader might reflect upon this discussion of present and past surveys and the observation, the interview and the questionnaire technics of approach, and consider what might happen. As the surveyor goes from the present to the past and from the observation to the interview and then to the questionnaire, his ability to control the data-collection process is diminished. It is probable that the different situations will vary in conformity to the problem statement in the order named. When he can observe an ongoing situation, he can determine whether or not the observation fits the requirements of the problem. When he interviews some one in regard to past observations, his information is secondhand, but at least he can inquire about specifics. When he acquires his information by questionnaire only, he usually must accept what the respondent has to say; he has little opportunity to verify the information.

In general, any survey is difficult to control. Whatever control can be developed is exercised through selection. However, it is highly unlikely that the researcher will be able to choose exact matches or pairings.

On the other hand, perhaps the survey situation can be closest to the point of application. The situation is not created artificially to satisfy the requirements of the researcher. It is realistic in the sense that it actually has occurred or will occur. It could be the point of application itself.

The survey approach to data collection may offer more readily available access to bulk information. It is a fact-collecting mechanism for depicting essentially what is or has been. However, it also may provide a crude and rather primitive testing device. The various conditions of a test can seldom be satisfied in a general exploration of the world at large.

The survey approach may be useful during the early exploratory stages of research. It may feed the descriptive cycle at a time when the coffers of knowledge are bare. The fruits of the survey may stimulate the thought processes of the researcher and enable him to formulate more hypotheses. But when the time comes to establish more exact relationships and to separate the truth from the bulk, this methodology may be found lacking. It should not be employed as the final test.

The Experimental Approach

If the researcher is not satisfied with the conditions that the world at large presents to him, then possibly he may erect his own world on his own terms. That is, he may reconstruct the model according to the paper specifications, employing real subjects in a real situation, and determine what happens.

This approach has been called the experimental method. Perhaps it has been designated as such because the researcher experiments with the world. He does not, as in the survey, simply describe what he sees. He interposes his own conditions and makes the changes demanded by his hypothesis. In other words, the researcher has the opportunity to do something differently.

It also has been termed the laboratory or the controlled method. The researcher finds an appropriate setting and evacuates the existing contents. In a sense, he filters the situation of extraneous matter and creates a vacuum devoid of the irrelevant. And, into this purified world, he may introduce and test the relationship between the explanatory variables.

Let the reader picture a bare room with four blank walls and a bed. A patient with certain well-defined characteristics is placed in this bed. He is requested to remain in the bed for a specified period of time, during which he is given certain select services. His reactions are observed throughout the period. At the conclusion of the test interval, he is replaced by another patient with the same well-defined characteristics. The second patient receives similar services but is required to remain in bed for a somewhat longer period. And this patient, in turn, is replaced by another patient, and that one by another. On each occasion the treatment remains the same, but the interval of confinement to bed is lengthened.

In the experimental setting, each entity may be selected independently to conform with its own specific requirements. Thus, the researcher does not need to accept the situation in order to obtain the particular subjects, or the subjects because they happen to be in the situation. Instead, a setting may be established to match the problem situation. Subjects are chosen from a defined universe in accordance with appropriate sampling procedures. Then the plan may prescribe that the one will be introduced into the other.

Since the experimental approach is an active process, i.e., the situation is ongoing, observational technics usually are employed. The researcher will use materials that clearly describe what happens. In addition, he may be interested in securing measures of change. He may desire to determine the degree to which the subjects react or fail to react as a function of the conditions that have been introduced into the setting.

If the optimal requirements of the experiment can be satisfied, then the researcher may effect a model test. It will be designed to conform to the problem statement. It will reduce the extraneous variables to a minimum and exercise some measure of control over the remainder. It may be considered that the experimental method is an example of how the researcher can manipulate the test to satisfy the study's needs.

However, model experiments seldom are effected. There are very few vacuums available to the researcher in this world. There are very few situations that the researcher can create to his exact specifications. While the illustration may serve as a model example, it is also hypothetic and unlikely to occur as stated.

Instead, the experimenter must compromise with the world. He will either accept what is available or wait for something better to come along. Rather than experiment with people, who have innumerable characteristics, he may study animals. Rather than work with adults who may question or resist the kind of treatment that is to be interjected, he may resort to available groups of children.

This discussion leads to a second objectionable quality of the experimental approach, its artificiality. The experiment tends to depart more radically from the point of application. Practitioners are apt to remark that they do not work in a vacuum or that what happens to rats may not be applicable to patients. So the results of the experiment may not be exactly applicable to specific situations that are uncontrollable.

Both the researcher and the practitioner are correct in this respect. However, each represents a different point of view. It is the primary purpose of the researcher to acquire knowledge or to ascertain relationships, but not to solve the problems of the practitioner. Therefore, he may establish an experiment to test his understanding of the relationship, but not to apply his conclusions. It remains for the practitioner to interpret and implement the results of the study. In some cases, they will be somewhat satisfactory; in other cases, they may be entirely useless. They never will be completely applicable.

The experimental approach represents an advanced stage in the accumulation of knowledge. It signifies man's attempt to control the test environment. It typifies his ability to do something different, to experiment with the world and to create new responses. It is most useful during the predictive and explanatory phases of research, when the researcher has solidified his thinking and has developed a fruitful network of hypotheses. It is a step closer to truth.

The Demonstration Approach

The previous discussion suggests that a paradox seems to exist between practice and research. One implements the other, yet they seem at odds. Research problems often arise from incidents on the job. And frequently the practice situation becomes the proving ground for research. But practice comprises an uncontrollable multitude of factors, while the research problem generally is restricted to the controlled manipulation of one pair of events at a time. Thus, the outcome of research, especially of the more specialized studies, may not be directly applicable to practice.

When a researcher looks at reality, what does he see? Out of myriad events, he selects and focuses upon a pair. Everything else is inconsequential—either irrelevant or an impediment to concentrated effort. He has an idea about the pair of events and seeks a mechanism to test his idea. The total situation is not important to him for its own sake; it is a means to an end. The objective is the validation of the idea. His idea states that confinement to bed for X days leads to irritable behavior. The researcher feels that the idea is logically sound, but that it cannot be tested properly if other conditions interfere. Thus, he deliberately arranges the situation so that interference will be minimized and the idea has the best possible opportunity to have a fair test. The result of his efforts may be a statement that the idea is sound when qualified, perhaps severely, by the conditions of the test. What happens to the remaining events in the situation may be ignored.

When a practitioner looks at reality, what does he see? Several things happen simultaneously; each will affect his work. He has an assignment that may involve a multitude of activities. If he concentrates upon one to the exclusion of the others, then he will fail to perform his complete assignment. His aim is to bring the total situation into harmony. The individual activities contribute toward this end. His assignment requires him to satisfy the nursing care needs of a group of patients. While the patients have common requirements, they differ sufficiently to necessitate individual care plans. The practitioner must be prepared for divergencies. He cannot dictate that conditions are to be arranged to his specifications or that they will remain constant. The researcher may suggest what will happen when certain conditions arise; but he may not relate what will happen in the event that other conditions arise. The practitioner must act under any circumstance.

When is the transition made from research to practice? Does the researcher who has acquired knowledge in a so-called purified atmosphere stop short of application? Does the practitioner who is enmeshed in the realities of the job gloss over the products of research as interesting but impractical? Who intervenes, and by what mechanism?

The demonstration is an approach linking research to practice. It represents an application of a research series. The research effort culminates in a demonstration to the practitioner of how the results may be employed in an actual situation.

The purpose of the demonstration is to make the output of research workable. That is, someone generates a model practice situation featuring the newly developed concepts. A technician or a professional worker who is familiar with the needs of the practitioner and can understand and appreciate the intent of the researcher often assumes the role of demonstrator. This person is not necessarily a researcher, although familiarity with research methodology is helpful.

The demonstration is generally a global or multifactorial approach. The technician does not merely concentrate upon one small aspect of the situation, such as demonstrating that people confined to bed for X days will become irritable. The researcher has already verified this relationship. Instead, the demonstrator may display a variety of things happening as they relate to a variety of causes. In addition, he even may intervene in the situation to produce more favorable consequences, e.g., he may permit the patient who becomes irritable to get out of bed. What is done is done in accordance with some other derived relationship.

There are many examples of demonstrations. Each year major automobile manufacturers display new models in which the principles developed in previous years have been incorporated. Drug companies may demonstrate the effectiveness of new compounds in the treatment of various ailments; surgeons reveal new operative technics; and nurses exhibit new procedures for the care of particular types of patients. When this nation sent a man into a suborbital flight beyond the earth's atmosphere, it demonstrated publicly the culmination of a large number of individual efforts. It tested the man, the capsule, the rockets and the release and descent mechanisms in their responses to actual changes in speed and atmosphere conditions. The total flight was made up of a series of independent relationships, formulated and tested beforehand under the simulated circumstances of a laboratory. The demonstration was a workable display of the relationships interacting together.

The demonstration may be viewed as a series of successive acts that culminate in the attainment of the ultimate objective:[1]

1. Suited-up and carrying a portable air-conditioner to cool the inside of the sealed pressure suit, the astronaut left his quarters and entered a van which took him to the missile gantry.

2. The astronaut walked to the gantry elevator which lifted him to

the launching platform. Technicians assisted him through a hatch into the capsule situated on top of the Redstone rocket. The astronaut was strapped onto a contour couch and connected to a multitude of wires and tubes.

3. When the count-down reached T-minus 30 seconds, the cord through which electricity and liquid oxygen had been supplied was disconnected. At the last count, the rocket's engine was ignited and the capsule was in flight.

4. Two and a-half minutes later the Redstone's power was cut off and the capsule was separated from the rocket.

5. As the rocket climbed through space, the capsule was automatically controlled; the astronaut later maneuvered the capsule and performed other operations. (During this time he experienced 5 minutes of weightlessness.)

6. The retro-rockets were fired.

7. The retro-package was discarded and the astronaut maneuvered the capsule for re-entry from space. The periscope was retracted and the capsule entered the atmosphere.

8. The capsule descended, whirling on its chute (which opened in flight), down to the water, where the helicopters waited to approach it.

9. The capsule was steadied as the astronaut was lifted to a helicopter which took him to the carrier Lake Champlain.

Each act can be considered as a separate test, requiring distinct subjects and measures. In some instances in the above example the rocket is the source of the test; in other instances, the man becomes the vehicle for study; and, more often, the same subjects will appear in different phases of the total demonstration.

The demonstration has features in common with both the survey and the experiment. In dealing with the actual situation rather than laboratory artificialities, it is similar to the survey. However, this approach is also a living series of acts concocted by the demonstrator with definite controls and periodic tests. The subjects and the materials may be selected with deliberation, apart from the situation. These are qualities of the experiment.

In other respects, the demonstration may be considered as a distinct entity. It is a multivariable approach in which all the factors are treated as explanatory variables and are permitted to interact. Anything that impinges upon the final outcome cannot be regarded as extraneous to the study. Thus, the kinds of controls necessary for the establishment of clear-cut relationships may be lacking. But the demonstration is also an application, and it may be assumed that the clear-cut relationships had been established beforehand in controlled settings.

Because of these features, the reader may question that the demonstration is a research procedure. And it may not be, if some of the attributes already discussed are considered. However, the approach may be part of the research process that has not been discussed. It may comprise the implementation step: the necessary link between knowledge and practice.

COLLECTING INFORMATION IN NURSING RESEARCH

There has been a history in nursing research of the utilization of the various approaches to the collection of information. A pattern can be traced that conforms to the nature of nursing, its practitioners and the requirements for knowledge. It reveals that some approaches have been used more extensively than others; they seem to comply more readily with the established pattern.

The orientation that has predominated in research in nursing has been directed toward the requirements of practice rather than toward the resources of knowledge. The problems of the practitioners became the problems of research. And it was often the practitioner who was the researcher.

Many of the early studies reflect this pattern. They consist primarily of demonstrations of how specific nursing problems could be solved by nurses. In a sense, it was like the merchant displaying his wares. In this case, it was the nurse or the nurse consultant offering another technic for effecting care.

Hypodermic Technics That Save Time[2]

This report detailed a time-saving and safe method for sterilizing hypodermic syringes and needles and administering hypodermics. Three wooden blocks were employed as equipment. There was a block for used and one for unused materials; the third block was set aside for narcotics.

The following procedure was suggested:[3]

Read order.

Wash hands.

Remove block, containing narcotics, from locked cupboard to medicine cupboard.

Remove vial containing desired drug from block; drop tablet from vial to lid, leaving lid directly in front of open vial.

With forceps, remove two alcohol sponges. . . .

Sponge off rubber stopper of sterile distilled bottle. . . .

Remove hypodermic syringe from container; attach needle. . . .

Place syringe container in block for used syringes. . . .

Separate syringe, holding barrel between thumb and index finger. . . .

Cleanse site of injection with alcohol, sponging outward. . . .

Grasp flesh with thumb and forefinger of one hand; insert needle. . . .

After all seven syringes have been used, the used syringe block is taken to the central-supply room and exchanged for one with sterile syringes. . . .

An average time of 1 minute was required for the procedure.

Simplified Breast Care[4]

A plastic nipple shield resulted from a series of attempts at the Minnesota General Hospital to simplify the nursing procedure in breast care of the postpartum patient. A technic for applying the shield was developed that reduced the nurse's time from 30 to 5 minutes.

Before each breast feeding, the mother is given two cotton balls saturated with alcohol or Zephiran Chloride for cleansing the inside of the shield. The shield is removed, cleansed, and set clean side up on the bedside table when the baby is brought for a feeding. The shield is reapplied and the breast support pinned after nursing. Ointment is not used, nor are the nipples cleansed before or after nursing.[5]

The above examples were practice-oriented projects. They were presentations of technics to solve nursing problems. The critical element of the test to control and limit the number of factors and to define exact relationships was essentially absent. Instead, each technic encompassed a number and a variety of steps that contributed to the final solution. The reports seemed to say "see how it works."

Nevertheless, demonstration still has a prominent place in nursing research. It has become a useful means to feed back information from research to practice. Newly discovered relationships that have been described in the annals of nursing research as well as discoveries in other fields of endeavor are introduced to the practitioner in this way. The concepts are translated into nursing procedures and offered as another mode of practice.

Handwashing—An Important Part of Medical Asepsis[6]

This is a report of a handwashing technic that was developed to conform with bacteriologic, physical and psychological principles. It consisted basically of a 1-to-2-minute handwashing with a liquid nonalkaline detergent containing hexachloraphene. The task was to be performed without a brush, utilizing only the principles of mechanical motion, friction and rinsing. The following instructions were given:

The nurse should use good body mechanics so that she assumes a position at the sink which can use foot pedal controls comfortably, bend so that her uniform does not touch the sink rim, and wash so that the water and suds fall into the bowl.[7]

Detailed directions for the actual washing procedure are provided.

Unity of Nursing Care: A Report of a Project To Study the Integration of Social Science and Psychiatric Concepts in Nursing Education[8]

Purpose:

1. To identify mental health concepts from the social sciences and psychiatry that are relevant to nurse-patient relationships.

2. To demonstrate how the concepts can be employed to foster a better understanding of nurse-patient relationships.

Procedure:

1. A team of experts identified concepts as a result of extensive observations of class and clinical instruction and student behavior in hospital wards.

2. An experimental teaching program consisting of lectures, discussion and concurrent clinical experience was established to integrate understanding of the concepts. An experimental group of 20 students participated in the program. A matched control group of 20 students took an elective course during the same period of time. The groups were observed, evaluated and compared.

Conclusions:

1. The project staff and the faculty felt that they had achieved their purpose. They learned more about the relevance of social science and psychiatric concepts to nursing. They became aware of the procedures implementing the concepts in a teaching situation.

2. The students felt that they had obtained a broader concept of the nursing role.

3. The patients seemed to appreciate and accept the changes in student behavior and understanding as they progressed through the experimental program.

The drive for information after World War II forced considerable reliance upon the survey technic. It may be reasoned that the most accessible means to replenish the stockpiles of knowledge is to examine what is or what has been. The answers to some of the problems on staffing, for example, can be obtained readily by investigating the past and the present approaches to staffing.

A Survey of the Social and Occupational Characteristics of a Metropolitan Nurse Complement[9]

The purpose of this survey was to describe the nurse complement in a selected metropolitan area. This included the number of graduate nurses, their social and personal characteristics, where they worked, what they did with their time, what their occupational characteristics were, how the nurses differed from one another, and lastly, what graduate nurses believed to be some of the major issues confronting professional nursing today.

Questionnaires were mailed to 3,809 graduate nurses, both active and inactive. A total of 2,441 graduate nurses responded and were included in the tabulation of results. The data were analyzed under the following categories:

1. *Personal and family characteristics:* sex, age, place of birth, marital status, religious affiliation, off-duty activities, sibling status, ethnic group, socioeconomic status and occupation of parents.

2. *Occupational characteristics:* labor-force status according to income, hospital employment, type of position, job mobility, fields of nursing and membership in professional nursing clubs and organizations.

3. *Educational characteristics:* high school, type of nursing school, and postgraduate education.

The study concluded by suggesting that: There are many kinds of nurses, who differ from each other both in terms of their occupational and their social characteristics . . . the kind of training they have had, the setting they work in, and, most important, the field of nursing in which they practice. It is almost possible to conceive of private-duty, office-nursing, public health, general-duty, industry, and the other fields as different occupations.[10]

Change and Dilemma in the Nursing Profession. Part II. Studies of a Premature Center[11]

A survey was made of a premature center in a selected medical center to ascertain the role of the nurse. A variety of technics and materials—questionnaires, interviews, tests, observation schedules and check lists, tape recordings and verbal job descriptions—were employed to collect data.

Two sources of descriptive information evolved from this report. One presented the physical and social setting of the premature center, which included:

1. The formal organization structure of personnel and their relationships to other units in the center and to other agencies.

2. The formal functions in the care of infants and the training of personnel.

3. The informal organization structure comprising diverse groupings of nurses, such as "old guard," "care group," "education group" and "service group."

In addition, the tensions and the conflicts arising among the formal and the informal groupings were described and compared with those in other departments of the medical center.

That the survey has been an acceptable approach can be inferred from its widespread use among the collectors of nursing data. The journals are filled with survey reports. Literally tons of information have been thrown upon the nursing public in a relatively short period of time.

But can growth be measured by volume alone? How useful are the fruits of the survey? How many principles actually have been extracted and set forth from the vast amount of information secured? How authentic are the results? Where are the hypotheses? Where are the empiric tests?

As the survey approach was adopted, the experimental approach was avoided. The nurse researcher generally has been reluctant to take the step forward. How can those who deal with people establish vigorous controls? How can a practice area be turned into a laboratory? How can we tamper with conditions of life and death? Why work so hard and wait so long to achieve so little?

Notwithstanding these comments, the experiment has been tried in nursing research. Here is an illustration:

A Comparative Study of Temperature Readings[12]

Purpose: To study the variability in readings of oral and rectal temperatures in normal test subjects.

Hypothesis: none stated.

Procedure: Ten men were subjected to five periods in which the environmental temperatures and the amount of exercise were varied. The periods were controlled to maintain average environmental temperatures of from 67 to 100.6° F. Set exercises were performed in all but one of the periods. The water intake was weighed throughout the study. Oral and rectal temperatures were taken simultaneously for 3 minutes each, three times a day, by one of the two nurses, who also prepared the thermometers and recorded the readings.

Results:

1. There was marked variation in the differences between the oral and the rectal readings.

2. Oral temperature changes did not show a close relationship to rectal temperature changes.

3. Neither the environmental temperature nor the exercise appeared to influence the degree of difference between the oral and the rectal temperatures.

Some of the studies mentioned before also can be scrutinized from this point of view.*

These were some isolated attempts made to establish more effective controls over the testing situation. Oddly enough, they were not wholly successful. In some instances, the researcher could not develop or maintain the necessary controls. In other instances, the more elaborate controls did not contribute substantially to the end-products. The results were in-

* Wilcox, Jane: Observer factors in the measurement of blood pressure, Nurs. Res. *10*:4-17, 1961; Struve, M., and Levine, E.: Disposable and reusable surgeons' gloves, Nurs. Res. *10*:79-96, 1961; Courtney, M. E.: The effectiveness of the classroom laboratory in the teaching of nursing arts, Nurs. Res. *8*:148-154, 1959; An Investigation of the Relation Between Nursing Activity and Patient Welfare, Nurse Utilization Project, Ames, Iowa, State Univ. Iowa, 1960.

conclusive or so narrowly limited by the study design as to be rendered virtually useless in practice.

Do these statements imply that the experimental approach is not suitable to research in applied areas such as nursing? Do they indicate that we cannot or should not expect to develop truly adequate tests of hypotheses and must be satisfied with the less stringent but more available returns from survey-type technics? The expected frustrations derived from experiment, as opposed to the more immediate rewards from the survey, may have persuaded many would-be nurse researchers to select the survey mode of approach.

However, it must be realized that the end-products of research are no better than the procedures employed to secure them. The authors have proposed the point of view that considers research as distinct from other forms of problem-solving; it is to derive solutions from the total process of reasoning and empiric testing. Any partial solution must be evaluated accordingly. A hypothesis, not fully tested, remains only a hypothesis and not a factual statement.

The idea of a laboratory should not signify merely an isolated corner full of test tubes. A laboratory can be regarded as a living thing: a nursing unit, a classroom or a series of homelike situations. However, the specifications for an appropriate testing sequence may necessitate the same type of mental demands upon the researcher that are required in formulating a hypothesis, designing a test or developing instruments. She may have to use her imagination to create or concoct appropriate settings to maintain the necessary controls that otherwise might be lacking in a normal situation.

The idea of a laboratory is also a frame of mind. It represents a disposition on the part of the researcher to give each piece of newly derived knowledge the full measure of treatment. She will not merely offer untested hypotheses, regardless of the support given by authoritative evidence. She will not merely be satisfied with solutions verified partially in amorphous settings. They tend only to confuse issues. She will persist until each step in problem-solving has been completed.

She will attempt to present an offering that can stand in the "teeth of irrefutable fact."

THE METHOD OF ANALYSIS

Data may be construed as descriptive materials. In the restricted sense, we refer to data as facts. More realistically, they may represent the means to identify objects, persons, situations, events or observable qualities. In essence, data are the products of the information collection process.

The objective of the procedure that includes data collection is to determine the tenability of the hypothesis. The researcher must decide whether to accept or reject his hypothesis or that there is not sufficient evidence to make a decision. The evidence consists of the data that are secured. These materials are to be examined and evaluated for decision-making purposes.

The decision-making process is not necessarily a simple one. Ideally, the researcher desires to arrive at a precise statement. At the conclusion of an observation, he would like to accept or reject the hypothesis with an unqualified "yes" or "no" answer. However, such a statement of finality is seldom attained. The researcher usually is not concerned with a single stimulus-response relationship. He must be aware also of other extraneous stimuli or responses. The researcher normally cannot make judgments from one observation. He must consider the results of many observations, of many "yes" or "no" responses.

Suppose the researcher wished to verify the "confinement to bed" hypothesis as it may be related to "irritable behavior," independently of "age." Three days of confinement was determined to be the critical point. Data were collected by a survey. The researcher selected randomly a sample of 20 male patients, stratified by age, who had been hospitalized for 2 days. The behavior of the subjects was observed and recorded during the 3rd and the 4th days of hospitalization (before and after the critical point).

As a result of this endeavor, the researcher could have accumulated data in the following form:

Prior to the observations, Patient R, a middle-aged male, had been confined to bed for 2 consecutive days. He was permitted to get up briefly during the 1st day of observation, but was confined again the next day. At first he appeared pleasant and highly co-operative. However, as time went by, he became moody and abusive.

or

Patient M was highly excited during the 2 days of observation. He refused food and medication, yet demanded constant attention from the nurses. This 43-year-old male patient had not been out of his bed for 4 consecutive days.

The examples are case studies organized about the affairs of the individual patient. But how do they assist the researcher? He has 20 such descriptive passages that literally consist of hundreds of pieces of data. They are to be compressed for decision-making into a single statement that "confinement to bed" independently of "age" does or does not lead to "irritable behavior."

Usually, the researcher cannot deal directly with the observations as they are recorded. He is required to condense the bulk information to a more comprehensive state that can be evaluated in terms of some pre-established standards. These may be treated as problems of data reduction and comparison. They will compose the method of analysis.

The reader soon may observe that the method of analysis is another essential part of the procedure. It is tied hand in hand with the method of collecting information; one without the other is not wholly useful. Analysis refers to the treatment of the information that is collected. Without analysis, the investigator merely has stockpiles of materials. Without data, there is no need for analysis.

DATA REDUCTION

Analysis may be conceived of as the continual and repetitive reduction of materials to attain a manipulative order. First, the numerous descriptions of the individual must be reduced to a small number of statements: that the patient has or has not been confined to bed for 3 days; that the patient is of a particular age level; and that the patient has or has not become irritable. Second, the various statements regarding individuals should be condensed into classifications descriptive of the independent variables: "confinement to bed" and "age." When several such groupings are formulated, they may be characterized further by the dependent variable, "irritable behavior," and compared.

Data-reduction procedures entail the processes of identification, organization and transformation. First, the analyst identifies the common properties among the materials. Then they are organized by property and transformed to a reduced set of values.

Common properties should be prescribed by the hypothesis. The researcher wishes to identify data that are common to each of the independent variables and to group the materials accordingly. For example, the researcher could select data from the case-study materials that signify the properties of "confinement to bed" and "nonconfinement to bed." He may stipulate that patients whose observational records signify confinement for 4 consecutive days should be categorized under the first heading. Any other patient would fall into the second classification.

However, materials such as case studies may be gathered in several forms. They may consist of numbers, words or some symbolic or coded referents. Age, for example, was depicted by a numerical value in one case study and a descriptive term in another. This lack of consistency can hamper identification. A systematic coding sequence to establish equivalency between the numerical and the verbal information often is a preliminary requirement.

The organization of data to bring order to some of the chaos is a second step in data reduction.

Masses of observation taken by themselves are bewildering and almost meaningless. Before we can see the forest as well as the trees, order must be given to the data.[13]

The information may be received in raw or unorganized form or in various stages of organization. Any independent array of observations, such as the case-study materials or responses to a pile of unassembled items, describes a raw form of data. Some organization occurs when the item responses are assembled in an instrument that ultimately yields a measure or a score.

Instruments incorporate many of the requisites for analysis. As record forms, they may force observers to report what is seen in a systematic and uniform manner. The categories are identified beforehand, and the observations are channeled into appropriate boxes. As measuring devices, they may require the data for the individual to be organized in a particular fashion. Any resultant score can be regarded as a transformation of items to a reduced index of the person.

Regardless of how the initial data is collected, it must be organized before analysis can start. Table 4 represents the organization of the individual materials into identifiable categories. The table assumes that instruments were employed during data collection. The assemblage of information in this fashion marks the beginning of organization. Here are fairly concise and orderly records of what happened during each observation. Each variable is represented in the same way for each subject. These records should be compared with the varied descriptive passages of the case studies.

Yet the table only tells a story of individuals, and says little about the total group. The researcher may skip from subject to subject and make cursory judgments of the group. However, a more precise approach would have reorganized the individual data further in the manner depicted in Table 5. The materials have been reassembled into four groups, characterizing the independent variables.

Observe that the bulk information has been reduced considerably. Confinement groups were organized in accordance with the criteria stipulated above. Days of confinement were transformed and reduced to one of two classifications. Two age groupings within each of the confinement groups also were developed. The procedure for transforming the age data into these categories should be obvious to the reader.

TABLE 4. THE INITIAL ORGANIZATION OF INDIVIDUAL MATERIALS INTO IDENTIFIABLE CATEGORIES

| | | DAYS OF CONFINEMENT | | OBSERVATIONS OF IRRITABLE BEHAVIOR | | | | | | | |
| | | | | BEFORE CRITICAL DAY | | | | AFTER CRITICAL DAY | | | |
PA-TIENT	AGE IN YEARS	BEFORE	AFTER	D*	A*	C*	E*	D*	A*	C*	E*
1	54	3	2	4	3	1	2	4	4	2	4
2	23	3	3	2	3	1	1	3	3	2	1
3	37	2	3	2	3	4	3	2	3	3	3
4	61	3	1	3	3	2	4	4	4	3	4
5	30	1	0	4	2	2	1	4	3	2	1
6	48	3	0	3	3	2	4	3	3	3	4
7	62	0	0	2	1	1	2	2	2	1	2
8	25	3	1	3	1	1	3	3	2	3	4
9	33	3	0	2	1	2	1	2	2	2	2
10	36	2	1	2	2	1	1	1	2	1	1
11	47	3	2	4	2	4	3	4	3	4	4
12	28	0	2	3	2	2	4	3	2	3	3
13	59	3	3	4	1	2	2	4	3	3	4
14	56	2	1	3	2	1	2	3	1	2	2
15	50	3	1	2	3	4	2	4	4	4	4
16	43	1	3	2	1	1	1	2	3	1	2
17	39	3	3	3	2	4	2	4	3	4	3
18	45	1	0	4	3	1	2	4	3	2	3
19	41	2	1	2	4	1	1	2	3	1	1
20	37	3	2	1	2	1	2	2	3	2	3

* D—Demandingness
A—Abusiveness
C—Co-operativeness (Lack of)
E—Excitability

TABLE 5. THE REORGANIZATION OF INDIVIDUAL MATERIALS BY GROUPS

| CONFINEMENT GROUP | | | | NONCONFINEMENT GROUP | | | |
| LESS THAN 45 YEARS | | 45 OR MORE YEARS | | LESS THAN 45 YEARS | | 45 OR MORE YEARS | |
BEFORE	AFTER	BEFORE	AFTER	BEFORE	AFTER	BEFORE	AFTER
7	9	10	14	12	11	12	13
8	12	12	15	9	10	6	7
11	14	13	15	6	8	8	8
6	10	9	14	6	5	10	12
		11	16	11	11		
				5	8		
				8	7		

It should be noted that a basis for comparison has emerged. Confinement for particular age groups may be compared with nonconfinement. If behavioral data is introduced, predictive criteria arise. The irritability observations, before and after the critical point, have been transformed and appear as scores.*

The organizational process for this analysis is essentially complete. But the transformation process must continue. The individual behavioral criteria must be compressed further into a small number of values descriptive of each group. This can be accomplished in several ways.

An enumeration or count is one of the simplest methods for transforming a series of individual events to a value for the group. The data are treated as discrete variables: they will either occur or fail to occur. For example, the researcher will predict a greater incidence of irritable behavior among the confinement group of subjects. In this respect, he is interested in displaying the change in behavior before and after the critical point. An increase or a gain in score may be denoted as a sign of greater irritability. Therefore, he may list the number of times a gain or no gain is recorded among the various groups. As seen in Table 6, the incidence of gain or no gain appears as descriptive of the groups.

The reader may have noted the disproportionate totals among the groups and wondered: Will the group having the

TABLE 6. A COMPARISON OF THE INCIDENCE OF GAIN IN "IRRITABILITY" AMONG GROUPS CLASSIFIED BY INDEPENDENT VARIABLES

| | CONFINEMENT GROUP | | NONCONFINEMENT GROUP | |
	LESS THAN 45 YEARS	45 OR MORE YEARS	LESS THAN 45 YEARS	45 OR MORE YEARS
Gained	4	5	3	3
Failure to Gain	0	0	4	1
Total	4	5	7	4

* A score was derived by summing the parts.

greatest number of subjects be favored? The answer, of course, is "Yes." However, the values in Table 6 can be corrected by converting the tallies to the percentages exhibited in Table 7. In this case, each group value is derived as if it were based upon a total of 100 observations.

TABLE 7. A COMPARISON OF THE PER CENT OF GAIN IN "IRRITABILITY" AMONG GROUPS CLASSIFIED BY INDEPENDENT VARIABLES

PER CENT	CONFINEMENT GROUP		NONCONFINEMENT GROUP	
	LESS THAN 45 YEARS	45 OR MORE YEARS	LESS THAN 45 YEARS	45 OR MORE YEARS
Gained	100	100	43	75
Failed to Gain	0	0	57	25
Total	100	100	100	100

When data are condensed in this fashion, the researcher may experience the feeling of having omitted vital pieces of information and even of having misrepresented the true state of affairs. This is particularly so when discrete data are employed. They often represent very limited descriptions of what actually transpired. The tallies or percentages, for example, reveal nothing about the size of the gain in irritable behavior. Thus, a patient who became highly irritable was treated equivalently with another patient who exhibited a very slight gain. Furthermore, no-gain patients were not differentiated from patients whose degree of irritability actually was diminished.

The behavior score could have been employed also as scaled or continuous measures.* In such cases, the material becomes more flexible. The analyst can deal with more of the data and, in the process of transforming individual scores to group values, provide a greater variety of descriptive information.

The criterion scores have been treated as continuous measures in Table 8. A convenient summary is furnished first,

---

* See pages 343-344 for a definition of a continuous score.

simply by adding the individual scores in each group. However, these totals also suffer the disadvantage of disproportionate numbers. It can be overcome by dividing each summation by the number of subjects in the group to produce an arithmetic average or mean.

TABLE 8. A COMPARISON OF "IRRITABILITY" SCORES AMONG
GROUPS CLASSIFIED BY THE INDEPENDENT VARIABLES

	CONFINEMENT GROUP				NONCONFINEMENT GROUP			
	LESS THAN 45 YEARS		45 OR MORE YEARS		LESS THAN 45 YEARS		45 OR MORE YEARS	
	BEFORE	AFTER	BEFORE	AFTER	BEFORE	AFTER	BEFORE	AFTER
The Sum of Scores	32	45	55	74	57	60	36	40
Number of Subjects	4	4	5	5	7	7	4	4
Mean Score	8.0	11.3	11.0	14.8	8.1	8.6	9.0	10.0
Range	5	5	4	2	7	6	6	6
Standard Deviation	2.5	2.6	1.8	.9	2.9	2.4	3.0	3.4

The mean is one of several measures of central tendency. As the name implies, the measures are used as estimates of what is most central to a group of scores. It is reasoned that what is central is also the most common property of the group. The median, another measure of central tendency, is actually the central score of a group of values that have been ranked in order. The mode, a third index, is the point or score achieved by the greatest number of subjects within a group.

Measures of central tendency are supplemented normally by measures of variability or dispersion. These values are indices of the spread of the scores within a distribution. One such measure, the range, is easily obtainable. It signifies the difference between the two extreme scores of the distribution. The most commonly used indicator of variability is the standard deviation. This measure is defined roughly as a kind of average of the numerical differences between each score of a distribution and the mean score. It is the most difficult measure to compute.

Measures of dispersion tend to complete the analytic picture of a display of reduced values. A mean score provides only a single description of the group. It relates nothing of the spread of scores. Two independent groups could have identical means of 50 but differ widely in range. The scores of one group can range from 40 to 60, while the other is spread from 10 to 90. An analyst would hesitate to describe the two groups by their mean values alone.

Comparative Analysis

The data are displayed now in manageable form. The materials have been arranged concisely and according to the conditions of the test in Tables 6 to 8. Is the researcher ready to verify his hypothesis? Upon what basis does he make a decision?

The survey was designed deliberately to provide standards for judgment. Control groups were established primarily as points of departure or bases for comparison. Consider the arrangement of Table 8. Several comparisons can be made. Confinement can be contrasted with nonconfinement, confinement for those less than 45 years old (or 45 or more years) with nonconfinement for those less than 45 years old (or 45 or more years), or the four conditions of confinement and age with one another.

For ease of discussion, the data have been compressed in Table 9, and a limited condition of comparing confinement with nonconfinement, irrespective of age, has been assumed. A mere inspection of the table would lead the researcher to support the hypothesis—larger irritability scores were recorded during the 2nd day of observation among the subjects of the confinement group.

Before a decision is made, however, we should reflect again upon the nature of the hypothesis and the conditions of the test. The hypothesis stipulates a relationship for a total population or universe. This is characteristic of knowledge. Yet

TABLE 9. A COMPARISON OF "IRRITABILITY" SCORES BETWEEN
"CONFINEMENT" AND "NONCONFINEMENT" GROUPS,
IRRESPECTIVE OF "AGE"

| | CONFINEMENT GROUP | | NONCONFINEMENT GROUP | |
	BEFORE	AFTER	BEFORE	AFTER
The Sum of Scores	87	119	93	100
Number of Subjects	9	9	11	11
Mean Score	9.7	13.2	8.5	9.1
Standard Deviation	2.5	2.5	2.7	2.6

only a small portion or sample of that population actually was observed. We must make judgments based upon the results of a limited segment of the total population: "we draw a sample in order to determine which *hypotheses* about the population are *tenable* in the light of what is learned from the sample."[14]

The technics of statistical analysis are provided to treat problems of this type. The specific application often is termed statistical inference. We infer from the sample observations about the universe and draw conclusions about the hypothesis. The discussion that follows will deal with this subject. It will be presented as an essay on the meaning, the usefulness and the limitations of statistics rather than as a discourse on statistical applications.

The descriptive denotations or scores for a universe of subjects, like any other distribution, may be spread along a continuum. A measure of that distribution, such as an arithmetic mean, is termed a parameter. It is considered to be an exact and true description of the population. It is seldom obtained.

When sampling occurs, subjects are selected from various parts of the total distribution. A measure of the sample is known as a statistic. It is an estimate of the parameter. Since the statistic can be observed or obtained, it usually is employed to represent the parameter.

The sample estimate or statistic normally can be expected

to differ or deviate from the parameter. The differences may arise solely as a result of the selection process. The subjects may be chosen purposely or accidentally to represent a limited portion or the entire distribution of the population. In random sampling, for example, where everyone has an equal opportunity to be selected, it is possible to draw subjects from the various segments only. To the extent that this occurs, the derived statistic will depart from the true measure of the universe.

The differences between a parameter and obtained statistics are known as sampling errors. A distribution of sampling errors will result when successive samples are drawn from the same universe. If an infinite number of samples are drawn randomly from an actual population, the sampling errors will be distributed along a chance continuum. This is a very important concept. It suggests the availability of an index of the probability or the chance of securing errors of various sizes by random-selection processes.

A random distribution of sampling errors is depicted in Figure 8. The height of the curve is directly indicative of the probability values. The center of the distribution is estimated to be the point of zero distribution or no error. It will have the highest probability of occurrence. The errors will increase in size as they depart on either side of the zero point, while the probability of occurrence is diminished. Thus, the researcher may reckon the probability of securing the sampling error at point X as by chance alone.

But how does this discussion relate to the problem of testing a hypothesis such as the one in the illustration? Here, dif-

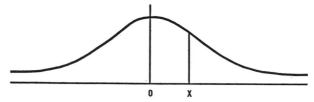

Fig. 8. A random distribution of sampling errors.

ferences between two or more groups are being compared with one another rather than with a hypothetic universe. Here, it is stated deliberately that any differences among group measures result from the presence of the explanatory variable rather than from chance selection factors.

The table of values comparing confinement with nonconfinement evolved after a series of data-reduction steps. The initial sample of 20 subjects was selected by chance from a hypothetic universe of male patients who had been hospitalized for 2 days. Theoretically, any differences between the mean irritability scores of the total sample and the universe on the 1st day of observation could be denoted as a sampling error. However, since the universe score is unknown, let us assume that it is represented by the sample value. This value is the zero point in Figure 9. For comparative purposes, the sample was split into a confinement and a nonconfinement group and two pairs of mean values were derived: one before and the other after the critical point. Each value could be depicted on the chart as an error or a deviation from the estimate of the universe. They also may be considered as departures from one another.

Several logical deductions can be made regarding the dif-

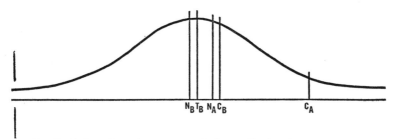

T_B—Deviation of total mean score before critical point
N_B—Deviation of nonconfinement mean score before critical point
N_A—Deviation of nonconfinement mean score after critical point
C_B—Deviation of confinement mean score before critical point
C_A—Deviation of confinement mean score after critical point

FIG. 9. Distribution of sample deviations before and after the critical day of observation.

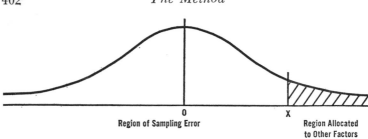

Region of Sampling Error 0 X Region Allocated to Other Factors

FIG. 10. The demarcation of the distribution of deviations.

ferences in the scores. First, let us consider the scores attained on the initial day of observation. According to the hypothesis, there is no reason to believe that the deviations represent anything other than sampling errors.* However, the hypothesis stipulates that the differences on the 2nd day of the observation may be attributed, in addition, to the presence of the explanatory variable, namely, that one group of subjects was confined to bed for 4 consecutive days.

This discussion lays out the rationale for testing a hypothesis by statistical analysis. The researcher will segment the distribution of deviations beforehand into two regions demarcated by probability values (Fig. 10). Any derived differences lying within the probability values may be attributed to sampling or to chance. All other differences can be allocated to other factors. In testing a hypothesis the researcher will determine the position of the obtained deviations and make judgments accordingly. Thus, the probabilities become yardsticks or standards for gauging differences among groups.

In essence, the researcher is guided by a set of rules for evaluating data. First, he must reformulate the research hypothesis in statistical terminology. Second, he must choose an

---

* It may be argued, correctly, that the split did not result in two randomly distributed samples. While the subjects were selected initially by chance, they were regrouped in accordance with the confinement criteria and not by chance. It is quite possible that the mean scores would represent two distinct segments of the distribution that could not be attributed logically to a sampling error. However, for the sake of the discussion, let us assume again that the groups remained in random form.

appropriate statistical test and perform the analysis. Third, he must establish the conditions upon which he will evaluate the statistical hypothesis. Finally, he will pass judgment upon the research hypothesis itself.

The research hypothesis is tested indirectly. It generally is restated in a negative way. The researcher begins by stipulating that there are no real differences in criterion values between the groups, and then sets out to disprove this statement. That is, he implies that the sample statistics actually are similar, or that the samples were drawn from the same universe, or that any differences in the group data are due to sampling errors. These statements usually are referred to as null hypotheses. In order to verify the research hypothesis, the null hypothesis must be disproved or rejected.

In the example, it is the researcher's purpose to demonstrate that the "irritability" scores of the 2nd day were substantially greater for the group of subjects confined to bed for 4 consecutive days. However, he will proceed with his task by stating first that there are no real differences in scores between the confinement and the nonconfinement groups. This is his null hypothesis. By implication, he ascribes the obvious differences in the table to errors in sampling. Nevertheless, he will determine the probability of securing such differences and will evaluate the null hypothesis accordingly.

There are many statistical tests of a hypothesis. Each test will result in a statistic that is a measure of differences and can be evaluated in a table of probability. Which test to employ will depend upon the nature of the data and the design of the study.

The various tests are constructed about unique statistics that are employed as standard expressions of sample differences from the population parameter and that have known or estimated sampling distributions. In addition, there is provided a formula to derive the statistics and the probability tables for the various values of the statistics.

Different kinds of tests are needed to accommodate the requirements of the data. For example, two kinds of data were generated and presented in the preceding analysis: frequencies and mean scores. The former represents discrete or discontinuous materials and has a different set of requirements than the latter, which was derived from continuous measures. Special statistics have been devised for each type of variable. They also are accompanied by a set of conditions and/or assumptions regarding the characteristics of the data and the underlying population. The tests cannot be used interchangeably.

The design of the test also will influence the selection of the statistical technic. Some forms of analysis have been developed to test differences between only two groups of subjects at a time. Some technics can be used to compare more than two groups. In addition, there are procedures to determine the interrelationship or the interaction of two variables upon a third, e.g., confinement and age upon irritability. These are but a sample of a wide variety of statistical developments derived over the years that are adaptable to an equally large assortment of research designs.

The ultimate product of a statistical test is a probability value. It is indicative of the likelihood of obtaining differences as large as those resulting in the study. This value also is known as a level of significance. That is, it specifies the level of probability at which the researcher considers the differences to be significant, i.e., due to factors other than selection. The level of significance is the point at which he is willing to reject the null hypothesis.

The probability value can be interpreted in still another way. It can be considered as an error of estimate or prediction. For example, if the probability has been set at 1 per cent, it is implied that the chances of obtaining a sampling error beyond this point would be less than 1 in 100. But there remains the possibility of being wrong that one time.

The level of significance is, therefore, an index of the confidence that a researcher places in the analysis. He evidently would have more confidence in a 1 than a 10 per cent error. At the same time, real differences may be obscured by ultra-conservative requirements. Where the level of significance is to be established is an aribtrary decision and often depends upon the amount of error that the researcher is willing to tolerate.

The error term in the above reference may be described as the error of rejecting a null hypothesis when it actually is true. There is also a second type of error, that of accepting a hypothesis when it is false. Most statistical formulas provide a measure of the former type of error; very few can describe the latter. The difficulty lies in restricting the boundaries for accepting a hypothesis. The region of acceptance may be anywhere beyond the rejection point, i.e., from the 1 per cent level of significance on.

Thus, the researcher may reject the null hypothesis, but he hardly ever accepts it. This statement implies that the researcher either has or has not sufficient evidence to conclude that the statistical differences between groups are due to factors other than chance. He cannot state that the differences actually are due to chance.

Under these circumstances, a statistical test of a hypothesis is more definitive than mere inspection. Each procedure involves a comparison of group measures. In inspection, the researcher simply looks at the data and makes a judgment. In statistical testing, however, the judgment is delayed until the effect of the sampling error is estimated and, in a sense, extracted from the differences in score values. Whatever remains may be attributed to other factors.

And what can the researcher state about the other factors? Can he attribute the differences to the conditions set forth in the hypothesis? Lindquist says the following:

> to prove the difference significant does not establish the *cause* of the difference. In rejecting the null hypothesis we have only rejected *one* possible cause—chance fluctuation due to random selection. What really accounts for the difference—whether it is a real difference in effectiveness of the methods, or some extraneous factor which was not adequately controlled in the experiment—is quite another matter.[15]

In essence, the researcher may have advanced just one more step toward truth. He has yet to attain the apex.

A FINAL WORD ABOUT THE PROCEDURE

The parts of the procedure are intimately related. They have been treated as separate entities for discussion purposes only. In reality, we cannot plan any single segment without regard to the others.

Design is influential throughout. It is suggestive of the different kinds of subjects to be selected, the need for descriptive materials, and the method for collecting data. In many instances, the design and the method of analysis even may be the same mode of expression. The various tables presented in this chapter actually feature different patterns of design.

Nor can the researcher readily divorce subjects, materials and data-collection processes from one another or from the analysis. The reader has observed how the number of subjects chosen, the selection processes and the type of measures, whether discrete or continuous, influenced the development of an appropriate statistical test. He has noted how the record-keeping processes and the limitations of the survey approach either help or hinder analysis.

In view of these considerations, the issue of planning can be raised again. We cannot expect the various parts to fall into place accidentally. For example, all too often the method of analysis is left to the whimsies of the data-collection process, which, in turn, falls prey to whoever happens upon the scene and whatever materials are available. Analysis becomes a means to unscramble some garbled information rather than a step in a systematic plan to test a clearly defined relationship. It need not happen this way. Planning is the key to success in research.

REFERENCES

1. Time, The Weekly Magazine, Vol. LXXVII, No. 20, pp. 52-56, May 12, 1961.
2. Buechell, P. S.: Hypodermic technics that save time, Amer. J. Nurs. *44*:1033-1034, 1944.
3. *Ibid.*

4. Hoffert, Frances: Simplified breast care, Amer. J. Nur. *48*:372, 1948.
5. *Ibid.*
6. Benson, M. E.: Handwashing—an important part of medical asepsis, Amer. J. Nurs. *57*:1136-1138, 1957.
7. *Ibid.*, p. 1138.
8. Gifford, Alice (ed.): Unity of Nursing Care: A Report of a Project to Study the Integration of Social Science and Psychiatric Concepts in Nursing Education, Chapel Hill, N. C., Univ. North Carolina, 1961.
9. A Survey of the Social and Occupational Characteristics of a Metropolitan Nurse Complement, Kansas City, Mo., Community Studies, Inc., 1956.
10. *Ibid.*, p. 135.
11. Reissman, Leonard, and Rohrer, J. H.: Change and Dilemma in the Nursing Profession, pp. 181-279, New York, Putnam, 1957.
12. Sellars, J. H., and Yoder, A. E.: A comparative study of temperature readings, Nurs. Res. *10*:43-45, 1961.
13. Guilford, J. P.: Fundamental Statistics in Psychology and Education, p. 3, New York, McGraw-Hill, 1942.
14. Lindquist, E. F.: Statistical Analysis in Educational Research, p. 10, New York, Houghton, 1940.
15. *Ibid.*, pp. 15-16.

CHAPTER 10

Discussion and Conclusions

The researcher occupies a unique position in the society of men. He stands on the bridge of time and scans the passing world. His work may have been started in the remote past and may be shared in the future by people as yet unborn. And he is wary of the present, which underwrites his activities, prods him for solutions, is offered as his guinea pig, and is critical of his indecisive character but will quickly absorb the fruits of his labors.

Thus, the researcher communicates with three worlds: the past, the future and the present. He interrelates his findings with those of the past and perhaps remodels old structures. To the future, he suggests new food for thought, another inlet to the way of knowledge. For his contemporaries, he may provide a useful solution to a persistent problem. These communications comprise the end-products of the research study.

However, the reader may question that the researcher really is ready to draw any conclusions at this point in his study. A feeling of incompleteness could have been engendered by the discussion on analysis. The researcher was left dangling on the ledge of uncertainty. He passed through a series of exacting tests. Each step was planned with considerable forethought to avoid the confusion and the torment of doubt. Yet the only conclusion that could be drawn was the likelihood that chance did not markedly influence the results of his test.

Actually, we have reached another time for deliberation. The researcher does not jump to reckless decisions now. He must sit in judgment of what has been done. He will weigh his actions carefully and decide upon his statements to the past, the present and the future. This intervening step, termed a discussion, is designed to integrate the logical and the statistical findings and serve as a springboard for his conclusions.

DISCUSSION

There are three pathways to a conclusion. Each centers about a solution to a problem. The first avenue of thought considers the possibility that an adequate solution has been revealed. The second may recognize that the proposal is not sound. The third may acknowledge that the evidence is insufficient to support or to refute the proposal.

A POSITIVE CONCLUSION

How can the researcher explain or account for the results? When the null hypothesis is rejected, one possible explanation—that they arose by chance—can be eliminated. The results are to be attributed to other factors. But the question remains: What other factors?

A reasonable explanation is offered by the hypothesis. A number of possibilities could have been considered during the formulation procedure. However, each alternative purportedly was scrutinized in the wake of the available evidence, and the most acceptable proposal emerged.

It also was reasoned that other factors, in addition to the explanatory variables, might be present in the situation and influence the outcome. Therefore, the test was designed deliberately to maintain control over or, at least, to determine the contribution of these extraneous variables to the final results. An appropriate design will restrict the range of extraneous factors and focus attention upon the explanatory variables. For example, when the variable "age" was merged with "confinement to bed" in Table 9 (p. 399), the researcher could conclude only that apparently both factors were influential. He would not be able to discern the contribution of each. On the other hand, the effect of "age" can be ascertained and controlled in the pattern displayed in Table 8 (p. 397). In pursuing an analysis along these lines, the researcher may reason with relative confidence about the sole influence of "confinement to bed" upon "irritable behavior."

This discussion may serve as a basis for reviewing and re-evaluating the conditions for accepting a piece of knowledge. Briefly, it has been stated that the researcher formulates a logical hypothesis that is submitted to an empiric test. And in consideration of this 2-fold analysis, first logical and then empiric, the researcher may or may not offer another contribution to knowledge.

Now there are some who contend that we should reason only after the fact. They state that we should observe and then provide an appropriate description and/or explanation of what has been observed. To this, the authors have replied: Lacking a hypothesis (stated formally or implied), what is to be observed? Lacking a hypothesis, what is to be designed? and Lacking a design, what is to be controlled? In other words, is the researcher truly prepared to isolate and adopt precisely stated relationships without some preconceived notions regarding the observations? Only by chance would he be in a position to allocate the effects of the other factors, "confinement to bed" and "age," upon "irritable behavior."

There are, of course, many instances in which the researcher cannot be wholly precise. He may not be able to formulate an adequate hypothesis, design an appropriate test, select sufficient subjects, develop valid materials or collect data in a situation in which all the relevant factors can be controlled adequately. His contribution will be limited in any or all of these respects despite the degree of significance revealed by the statistical test. He may be able to offer little more than another hypothesis.

The researcher should be ready and willing to discuss these matters freely. After all, he is but one of a vast and continuing network of problem-solvers and truth-seekers who may be engaged in similiar pursuits. He simply is saying to them: "Here is what I have found, and these are the conditions under which the observations were obtained. Examine and use the results at their face value." The implications of the study convey meaning to the output of knowledge and are governed partially by the limitations.

On the other hand, there also are some positive implications to be considered. Practically every study—no matter how inconclusive the results—is a step forward. The researcher should regard his findings as a contribution to previously obtained knowledge. He also should give some thought to the requirements for future knowledge, i.e., what follow-up studies are to be recommended as a consequence of this one. And to the practitioners he may suggest a series of applications to augment the scope of our present knowledge.

A NEGATIVE CONCLUSION

The researcher may feel inclined to discard his hypothesis when the results are negative in character or appear to be unrelated. Negative results would signify that the explanatory variables actually are related although the direction of the relationship has been reversed. This would be the case, for example, if "irritable behavior" was found to decline as "confinement to bed" increased. A condition of "no relationship" indicates that one term does not influence the other, regardless of the direction.

It is quite possible to secure a significant relationship that is a reversal of the hypothesis. That is, the researcher can obtain results that are negative in character and associated with factors other than chance selection. The question is: What do these results mean? The researcher may consider one or more of several alternatives. Some of these are considered below.

One obvious possible cause to consider is the hypothesis. Researchers do formulate erroneous hypotheses. The reasoning process could have been built upon faulty premises or handicapped by illogical determinations. Perhaps the newly developed areas of knowledge are vulnerable to such happenings. However, researchers from older schools of thought are not immune. The empiric test is provided to ensure against such contingencies.

Nevertheless, the researcher should not discard the hypothesis hastily. There are many other sources of error that the authors have attempted to depict throughout the development of this book. The research process is not as precise as we should like it to be.

The possibility may exist, for example, that unnoticed but relevant factors were present to influence the results systematically rather than randomly. Perhaps the patients who were confined to bed for longer periods were also more seriously incapacitated and received more attention and better nursing care than that accorded the other group. Perhaps the 4-day period of confinement is not sufficiently critical. These subtleties often are overlooked, especially in areas of study in which background information is lacking.

We should recall that the statistical treatment of data offers results that are not completely without error. The level of significance may be interpreted as an error in rejecting a null hypothesis when it actually was true. The occasion of this study may have been one of the few times when differences as large as those obtained actually can be attributed to the selection procedure.

The outcome of this discussion should be directed to other researchers rather than to the practitioners. There are grounds for rejecting the initial proposal. Further study appears to be warranted. The investigator will provide clues indicative of the next step to be taken. For instance, he might suggest that the negative hypothesis is a more appropriate statement than the one tested. It could be reformulated positively, e.g., "confinement to bed for X days reduces irritability," and retested under controlled conditions. On the other hand, the researcher may maintain credence in the original formulation and attribute the results to other conditions, e.g., the appearance of unnoticed but relevant factors. Under these circumstances, he may recommend that the study be repeated with modified controls. Therefore, the major contribution of the present study may be a proposal for additional research.

A "no relationship" result is more difficult to interpret than a negative relationship. This outcome really implies that observational differences may be attributed to random factors. However, it was indicated previously that statistical tests rarely are designed to accept the null hypothesis. The researcher usually is accorded the option to reject or to fail to reject but seldom to accept.

In this event, a close inspection of the individual data may be more suitable than a statistical test. The researcher can look simply for patterns of consistency or inconsistency among the raw observations. An obvious lack of consistency, e.g., the scores of irritable behavior rising and falling indiscriminately among the confinement and the nonconfinement groups, may lead the researcher to conclude that the pair of explanatory variables really are unrelated.

There is something to be learned from the discovery of a condition of "no relationship." The researcher, of course, would scrutinize the various aspects of his study for clues indicative of why this result was obtained. Any apparent discrepancy could be suggested as the focal point of the study replication. However, the researcher may determine that the variables are just not related. His report to the research field then may be something like: "We have considered the possibility that X may be related to Y. This does not appear to be the case. Let us consider another alternative." A negative conclusion can be regarded as a positive contribution.

An Inconclusive Outcome

There is another alternative to be added to the discussion of negative conclusions. The researcher may decide that he has insufficient evidence to draw any kind of conclusion. He can neither reject nor accept the null hypothesis. However, an inconclusive result also may comprise a positive contribution to knowledge.

An inconclusive result is useful if the researcher is forced to re-examine the total process and uncover any devious pathway. A discussion may serve that purpose. Several possibilities —the nature of the hypothesis, the controls, the interpretation of the analysis—already have been mentioned with regard to other types of conclusions. Each also may effect an inconclusive finding. In addition, other pertinent steps, such as the selection of subjects, materials or methods for collecting the data, may require attention.

Selection of Subjects

Any one or more of the many points discussed under this topic may be evaluated. For example, the researcher can question that the various groups of subjects were truly random selections from some underlying population or universe.* He may be concerned that his groups were not sufficiently pure. In choosing subjects, he may have matched by "age" and "sex" but failed to consider "family relationships" and "degree of illness." Some of the inconsistencies may be accounted for by the latter two variables. Furthermore, the possible presence and influence of these other relevant factors may lead the researcher to inquire about the size of his sample. How could he possibly relegate so many factors among so few subjects to the chance-selection process?

Materials

The problem may lie here. How valid is the index of irritable behavior? How reliable are the records? To what extent did the observer influence the findings? Perhaps the scores were not sufficiently precise to discriminate adequately between irritable and nonirritable behavior. The combination of indecisive measures and small samples can produce inconclusive results.

* See the footnote on page 402 in the section on Comparative Analysis.

Method of Collecting Data

The illustration depicted the characteristics of a survey. The researcher observed an ongoing situation. He really could not control the flow of events. He was not able to restrict the nurse's behavior or to limit outside visitors or contacts. Perhaps, for some patients, "confinement to bed" did not conform to the concept of "confinement," developed in the formulation of the hypothesis. Perhaps, for others, "nonconfinement" was more realistically "confinement." The former, though bedded, were unrestricted otherwise; the latter, though on foot or in bedside chairs, essentially were inhibited. Upon re-examining the test situation, the researcher may determine that the observed reality did not conform exactly to the intended reality.

It must be remembered that research moves slowly. It advances by inches rather than by tremendous leaps. Any questionable procedure may have a bearing upon the final outcome. Thus, each step in the total process may be considered for its own sake and with regard to its place in the complete study. All studies are useful, even if they only contribute the suggestion of an erroneous course of action. Possibly this procedure may be corrected the next time that the investigation is undertaken. A researcher often must proceed step by step or inch by inch toward a positive and over-all contribution to knowledge.

SUMMARY AND CONCLUSIONS

The discussion examined an array of possible conclusions in the consideration of a variety of contingencies. However, a final and definitive statement of accomplishment remains to be made. The researcher should make some type of decision regarding his findings. Normally this statement is preceded by a brief summing-up.

The summary includes a restatement of the various steps leading to a conclusion. In a research study, it would encompass the purpose, the problem, the hypothesis, the procedure and the discussion. This review should be presented in a concise fashion. It is not intended to be a substitute for the actual and detailed presentations. (The reader might refer to the original statements for a complete understanding of what was done.) Instead, the summary is offered to preface the conclusions as a brief reference relating the means to the end.

The purpose of this study was to determine the relationship between days of confinement and irritable behavior. Accordingly, we inquired: What is the effect of confinement to bed for X days upon the behavior of hospitalized patients? It was hypothesized that confinement to bed for X days, independently of age and sex, would lead to irritable behavior.

A survey of hospitalized patients who had been confined to bed for X days was conducted to test the hypothesis. The behavior of male subjects, divided by age and confinement groups, was observed and compared.

The results of the study were limited by the small number of observations and the inability to control nursing services during the confinement period. The nurses appeared to devote more time to patients confined to bed.

The conclusion comprises the outcome of the total study. It stipulates whether or not the specific purpose has been served. It may provide the answer to the problem. It is offered in reference to both the logical hypothesis and the empiric test. Lastly, it suggests implications and/or requirements for future study.

As a result of the analysis, it would appear that hospitalized male patients who have been confined to bed for X days tend to become more irritable. However, more conclusive evidence may be obtained if the study is replicated with a larger sample of subjects and under more controlled conditions.

Thus, the study ended as it began—on a note from the past and an inquiry for the future.

THE PLACE OF RESEARCH IN NURSING—AN EPILOGUE

We will attempt to draw some conclusions about nursing and research. In the course of this endeavor, the numerous observations made throughout the book will be summarized and discussed. It will be a cursory kind of analysis because the observations were not gathered and organized in a systematic fashion toward a single end. Instead, they were selected primarily as illustrative of some other major points of discussion. We have gleaned from them the arguments for depicting the place of research in nursing.

DISCUSSION

In many respects, the following discussion of the place of research in nursing can lead only toward an inconclusive outcome. The statements already made with regard to the nature of the evidence point to this end. Furthermore, the question itself does not permit a definitive answer. It only can reflect the predominant views of the authors.

The very manner in which the issue is stated will affect the conclusions. If our concern is with the place of research in nursing, then arguments may be gathered to support the position of nursing. If, on the other hand, the issue deals with the place of nursing in research, then some counterproposals may be developed.

A discussion of the place of nursing in research may lead toward some negative conclusions. In this instance, we are inquiring about the contribution that nursing can make to research. We are concerned with the position of the nurse practitioner who is cast in the role of nurse researcher.

Would she not have a conflict of purpose? As a nurse practitioner, she is problem-oriented. It is her function to apply whatever specialized skills or resources are at her command to the development of the solutions to problems as they arise. She cares for patients who require her services. It is her purpose to satisfy their needs for nursing care.

As a researcher, she is knowledge-oriented. It is her function to derive relationships that depict a state of affairs and that may be applicable to some common group of problems in the future. The solution to a specific problem is important only as a vehicle for her proposed knowledge. She does not cater to patients or their needs but uses them to further her own ends in research. It is her purpose to fill the voids in the resource of knowledge.

Would there not be a conflict of subject matter? As a nurse practitioner, she deals in concrete terms with specific issues. The subject matter is nursing or whatever pertains to the job of giving nursing care. She is interested primarily in such topics as the care of Patient A, who has undergone surgery for a heart condition, or of Patient B, a diabetic in a comatose condition, or in how to tube-feed Patient C.

As a researcher, she often has abstract thoughts. They may not have any direct bearing upon the job. They may not even relate to nursing per se. She is alert to such concepts as stress, tension, electrolyte balance, equilibrium and the reparative process. These are matters that may appear on the job but be discernible only to the researcher theoretician.

Would there not be a conflict of method? As a practitioner or a researcher, she may employ the general method of problem-solving. That is, in either case she may advance through a statement of the problems to the formulation of the hypothesis to an empiric test. Nevertheless, there may be a difference in the manner in which each step is approached and in how the task is completed.

As a nurse practitioner, she may not state a narrowly defined problem. She cannot limit the number of factors in the practical situation. There may not be any necessity to define terms. The situation contains only the specific and concrete elements that are encountered normally in daily practice. There may not be any necessity to formulate hypotheses. She usually has a fairly good notion of what is to be done. If not, she will ask her supervisor and will be directed accordingly. Lastly, there may not be any necessity for a stringent empiric test. She simply will try whatever she has in mind. If it works, she is satisfied; if not, she will try something else.

As a researcher, she is more severely limited. There is no choice but to state a definitive problem. The test to follow stipulates that she can investigate the relationship between only two factors at a time. The terms of the problem must be well defined. They are abstractions that point, on the one hand, to a wide area of practice and a body of available knowledge and, on the other hand, to the specific situation in which the test will begin. She may turn to the body of available knowledge and attempt to deduce a series of alternative relationships that may be applicable to the problem. Each will be scrutinized carefully in the face of evidence or fact, and the most acceptable alternative will be posed as the hypothesis for study. It will be evaluated further in a controlled circumstance that may exist already or may be contrived to satisfy the requirements of the test. The total investigation may result in a generalization with prescribed limitations or some recommendations for further study.

The practitioner and the researcher play two distinct roles at any one time. One is time- and situation-bound, while the other is restricted only by the cognizance of the nature of acquiring knowledge through research.

For the practitioner, the present is the thing. She is interested in an immediate solution, here and now. She may not be very concerned about applications other than those related most directly to her own job. But she probably is good at getting her job done. She can see what needs to be done and take direct steps toward this end. She has learned to satisfy the constituents who require her services.

For the researcher, time is endless. She is forever roaming through the past, the present and the future, searching for a better understanding of the nature of reality. She does not just accept whatever seems to work; instead, she continually seeks to understand how it works. She may play persistently at some seemingly inconsequential (to the practitioner) series of events until she has extracted the fullest description of what happens. To her constituents, the practitioners, she may appear not to be overly productive.

In reality, the products of the endeavors are not the same. One gets the job done while the other may provide knowledge that can be utilized for doing a better job. That the world needs both may be exemplified by the persistence of each throughout the history of man. However, the respective contributions of practice and research should be recognized as unique and not necessarily interchangeable.

Thus, we also may consider the place of research in nursing and its contributions to nursing and derive some positive conclusions. However, in order to do this, each practice must be conceived as a separate and distinct entity. They have their own purposes, are governed by their own sets of rules and have separate groups of technicians. In this respect, research can contribute to nursing as it does to other fields of endeavor.

Accordingly, there is a need to recognize the purpose of research in nursing. A 2-fold purpose was considered. It was suggested that research can contribute knowledge or generalizations applicable to common problems in nursing. Research in nursing also can make contributions to underlying or scientific knowledge. This is a source of knowledge derived through nursing that also may have applications in related areas.

There is a need for an integrated approach toward the acquisition of knowledge useful to nursing. The products of researchers should not be geared directly to the needs of practitioners—to put out the fires that arise on the job. Too many unfinished and diversified studies are generated, which seldom move the state of nursing knowledge beyond the present. In the final analysis, the acquirement of a long-range program concentrated upon the development of a unified body of knowledge may be most helpful. Individual researchers can participate to share experiences. Their limited contributions may acquire increased stature when seen in the context of the over-all purpose.

There is a need for a research atmosphere. Nursing must begin to appreciate the requirements of the researcher, his problem focus, his emphasis upon the abstract, the nature of his truths, his determination to limit the scope of his studies and to secure more exact measures and descriptions. Nursing might recognize and perhaps answer his requirement for a living laboratory in which he can effect his own controls rather than hope that they will occur by happenstance.

There is a need for research practitioners as distinguished from nurse practitioners. These are the people who have the characteristics of researchers and have acquired the technical skills of the process. They may be nurses. However, they will have become researchers if they have research aptitude and have secured training and experience in research. They also may be comprised of others from outside nursing. These people have come to lend their skills to the advancement of knowledge in nursing, and to derive knowledge from nursing that is applicable to their own spheres of interest.

There is a need to understand the matters that have been discussed. A field of practice does not take on a research function simply because it is fashionable or timely. Instead, it recognizes how and in what way research will serve. It can differentiate between and appreciate the purposes of research and practice. It acknowledges and is willing to accept the responsibilities incurred by a research program. With this understanding, we may derive some positive conclusions about the place of research in nursing.

SUMMARY AND CONCLUSIONS

The pursuit of research in the field of nursing has been used throughout the book primarily as a vehicle to illustrate our point of view about the nature of research. Nursing was put on display (perhaps unfairly at times) to demonstrate how the art of practice and the acquisition of knowledge sometimes are melded. It did not have to be nursing. Almost any other area of practice would have sufficed. No doubt the same general difficulties encountered in the attempt to mature would have emerged.

Our plan was to provide a rational basis for research in general and nursing in particular. It was not our intent to offer a source book of research technics. Instead, we sought to derive, through understanding, answers to such questions as:

Why do research? Why state a problem? Why define terms? Why formulate hypotheses? Why test hypotheses? Why design a test? Why are subjects and materials needed? and Why develop methodology? The requirements for meaningful answers seemed to be more important than the exposition of available methodology.

Thus, each step was explored systematically, first to answer "why" and then to suggest "how." We also attempted to interrelate the steps as parts of a total process rather than as separate entities. And, in the course of this development, we tried to establish meaningful connotations and to avoid using amorphous words. As the concepts were derived, they were applied to the research process in nursing. Thus, a 2-fold purpose was served. Another link to understanding was made possible by this transition from the abstract to the concrete. We also were afforded the opportunity to evaluate the practices and to describe further the place of research in nursing.

What can be concluded from this inferential analysis of research in nursing? It would be illogical to draw any conclusions from the illustrative materials and from the discussion of the place of research in nursing. (The materials were employed for a distinctly different purpose.) Instead, some broad proposals for the future of research in nursing may be proffered, rather than definitive statements.

1. There is a real purpose to be served by research in nursing. It may contribute knowledge or generalizations applicable to common problems in the area of practice. It also may make contributions to underlying or scientific knowledge that have applications in related areas.

2. An integrated and systematic approach to bind together the numerous efforts of individual researchers and establish the goals for a long-range program may be most effective.

3. The development of a research atmosphere in which to recognize and appreciate the requirements of the researcher and afford him situations for experimentation and control seems to be essential.

4. The maturation of a body of research technicians oriented in purpose, steeped in skill and understanding and cognizant of the practice and the problems of nursing may enhance the quality of the work considerably.

The acquisition of a meaningful basis of the nature of research in nursing could foster any of these recommendations. With understanding, each investigator would develop his own point of view and proposals regarding the place of research in nursing.

Index

425